AF712495

Provided as an educational service by Amgen and Pfizer.

Arthritis in Color

Advanced Imaging of Arthritis

Arthritis in Color

Advanced Imaging of Arthritis

Michael A. Bruno, MS, MD
Associate Professor of Radiology and Medicine
Director of Quality Management Services
Department of Radiology
Penn State University College of Medicine
Hershey, Pennsylvania

Timothy J. Mosher, MS, MD
Professor of Radiology and Orthopaedics
Chief, Musculoskeletal Imaging, MRI and Radiology Research
Department of Radiology
Penn State University College of Medicine
Hershey, Pennsylvania

Garry E. Gold, MSEE, MD
Associate Professor of Radiology
Stanford University School of Medicine
Stanford, California

SAUNDERS
ELSEVIER

SAUNDERS
ELSEVIER

1600 John F. Kennedy Blvd.
Ste 1800
Philadelphia, PA 19103-2899

ARTHRITIS IN COLOR: ADVANCED IMAGING OF ARTHRITISISBN: 978-1-4160-4722-3

Notice

Knowledge and best practice in this field are constantly changing. As new research and experience broaden our knowledge, changes in practice, treatment, and drug therapy may become necessary or appropriate. Readers are advised to check the most current information provided (i) on procedures featured or (ii) by the manufacturer of each product to be administered, to verify the recommended dose or formula, the method and duration of administration, and contraindications. It is the responsibility of the practitioner, relying on his or her experience and knowledge of the patient, to make diagnoses, to determine dosages and the best treatment for each individual patient, and to take all appropriate safety precautions. To the fullest extent of the law, neither the Publisher nor the Editors assume any liability for any injury and/or damage to persons or property arising out of or related to any use of the material contained in this book.

The Publisher

Library of Congress Cataloging-in-Publication Data

Bruno, Michael A.

Arthritis in color : advanced imaging of arthritis / Michael A. Bruno, Timothy J. Mosher, Garry E. Gold.—1st ed.

p. ; cm.

Includes bibliographical references.

ISBN 978-1-4160-4722-3

1. Arthritis—Imaging. I. Mosher, Timothy J. II. Gold, Garry E. III. Title.

[DNLM: 1. Arthritis, Rheumatoid—diagnosis. 2. Diagnostic Imaging—methods. 3. Magnetic Resonance Imaging—methods. 4. Osteoarthritis—diagnosis. WE 346 B898a 2009]

RC933.B785 2009
616.7′220754—dc22 2008050298

Acquisitions Editor: Rebecca Gaertner
Publishing Services Manager: Tina Rebane
Senior Project Manager: Linda Lewis Grigg
Design Direction: Steven Stave

Printed in China
Last digit is the print number: 9 8 7 6 5 4 3 2 1

To our parents, who made it possible—and to our children,
who make it all worthwhile.

Michael A. Bruno
Timothy J. Mosher
Garry E. Gold

About the Authors

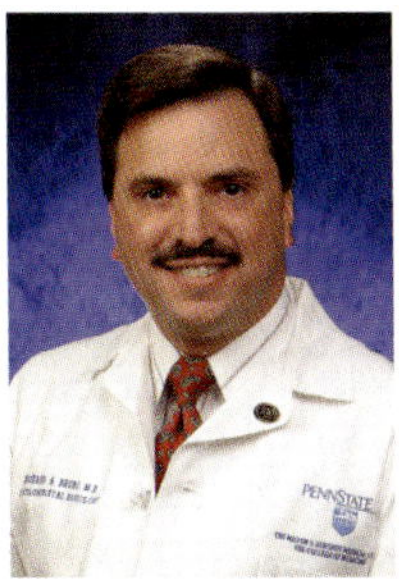

Michael A. Bruno, MS, MD, is Associate Professor of Radiology and Medicine and Director of Quality Management Services at Penn State University College of Medicine and the Milton S. Hershey Medical Center in Hershey, Pennsylvania, where in 2001 he initiated and served as the first program director of the Musculoskeletal Radiology Fellowship training program. Prior to that, Dr. Bruno was Assistant Professor of Radiology and Clinical Director of Emergency Radiology at Vanderbilt University School of Medicine, where he first developed his research interest in the application of Doppler ultrasonography for assessment of rheumatoid arthritis and related diseases. In 1998, he initiated the MSK Radiology fellowship training program at Vanderbilt and served as its program director until relocating to Hershey Medical Center in 1999. Dr. Bruno specializes in musculoskeletal imaging and nuclear medicine.

Dr. Bruno's research efforts over the past decade have been primarily focused on functional imaging, emphasizing quantified power Doppler ultrasonography. Dr. Bruno's arthritis imaging research has been supported by private foundations including a 1998 seed grant from the Radiological Society of North America (RSNA) and the National Institutes of Health (NIH). He is a frequent invited lecturer and keynote speaker on arthritis imaging and other musculoskeletal and practice quality improvement topics at national and international scientific meetings. He has written several scientific papers on these topics and serves as a reviewer for multiple medical and scientific journals. Dr. Bruno has also served on the editorial advisory panel for the American Journal of Roentgenology (AJR) and as a medical editor for the e-medicine online radiology textbook. He is a member of The RSNA Policy & Practice Committee, the "Examination of the Future" Development Committee for Musculoskeletal Radiology, the Research Committee of the Society of Skeletal Radiology and the RSNA's Roster of Distinguished Scientific Advisors. He lives in Hummelstown, Pennsylvania.

Ultrasound Evaluation of Rheumatoid Arthritis; MRI in Rheumatoid Arthritis

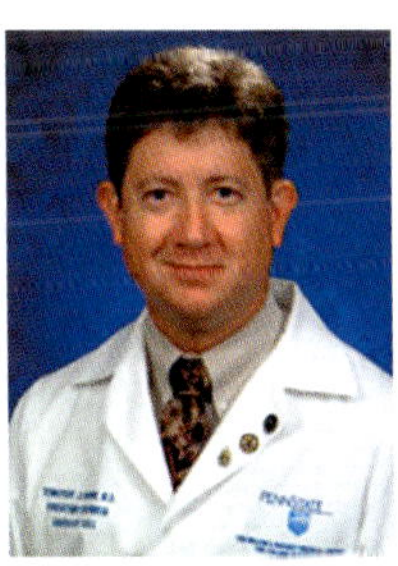

Timothy J. Mosher, MS, MD, is Professor of Radiology and Orthopaedics and Chief of Musculoskeletal Radiology, MRI and Radiology Research at the Milton S. Hershey Medical Center, Penn State College of Medicine in Hershey, Pennsylvania.

Dr. Mosher's research career has emphasized the use of MRI in cartilage imaging and osteoarthritis. He is an internationally recognized expert in high-field MR imaging of articular cartilage and pioneered the use of T2 mapping. His research has been supported by an RSNA Research Scholar Grant, Clinical Science Grants from the Arthritis Foundation, and R-01 Grants from the NIH. He has written or coauthored more than 25 original scientific articles, peer-reviewed electronic journal articles, and book chapters on the results of his extensive research. He has lectured extensively on MRI cartilage imaging nationally and abroad and has served on several national and international advisory committees and editorial boards, including the RSNA Distinguished Roster of Scientific Advisors, NIH Arthritis Imaging Study Sections, and ISMRM and RSNA Scientific Committees. He lives in Elizabethtown, Pennsylvania.

Functional Anatomy and Structure of the "Osteochondral Unit"; Clinical MRI of Osteoarthritis and Osteochondral Injury; New MRI Techniques for Osteoarthritis, Biochemical and Functional Techniques for Cartilage Imaging

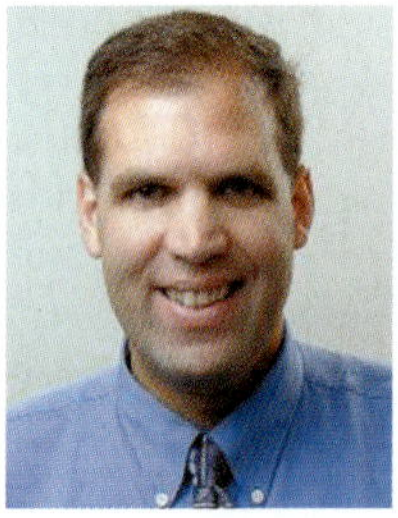

Garry E. Gold, MSEE, MD, is Associate Professor of Radiology and (by courtesy) Bioengineering and Orthopedics at Stanford University School of Medicine, specializing in musculoskeletal radiology.

Dr. Gold's research in rapid MRI for evaluation of osteoarthritis is funded by the NIH and emphasizes the development of new and optimal MRI sequences for the evaluation of articular cartilage and related topics. He has written or coauthored more than 60 articles in peer-reviewed journals, 2 book chapters and 15 invited reviews. He is on the editorial boards of two journals and has served on the Scientific Program Committee for the International Society for Magnetic Resonance in Medicine. He is a frequent invited lecturer and has made more than 120 scientific presentations of his research at national and international venues. In addition, he has won multiple awards for his work in cartilage MRI. He lives in Stanford, California, with his family, including new twins and a wonder-dog named Humboldt.

Technical Considerations for Clinical MRI of Arthritis; New MRI Techniques for Osteoarthritis

About the Contributors

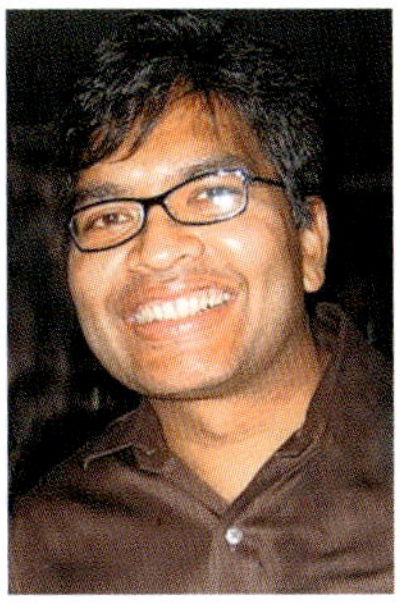

Sandip Biswal, MD, is Assistant Professor of Radiology, Musculoskeletal Division, and a Member of the Molecular Imaging Program at Stanford University School of Medicine, in Stanford, California.

Molecular Imaging of Rheumatoid Arthritis and Osteoarthritis

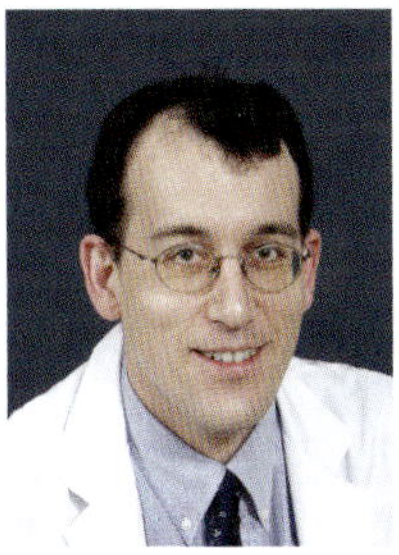

Roland Hustinx, MD, PhD, is chief of the division of nuclear medicine, University Hospital of Liège, Belgium. Dr. Hustinx's research has focused on PET imaging. His primary field of interest is the clinical validation of alternative radiotracers. He started his scientific career with a 2-year research fellowship at the University of Pennsylvania, Philadelphia. He is the current General Secretary of the Belgian Society of Nuclear Medicine and serves on the editorial board for the two major journals of nuclear medicine. He has written or coauthored more than 70 articles in peer-reviewed scientific publications and 12 book chapters.

Nuclear (Scintigraphic) Methods and FDG PET in Rheumatoid Arthritis and Osteoarthritis

Michael P. Recht, MD, is a musculoskeletal radiologist and serves as chairman of the department of business development for the Cleveland Clinic Imaging Institute. His main area of research interest is MRI of articular cartilage.

Surgical Approaches for Osteochondral Repair and Postoperative Imaging Considerations

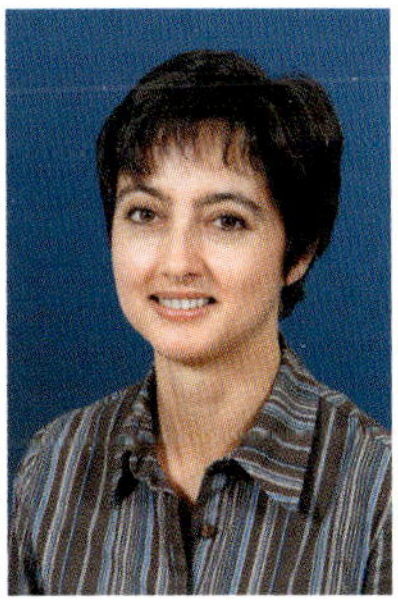

Clio Ribbens, MD, PhD, is Head of Clinic in the rheumatology department of the University Hospital of Liège, Belgium. Her main field of interest is rheumatoid arthritis. She started her scientific career as a fellow of the Belgian National Fund for Scientific Research and studied both in vitro and in vivo biomarkers of arthritis such as cytokines and matrix metalloproteinases. Her clinical work focuses on the assessment of inflammation in patients using imaging modalities such as ultrasonography and PET. She was the Scientific President of the Belgian Congress of Rheumatology in 2007.

Nuclear (Scintigraphic) Methods and FDG PET in Rheumatoid Arthritis and Osteoarthritis

Richard J. Wakefield, BM, MD, MRCP, is Senior Lecturer in Rheumatology, Academic Unit of Musculoskeletal Disease, University of Leeds and Leeds Infirmary, United Kingdom. He is also co-chair of the OMERACT Interest Group on the use of ultrasonography in rheumatoid arthritis. He is one of the foremost recognized experts in this topic and a frequent speaker at international meetings, as well as a regular teacher on national and international musculoskeletal ultrasonography courses. Dr. Wakefield qualified from Southampton University, UK in 1991. He began his rheumatology career in Leeds as a research fellow in 1997 when he first developed his interest in ultrasonography and early arthritis. In 2001, he became Lecturer / Honorary Registrar in Rheumatology at the University of Leeds and in 2004 became Senior Lecturer/Honorary Consultant. His major research interests include validation of ultrasound (MD thesis, University of Leeds 2006), ultrasound in early arthritis, and development of management pathways using imaging and training and education. In addition to his having been co-chair of the OMERACT Ultrasound Special Interest Group since 2004, he was also the coordinator for the ACR Musculoskeletal Ultrasound Group from 2002 to 2005. He organized the BSR ultrasonography course in Harrogate in 2004, the 2nd Advanced EULAR ultrasonography course in Leeds in October 2006, and coordinated the 7th BSR Musculoskeletal ultrasonography course in Leeds in 2008. Dr. Wakefield has been the author or coauthor of 60 peer-reviewed articles relating to ultrasonography and several book chapters.

Ultrasound Evaluation of Rheumatoid Arthritis

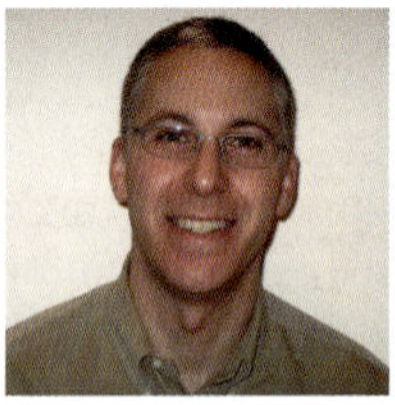

Lawrence M. White, MD, FRCPC, is Professor of Medical Imaging and Surgery (Orthopedics) and Head of the Division of Musculoskeletal Imaging at the University of Toronto.

Surgical Approaches for Osteochondral Repair and Postoperative Imaging Considerations

PREFACE

This book reviews the state of the art as well as current research and recent advances in the use of MRI, ultrasonography, computed tomography (CT), and nuclear and molecular imaging (MI) for the diagnosis and treatment of arthritis, especially rheumatoid arthritis (RA) and osteoarthritis (OA). The first section of the book focuses on the clinical state of the art, emphasizing methods that are currently available and in routine clinical use throughout the world; the second portion is forward-looking and emphasizes new and experimental methods and imaging strategies, including cutting-edge molecular imaging research, which is the topic of the final chapter.

Arthritis is a leading cause of disability worldwide. OA is the most common type of arthritis, affecting an estimated 20.7 million adults in the United States alone (U.S. Government data). RA is a generally more serious and debilitating disease, affecting more than 10 million persons of all ages in the United States. These diseases are among the most significant causes of disability in our society, with costs in lost work and productivity estimated at over $1 billion annually. As our world population ages, the impact of arthritis on the human condition, quality of life, and world economy will take on an even larger and increased significance.

In recent years, conservative management of arthritis has been replaced with new, aggressive drug therapies. These, in turn, have created an unprecedented demand for more rapid assessment of disease activity and response to treatment. Necessity is, as is often said, the mother of invention—but in a very real sense today's arthritis patients benefit from a lucky convergence of advances in imaging technology (that have coincidentally occurred in time to be of use) and new biopharmacologic therapies. More powerful drugs offer new hope for relief but have also created significant new challenges for physicians and pose some risks for patients. The pharmaceutical industry has invested heavily in developing new drugs for arthritis, and articles in the *Wall Street Journal** and other financial and business sources have speculated that drugs targeted to joint diseases—and especially RA—will become the premier growth market for the pharmaceutical industry, attracting considerable capital for research and development in both traditional and newer biotechnology firms.

These new disease-modifying and biologic response-altering drug therapies are extremely aggressive by historical standards in rheumatology; accordingly any sort of rapid assessment "feedback" that can be provided is of great value both to guide the clinician and to help justify the risks and expense involved in their use. Traditional radiographs, while still the mainstay of diagnosis and classification of disease, are insufficient for this purpose. Conventional radiography is limited in that it depicts the complex soft tissue changes in arthritis only in terms of the presence or absence of gross swelling and the bony changes only as the cumulative sum of the long-term effects of disease activity (e.g., the development of permanent bony deformities, such as osteophytes, joint subluxations, and erosions). To assess the severity of disease or response to treatment, radiographs essentially require a large number of observations (i.e., serial imaging at intervals), with painstaking comparison of the progression of small or subtle deformities observed over an extended period of time—and even when done meticulously and rigorously will provide only a very limited and incomplete portrayal of the dynamic disease processes involved in the complex, chronic disease entities as they affect an individual patient.

---

*For example, see "Enbrel Approved by FDA for Early Stage Rheumatoid Arthritis" in *The Wall Street Journal*, published April 12, 2000.

Because of these limitations, radiology researchers have turned their efforts toward adapting newer, advanced imaging methods and technologies toward the assessment of articular cartilage in OA and for assessment of disease activity by various means in inflammatory arthritis (mostly RA and related diseases). Gaining an understanding and mastery of these methods and their implications going forward is both a difficult challenge and a tremendous opportunity for the field of diagnostic radiology. Integrating these new methods rationally into the day-to-day management of patients is the 21st century challenge to the field of rheumatology.

This book is intended as a resource for both fields, and its goal is to efficiently and comprehensively educate diagnostic radiologists, rheumatologists, and other specialists as to the state of the art, current methodologies, and future research directions in this dynamic and rapidly evolving arena. In doing so, we have drawn from a huge and rapidly growing volume of clinical and research literature in the field—some quite recent and some published over the past 2 decades or more—in an attempt to provide a broad perspective on the field, as well as to distill a refined elixir of the most salient facts, organized in such a way as to make the topic as clear and as simple as possible. I am extremely indebted to my coauthors and the several outstanding contributors to this volume, all of whom are distinguished leaders in their respective fields, for giving so generously of their time and expertise to produce this textbook.

The title of this book was intended as an homage to the now classic radiology textbook from which so many of us learned the plain film diagnosis of the arthritides, *Arthritis in Black and White,* by Drs. Anne Brower and Donald J. Flemming, soon to be in its third edition. This landmark text, which to this day remains an intellectual staple and bedrock textbook for both radiologists and rheumatologists, is by no means diminished by our efforts here. To the contrary, we hope with our new textbook to build upon the solid foundation of *Arthritis in Black and White*, and we have attempted to provide in this volume a resource that will serve as a logical continuation on the topic of imaging in arthritis for the interested reader at all levels of professional training and experience. The ultimate goal in this learning and knowledge-distilling exercise is the benefit of our patients—those many, many people suffering from debilitating joint disease, who as a group have so often given of themselves so selflessly to be subjects for our research, in order that we might learn enough to help others in the future.

Michael A. Bruno

Contents

Part I

Advanced Arthritis Imaging in Clinical Practice

Chapter 1

Technical Considerations for Clinical MRI of Arthritis

Garry E. Gold

Inflammatory and noninflammatory arthropathies are a common cause of disability in modern society. MRI offers a noninvasive means of assessing the degree of damage to ligaments, muscle, bone, and articular cartilage. The keys to high-quality musculoskeletal MRI are as follows: (1) knowledge of tissue types and local joint anatomy, (2) selection of appropriate radiofrequency (RF) coils for a given clinical problem, and (3) selection of optimum pulse sequences to generate image contrast between normal or abnormal structures. With modern MRI methodology, it is possible to have *both* high spatial resolution and exquisite image contrast.

MUSCULOSKELETAL TISSUES AND ANATOMY

In the imaging of any body area, knowledge of tissue types and anatomy is critical. Musculoskeletal structures are composed of bone (cortical and cancellous), bone marrow, cartilage, ligaments, tendons, muscles, vessels, and nerves. Because of different proton densities and relaxation times, these tissues are well delineated with many MR pulse sequences, and combinations of sequences are usually used to cover a spectrum of image contrast regimens.

In general, tissues with a high amount of collagen and low water density have short T2 relaxation times and appear dark on common MRI methods that use an echo time (TE) in the millisecond range.[1,2] These tissues include cortical bone, the knee meniscus, the glenoid and acetabular labrum, and most ligaments and tendons. It is not unusual to see a slight amount of intermediate signal within these structures on short-echo TE pulse sequences; however, it is abnormal to see significant high signal with these structures on long TE (T2-weighted) sequences.

Arthritis causes predictable signal alterations on MRI. Inflammatory arthropathies cause bone marrow erosions and edema, which typically have long T2 relaxation times and enhance after administration of gadolinium. Synovial enhancement is also common in inflammatory disease but may also be seen in osteoarthritis. Degeneration of fibrocartilage, such as tendons and menisci, often appears as a T2 signal of intermediate intensity. Frank tearing or fissuring of structure appears as linear high T2 signal intensity on a background of short T2 or intermediate T2 tissue. To evaluate these changes, a mixture of contrast mechanisms is often helpful.

Protocols for evaluation of arthritis often include T1-weighted, intermediate-weighted, and T2-weighted images. Each of these weightings has strengths and weaknesses in the evaluation of certain joint structures. These different weightings are combined with fat suppression and contrast enhancement to give optimum images for each joint structure. Evaluation of a particular joint requires knowledge of the specific anatomy and disease process to design the best protocol to show abnormalities.

IMAGING PROTOCOL DESIGN

The fundamental tradeoffs in MRI involve image signal-to-noise ratio (SNR), acquisition time, contrast, and resolution (Fig. 1-1). In designing protocols for imaging of arthritis, a compromise much be reached between spatial resolution and keeping the examination times reasonable. For example, the Osteoarthritis Initiative decided on a maximum of 60 minutes of examination time for both knees in this large multicenter study (Available at www.oai.UCSF.edu). This resulted in compromises in the spatial resolution, acquisition plane, and contrast mechanisms used.

Protocols will vary on a particular MRI system, depending on field strength, coils, and imaging gradient hardware. Resolution that can be achieved depends greatly on the field strength, coil, and anatomy imaged (Fig. 1-2). For example, a 3.0T system with modern coils and high-performance gradients will be able to image faster or with higher resolution than a 1.5T or lower field strength system.

In terms of protocol selection, the field strength of the system will have a big impact on overall SNR. In general, a 3.0T system provides roughly twice the SNR of a 1.5T system; this means that images can be twice the resolution in one direction or up to four times faster and have the same SNR. Systems with stronger gradients will be able to image with longer echo train lengths with the same blurring, increasing imaging speed. Finally, good RF coils are essential at any field strength.

RADIOFREQUENCY COILS

Selection of appropriate RF coils is the most important aspect of optimizing image quality in musculoskeletal MRI.[3-5] The reason for this is that the signal seen by a coil is relatively constant, but the noise increases as the size of the coil increases. Hence, larger coils such as the body coil have a worse SNR than smaller coils such as a surface

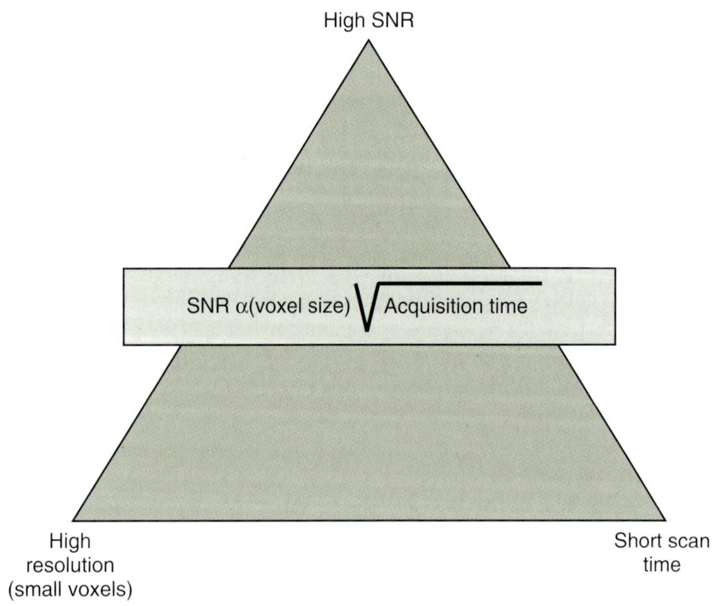

FIGURE 1-1. The relationship between signal-to-noise ratio (SNR), voxel size, and scan time in MRI. The signal in an MRI acquisition is proportional to the main field strength (B0) and the size of the voxel in each dimension (delta x, delta y, and delta z). The SNR may be increased by averaging and increases with the square root of the acquisition time. SNR is also a function of the contrast mechanism chosen and the T1 and T2 of the tissues being imaged.

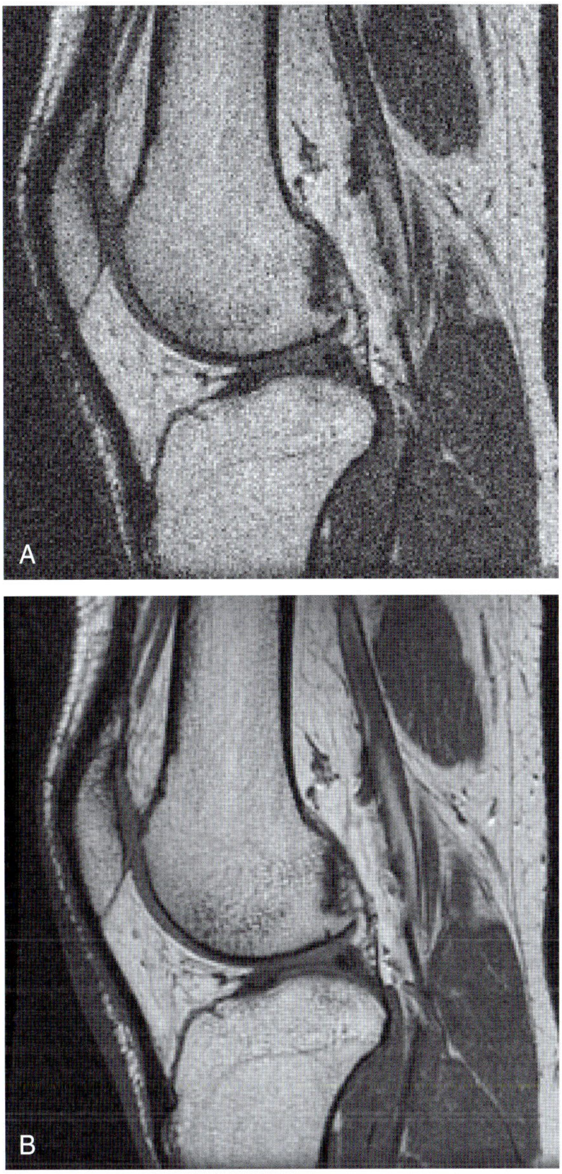

FIGURE 1-2. Example images showing the relationship between imaging time and signal-to-noise ratio (SNR). Two sagittal proton-density images are shown with identical scan parameters, except for the number of signal averages. **A,** Image acquired with one signal average has poor SNR. **B,** Same image acquired with four signal averages (4× the imaging time), with improvement in SNR by a factor of 2.

coil. So, in selecting the coil for a given body part or imaging area, one should select the smallest coil that will have sufficient field of view (FOV) and penetration for the area of interest.

Phased-array coils are combinations of surface coils that enlarge the effective FOV of the coil by combining the signal from many small coils (up to 32 coils).[6,7] Because each small coil sees only a limited area of tissue, the SNR remains as high as when using a surface coil, but because the signals from all coils are combined to form the image, the FOV is larger than that from one single surface coil. These coils are useful for parallel imaging, which can be used to decrease imaging times or shorten echo train lengths (Fig. 1-3). In general, the best SNR possible is achieved with a phased-array coil; however, if the area of interest is not deep within the body, high-quality images are achievable with a surface coil. General guidelines with descriptions of relative advantages and disadvantages of various coils are presented in the following sections.

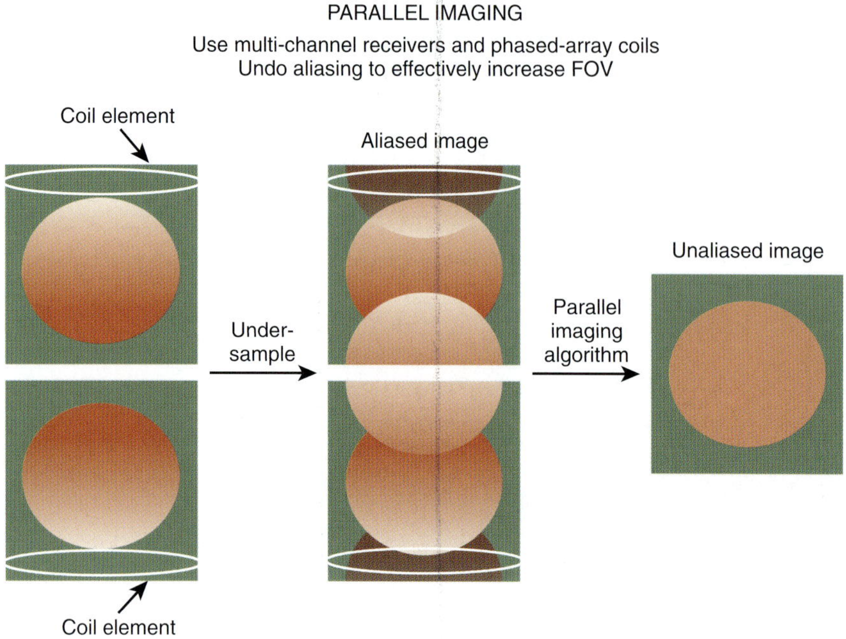

FIGURE 1-3. Parallel imaging. To speed up data acquisition, the object is placed in a phased-array coil with multiple elements. The object is then undersampled, leading to aliasing. The parallel imaging algorithm uses the coil sensitivity locations to create the final unaliased image. (Courtesy of Brian Hargreaves, PhD.)

Body Coil

Although the body coil is commonly used as the RF transmitter, its use as a receiver is rarely ideal, because better local coils exist for almost all body parts. For large FOV survey imaging, such as initial identification of areas of signal abnormality in an area such as the bilateral thighs or calves, the body coil is a good choice.

Torso Phased-Array Coil

The torso phased-array coil is the ideal coil for imaging of the pelvis and hips[8,9] and can in some circumstances be effectively used for more peripheral extremity imaging. Image SNR for this coil is considerably higher than that for the body coil, enabling improved spatial resolution. For patients with relatively normal abdominal girth, this coil has sufficient penetration of RF to provide uniform signal intensity in the hips. For extremity imaging, the torso coil can be used over the bilateral thighs, for example. Be aware that as the two elements of the coil get closer together, coil performance will diminish; similarly, as the coil becomes curved, imaging may degrade. This causes the coil's performance to be somewhat unpredictable in areas such as the bilateral calves or when placed off center in a smaller patient for imaging structures such as an upper extremity. If the torso coil is chosen for larger FOV imaging of an upper extremity such as a humerus, the coil should not be folded around the sides. Also, the coil should be kept relatively well centered in the magnet and the patient shifted eccentrically if possible. If the torso coil is not working well, these applications are probably best done initially with body coil imaging, followed by targeted imaging using a more dedicated coil.

As a rule of thumb, at 1.5T, the torso coil is adequate for 512-frequency matrix imaging with FOVs larger than 20 to 24 cm. At this large FOV the voxel size should allow ample SNR for these images; however, when one gets an FOV below this, consider switching back to a 256-frequency matrix. At FOVs below 20 cm, it is often possible to use a smaller coil with better intrinsic SNR.

Extremity Coil

This is a workhorse coil for standard imaging of the knee, ankle, and foot. In addition, this coil is used for imaging of extremities such as the forearm, wrist, and hand when a larger FOV is required, provided the patient is capable of positioning the arm above the head. Many extremity coils are transmit/receive coils that are mounted in the center of the scanner gantry and cannot be moved off center. To use an extremity coil, it must be closed, so those patients with extremely large extremities have to be imaged in an alternative coil. Phased-array coils are also available for the knee, foot, and ankle.[10,11] The maximum FOV coverage for the extremity coil is approximately 24 cm. The extremity coil is a reasonable choice for imaging of the elbow if a dedicated small extremity phased array is not available.

Wrist Coil

A dedicated wrist coil is optimal for imaging the hand and wrist and in some circumstances can be used for imaging the distal aspect of the foot. These are typically phased-array or quadrature receive-only coils that can be placed either in the center of the magnet or off center.[12] In the off-center situation, the most challenging aspect is to get good fat saturation. Coils may be oriented either with the long side parallel or perpendicular to the table. Note, however, that the coil should not be rotated with respect to the B0 axis because image quality will markedly degrade. Also, when 3D acquisitions are desired, remember that oblique prescriptions may not be allowed, so that having the wrist either perfectly parallel or perpendicular to the floor is necessary.

The wrist coil is also appropriate for use in imaging of the fingers and toes. Especially useful is high-resolution imaging of tissues such as the first metatarsophalangeal joint for sesamoid injury. Alternatively, a small surface coil can be used for these areas, with somewhat less signal uniformity.

Shoulder Coil

Shoulder coils are usually limited to use in the shoulder. Two different configurations exist. One is a traditional loop-type design. This is a single-element receive-only coil. The critical factor with this coil is that it needs to be positioned as perpendicularly to the B0 field as possible. Any flux from the main field traveling through the coil in the z-direction will decrease SNR. More recently, high-quality phased-array shoulder coils that have a fixed orientation relative to the scanner have become available, thus removing a variable that might degrade image quality.

Small Extremity Phased-Array Coil

This is a miniature version of an extremity coil that is ideal for imaging the elbow or for smaller extremities such as children's knees or ankles. This coil can also be placed off center in the magnet, which distinguishes it from the routine extremity coil.

General Purpose Surface Coils

Three-inch or 5-inch surface coils can be used alone or in pairs using a phased-array adapter. Such coils can be useful for imaging toes if they do not fit into the wrist coil. These coils are also useful for supplementary high-resolution imaging of joints. In general, superior dedicated coils exist for most situations.

Flex Coil

Flex coils can be used to image the elbow at the patient's side in the absence of a dedicated coil. Currently, most of the previous applications of the flex coil are better performed with more dedicated coils.

IMAGE CONTRAST

Pulse Sequence Selection

One of the major advantages of MRI is the ability to manipulate contrast to highlight tissue types. The common contrast mechanisms used in MRI are T1-weighted, proton-density (PD), and T2-weighted imaging (Figs. 1-4 and 1-5). The appearance of these has changed over time with the introduction of fast or turbo spin-echo imaging and the use of fat saturation.

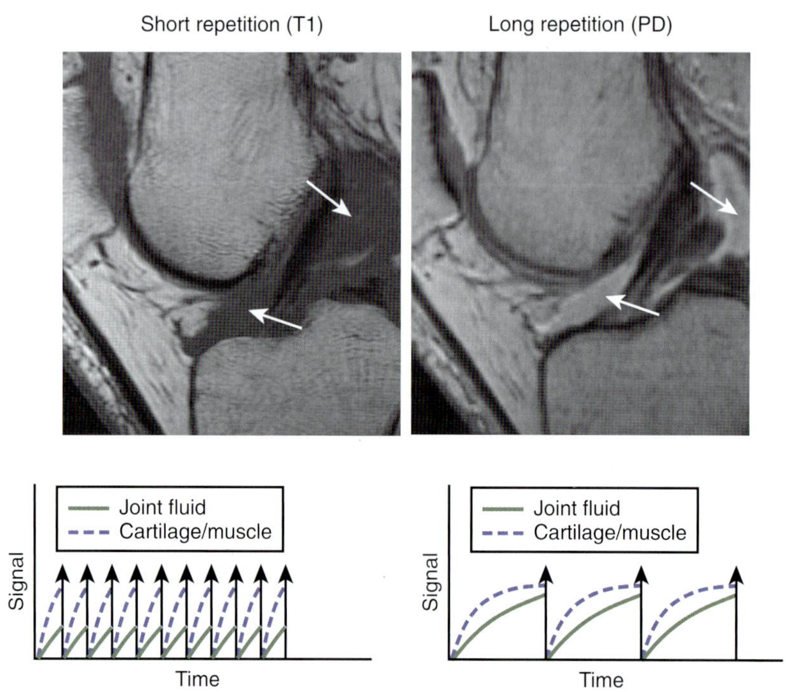

FIGURE 1-4. Image contrast generated by changing the repetition time (TR). The image on the left has a short TR, and cartilage and muscle (*dashed line*) are relatively bright compared with joint fluid (*solid line, arrows*). The image on the right is acquired with a long TR, allowing recovery of signal from joint fluid (*arrows*). The joint fluid is somewhat brighter than cartilage in this image owing to higher proton density (PD). (Courtesy of Brian Hargreaves, PhD.)

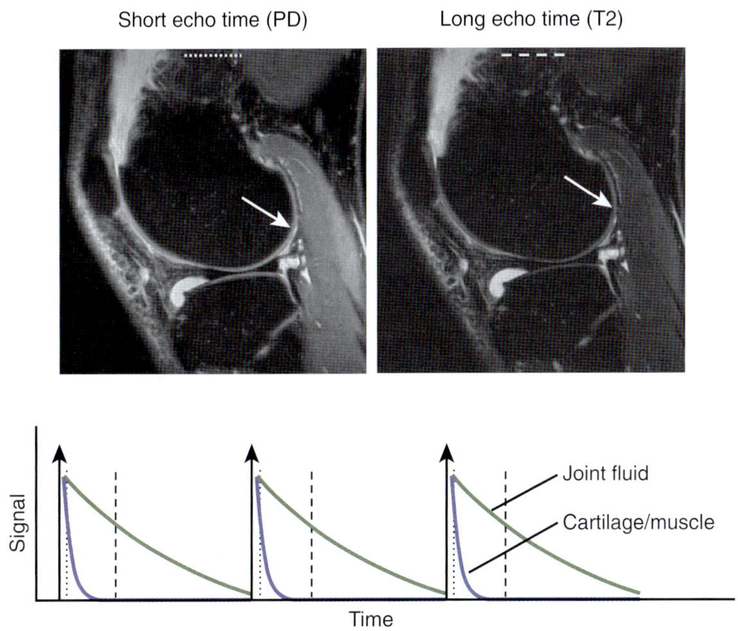

FIGURE 1-5. Image contrast generated by changing the echo time (TE). The image on the left has a short TE (*dotted line*), and the image on the right, a long TE (*dashed line*). In the short echo-time proton-density (PD) image, cartilage (*arrow*) and muscle are relatively close in signal compared with joint fluid. In the long echo-time T2-weighted image, the cartilage (*arrow*) and muscle are decreased in signal relative to joint fluid owing to shorter T2 relaxation times. (Courtesy of Brian Hargreaves, PhD.)

Spin-Echo and Fast Spin-Echo Imaging

T1- and T2-weighted spin-echo MRI allows depiction of joint structures and can demonstrate defects and gross morphologic changes. However, T1-weighted imaging does not show significant contrast between joint effusion and the cartilage surface, making surface irregularities difficult to detect. Fat suppression adds dynamic range and reduces the effects of chemical shift artifacts. T2-weighted conventional spin-echo imaging has largely been replaced by faster techniques.

Fast spin-echo (FSE) or turbo spin-echo (TSE) imaging is a technique that uses multiple echoes per repetition time (TR) to acquire data faster than conventional spin-echo imaging. Proton-density FSE (PD FSE) has a short TE, and the higher SNR echoes are placed at the center of k-space. T2 weighted FSE, with a longer TE, has the higher SNR echoes placed at the edges of k-space. One disadvantage of PD FSE is blurring of short-T2 species owing to acquisition of high spatial frequencies late in the echo train (Fig. 1-6).[13] The appropriate echo train length using FSE requires some knowledge of details about the given scanner in question. In general, increasing the echo train length decreases the imaging time, but the edge blurring effect increases in the images with short effective TE (Fig. 1-7). In longer TE (i.e., T2-weighted) sequences, there is actually an edge enhancement effect that occurs with FSE or TSE. The amount of blurring that occurs in the short-TE scans is a function of both the echo train length and inter-echo spacing, which depends on gradient hardware.

The key sequences for musculoskeletal MRI are spin-echo T1-weighted or PD-weighted sequences supplemented by T2-weighted images, almost always using fat suppression on high-field scanners. Conventional spin echo is used for T1-weighted scans, whereas FSE or TSE is used for PD- and T2-weighted imaging. On a 1.5T scanner, T1-weighted images are obtained with a TR of 600 to 800 ms, a TE of 9 to 17 ms, and 2 NEX, often with a 512 × 192 imaging matrix and 4-mm thick slices.

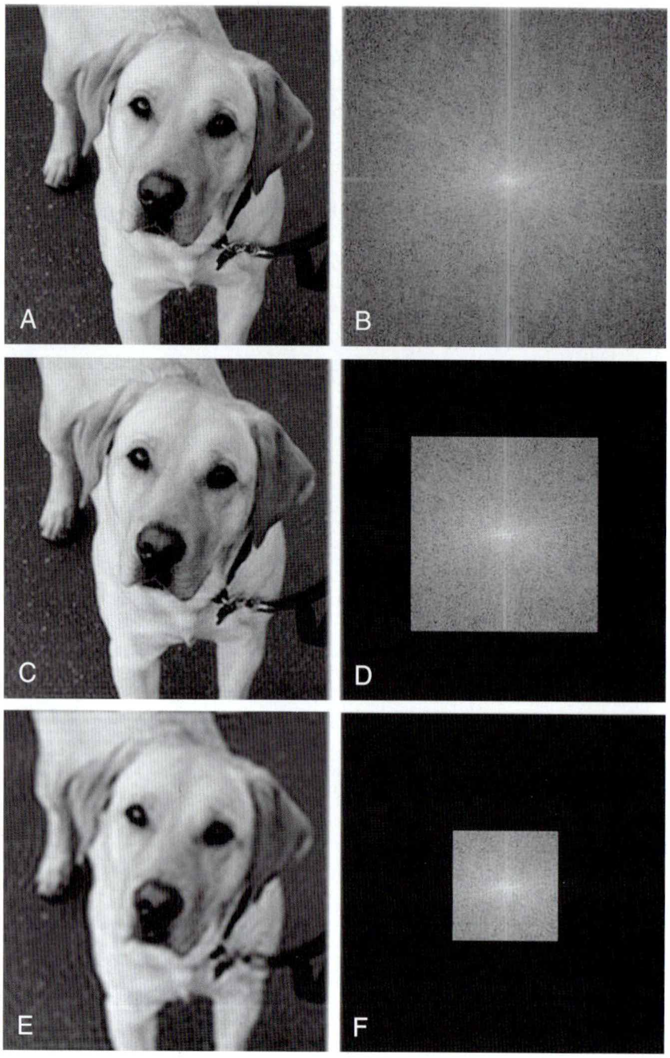

FIGURE 1-6. **A,** Gray-scale image of a 10-year-old yellow Labrador retriever. **B,** A k-space of the image in **A**, showing most of the image energy at the center, where image contrast is determined. **C,** Slightly blurred image, corresponding to **D**, in which the other portions of k-space are masked out. **E,** Even more blurred image, corresponding to **F**, in which even more high spatial frequency information has been lost. This is similar to what occurs in proton-density fast or turbo spin-echo imaging.

The long TR serves to improve the SNR in images typically obtained with a small FOV of 16 cm or less. PD FSE has been shown to be accurate in the detection of meniscal tears[14,15] and cruciate ligament tears.[16] T2-weighted FSE has also been shown to be accurate for detection of marrow edema and cartilage surface lesions.[17] Overall, FSE has replaced conventional spin-echo techniques for use in PD- or T2-weighted scans. For T2-weighted FSE imaging, I typically use chemical fat suppression and a TR of 4000 and TE of 54 to 72 ms, as long as the suppression is homogeneous. For PD FSE imaging, I again use a TR of 4000 ms and TE of about 15 ms.

Spatial Resolution

MRI of the morphology of joints requires close attention to the spatial resolution used.[18-20] With modern coils and gradient technology, at 1.5T, a matrix size of 512 is routinely achievable in the frequency encoding direction.[21] This matrix improves the appearance of the articular cartilage (Fig. 1-8).[22] This also improves overall image detail (Fig. 1-9) and allows for detection of small abnormalities. Whereas increasing the resolution in the phase-encoding direction can also improve image detail, imaging

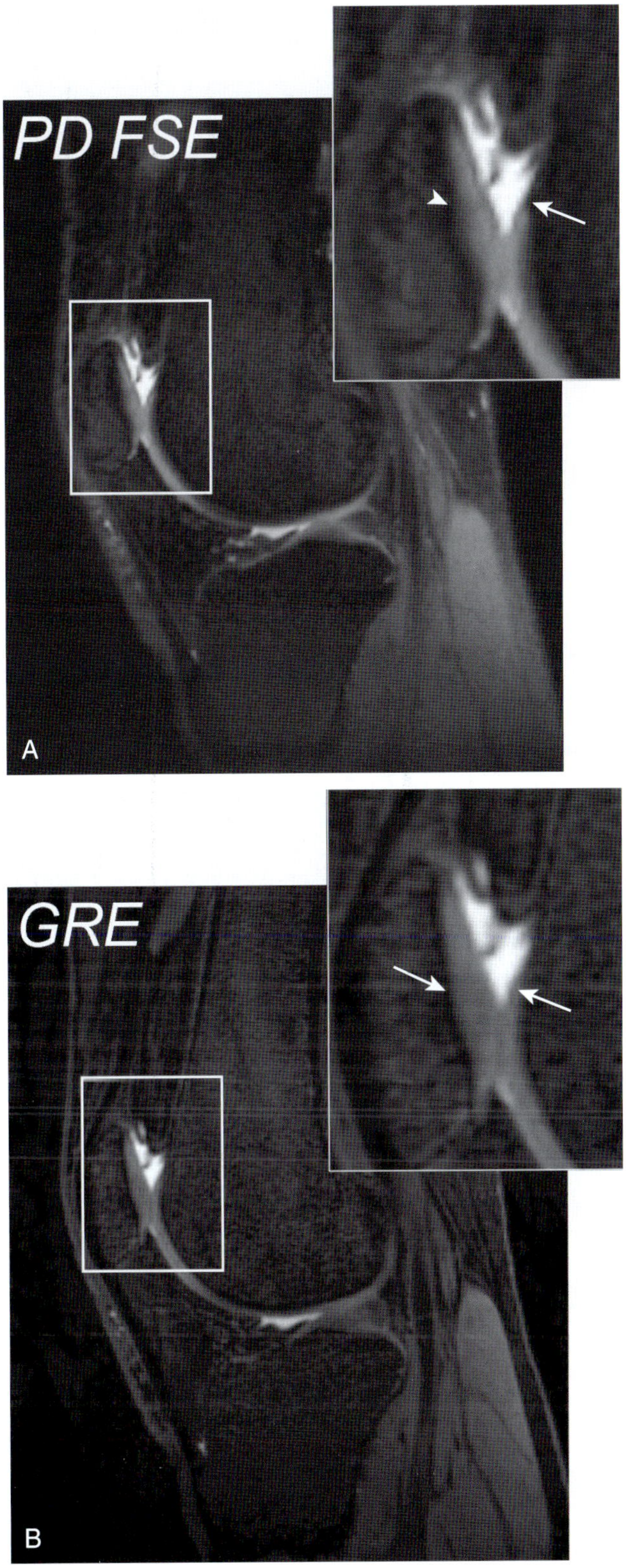

FIGURE 1-7. **A,** Blurring in proton-density fast spin-echo imaging (PD FSE). Blurring is seen at the fluid/cartilage interface (*arrow*) and bone/cartilage interface (*arrowhead*). **B,** No blurring is seen in the gradient-recalled-echo (GRE) image. (Courtesy of Brian Hargreaves, PhD.)

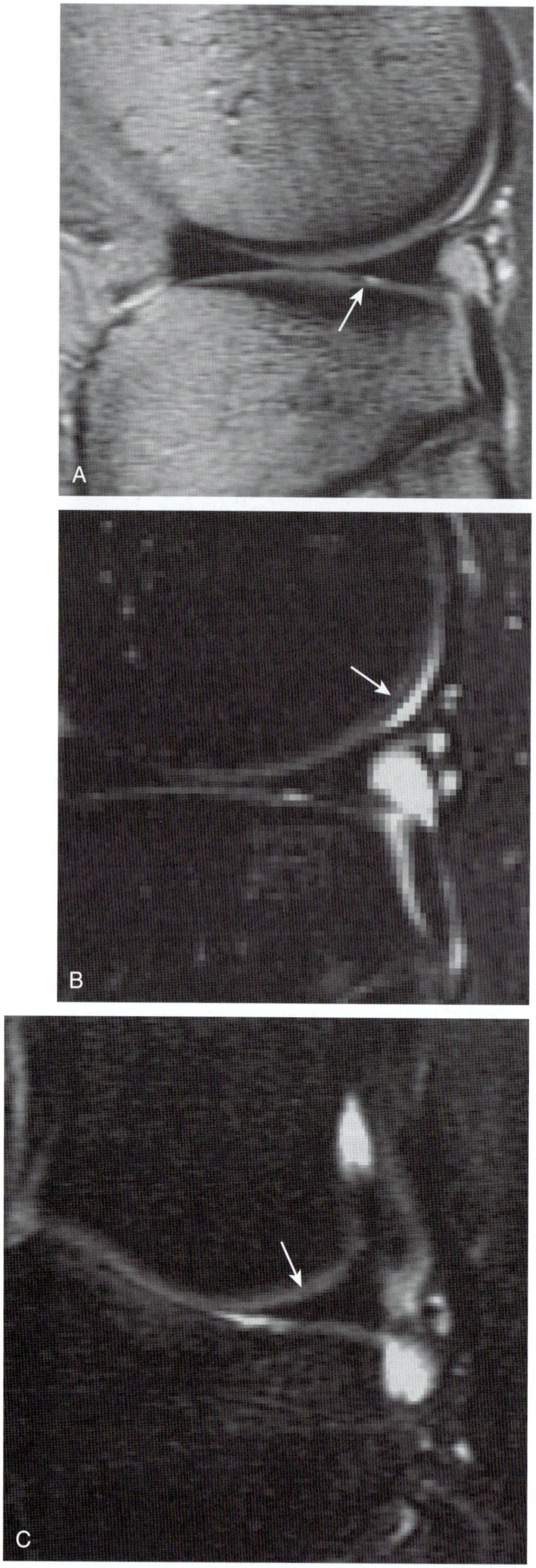

FIGURE 1-8. Importance of high-resolution imaging for articular cartilage. **A,** Sagittal proton-density image at a 512 × 192 matrix, showing a small chondral defect (*arrow*) on the lateral tibial plateau. **B,** Sagittal 256 × 192 image of the knee showing a jagged "stair step" appurtenance to the articular cartilage (*arrow*). **C,** Coronal 512 × 192 image of the articular cartilage, without the "stair step" artifact (*arrow*). The in-plane resolution on this image has been increased by a factor of 2.

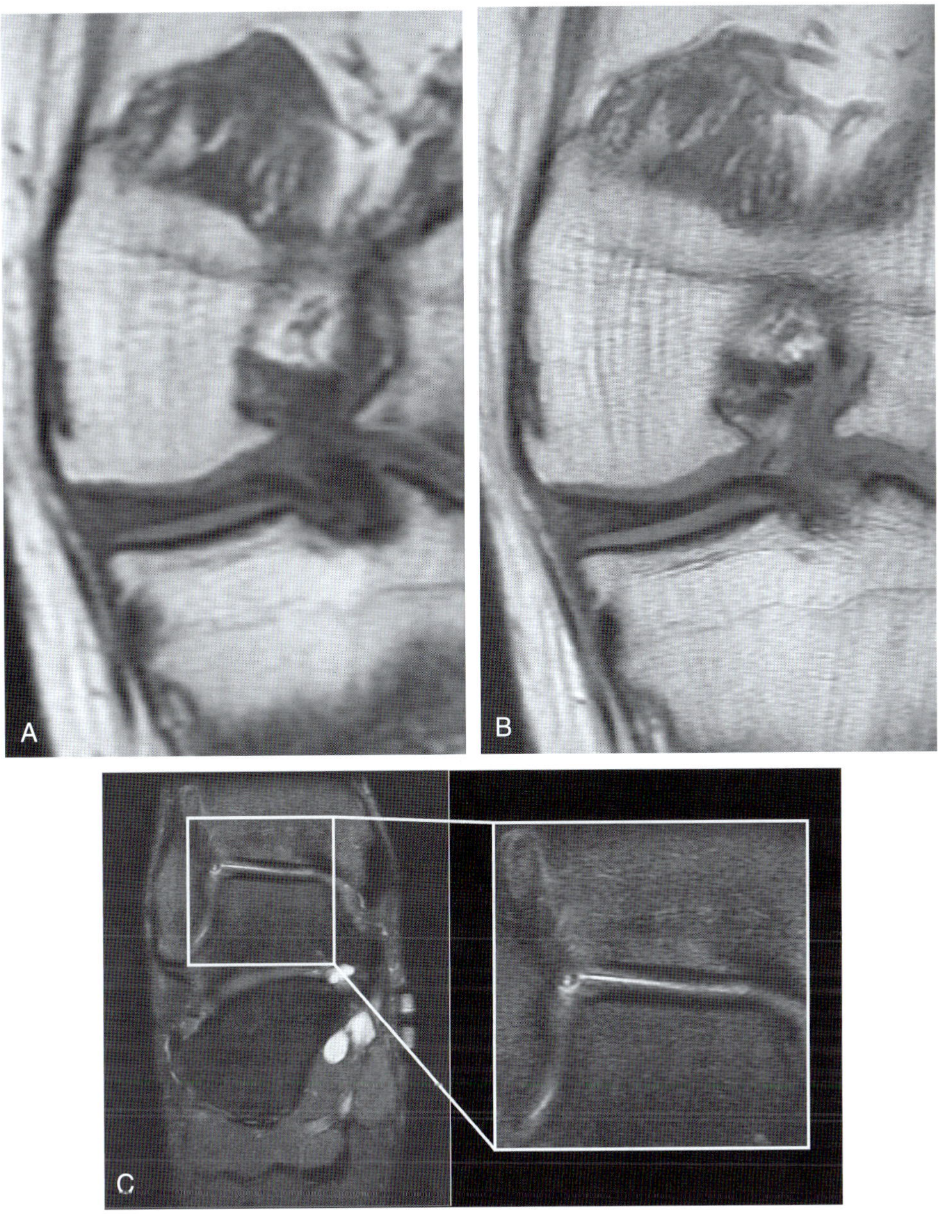

FIGURE 1-9. Usefulness of higher-resolution imaging. **A,** T1-weighted coronal image of the knee at 256×128 resolution. **B,** Same slice done at 512 × 192 resolution. Note the greater image detail seen, with still acceptable signal-to-noise ratio. **C,** Coronal T2-weighted image of the ankle, showing a small chondral defect (*box*) on the talar dome. High-resolution imaging enables visualization of small structures and defects.

time increases proportional to the number of phase-encoding steps. Thus, I typically do not use more than 192 phase-encoding steps.

At 3.0T, increases in T1 relaxation time mean that a longer TR can be used and still generate fluid that is dark relative to other structures.[23] To take advantage of the longer TR, and the higher SNR at 3.0T, more and thinner slices are acquired at 3.0T. It is often possible to use half the slice thickness at 3.0T that one uses at 1.5T. To avoid reaching RF power deposition limits at 3.0T, it is also possible to use T1-weighted FSE imaging, with a short echo train to minimize blurring (Fig. 1-10).

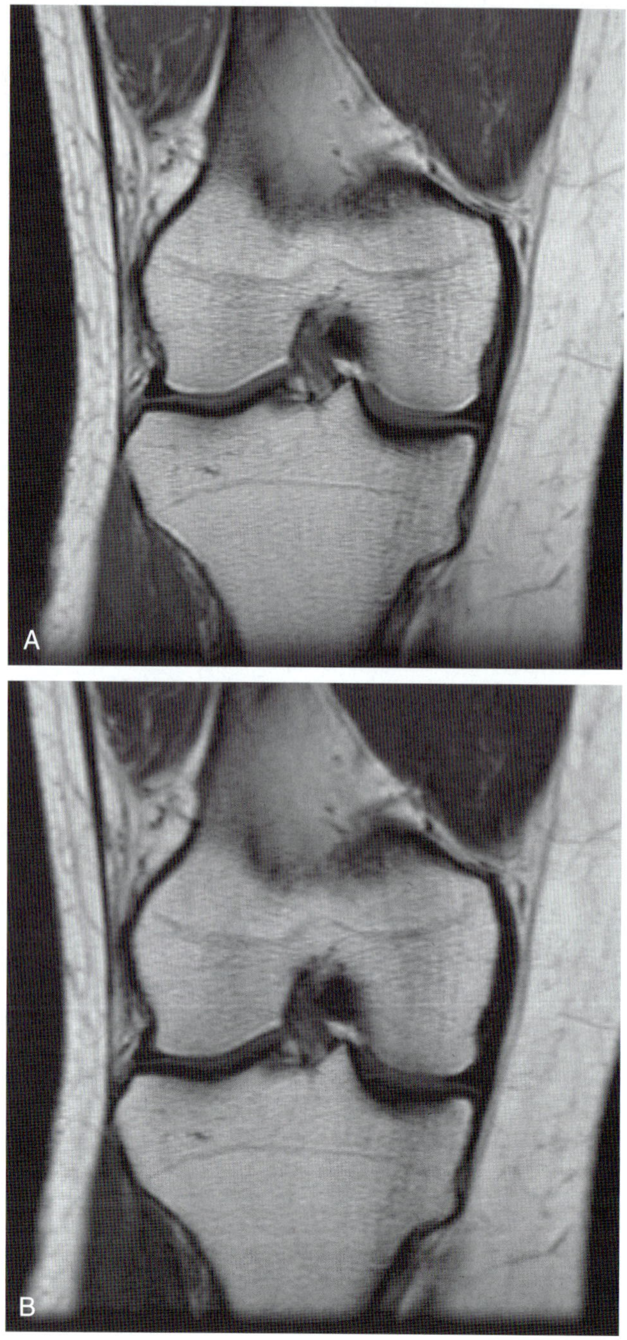

FIGURE 1-10. Coronal T1-weighted 3.0T images of the knee in a 42-year-old woman. Radiofrequency (RF) power deposition considerations at 3.0T suggest limited use of fast spin-echo imaging for short repetition time (TR) sequences. **A,** T1-weighted spin-echo image done with a TR of 800 ms at 3.0T. This image caused the power monitor to reach 66% of the limit for average RF power. **B,** T1-weighted fast spin-echo image using a TR of 800 ms and an echo train length of 2. The power monitor reached 33% of the average limit on this scan. Note a slight blurring resulting from the use of two echoes and a short echo train.

On non–fat-suppressed sequences, chemical shift artifact can interfere with evaluation of the bone/cartilage interface in a joint. Because fat and water protons precess at slightly different frequencies, fat is not placed in the proper location in the frequency-encoding direction. In a joint, this can result in the appearance of thin or absent cartilage on one surface with a thin bony cortex and an abnormally thick bony cortex on the other side (Fig. 1-11). Chemical shift increases linearly with field strength, so it is important to increase the receiver bandwidth at high fields on sequences without fat suppression to minimize this problem.

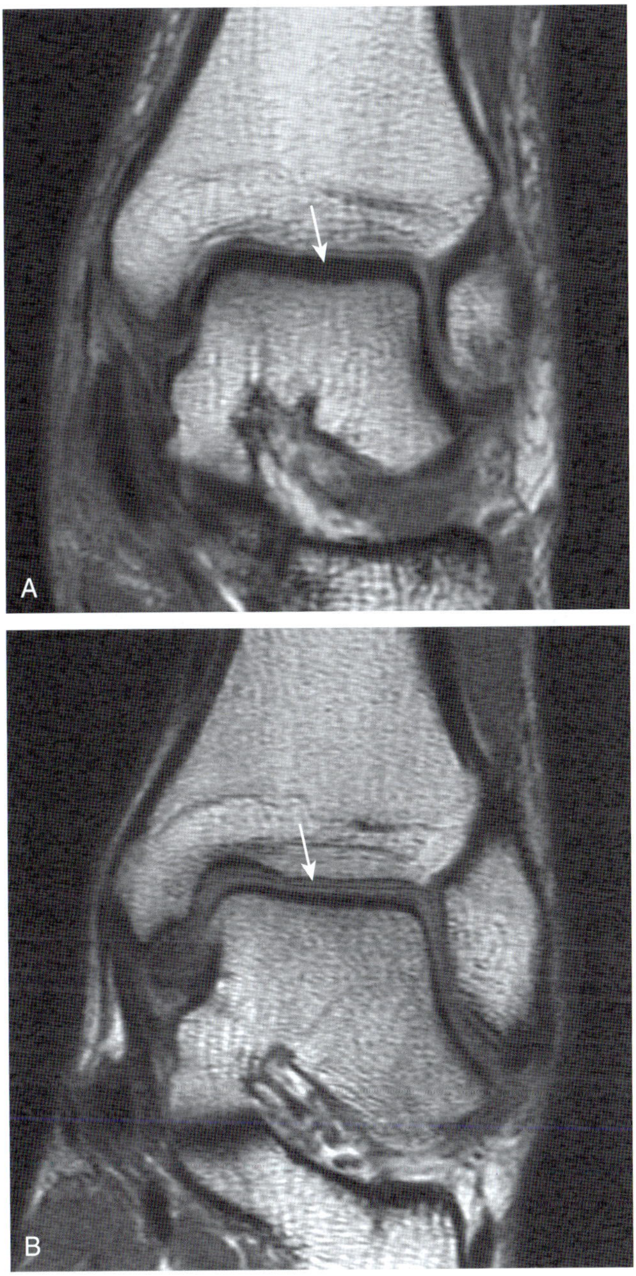

FIGURE 1-11. Coronal T1-weighted 3.0T images of the ankle in a 44-year-old woman, showing chemical shift. **A,** Readout bandwidth of ±16 kHz. The cortex of the talus appears thickened, and two layers of cartilage are not apparent (*arrow*). This is due to misregistration of lipid signal from the bone marrow into the joint. **B,** Readout bandwidth of ±64 kHz. The articular cartilage is clearly visible as are the normal thickness cortices of the tibia and talus (*arrow*). Increasing the receiver bandwidth by a factor of 4 in this case reduced the chemical shift artifact by the same amount.

Fat Suppression

The use of FSE and TSE techniques in musculoskeletal imaging has made fat suppression a requirement. The FSE technique uses a number of 180-degree refocusing pulses, which maintain the signal from fat (the J-coupling effect),[24] in comparison with conventional spin-echo techniques. The very high signal from fat on FSE images requires some type of fat saturation for detection of fluid and, hence, a pathologic process.

Although the tissue relaxation times and imaging parameters are the major determinants of contrast between joint structures and fluid, lipid suppression increases contrast between non–lipid- and lipid-containing tissues and affects how the MR scanner sets the overall dynamic range of the image (Fig. 1-12). The most

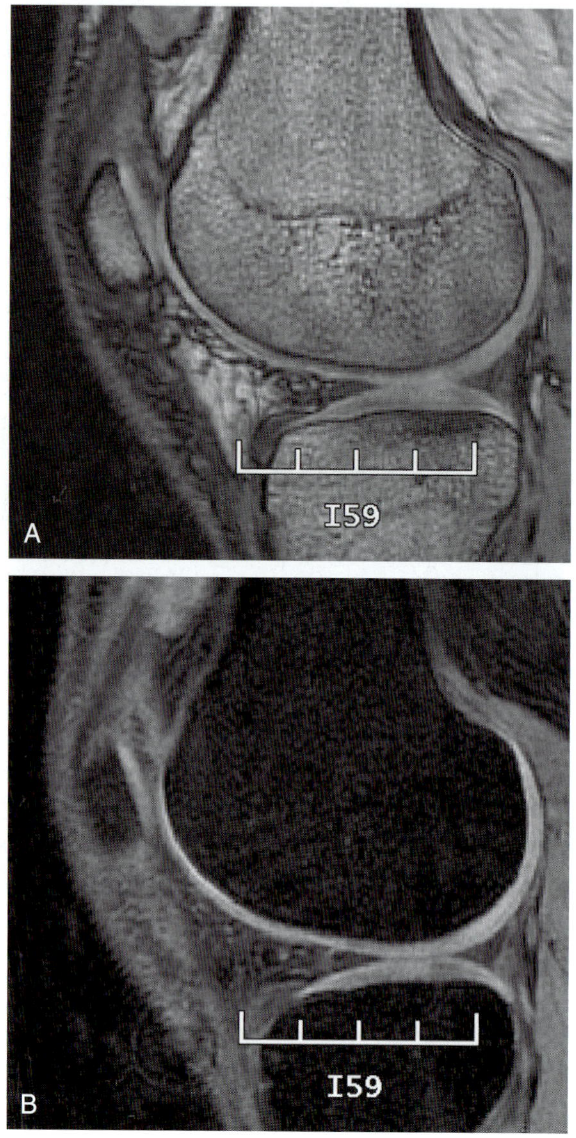

FIGURE 1-12. Examples of fat suppression imaging. **A,** Sagittal gradient-echo image of the knee without fat suppression. **B,** Sagittal gradient-echo image of the knee using chemical fat suppression. The fat suppression here is very homogeneous and improves the dynamic range in the cartilage.

common type of lipid suppression is chemical fat saturation, in which fat spins are excited and then dephased before imaging. In areas of magnetic field inhomogeneity, inversion recovery provides a way to suppress lipids at the expense of signal to noise.

If fat suppression is inhomogeneous or metal is present, as in an anterior cruciate ligament reconstruction, fast short tau inversion recovery (STIR)[25] is used with TR of 5000 ms, TE of 54 to 72 ms, and inversion time (TI) of 150 to 160 ms (1.5T scanner) (Fig. 1-13). In general, chemical saturation or water-selective excitation is preferable to inversion recovery imaging because of a higher SNR and generally superior image quality.[26] However, reliance of chemical fat saturation in areas of the body where the main field is inhomogeneous, such as the foot, can cause mistakes, because the fat saturation pulse can actually saturate water signal.

Because the difference in resonance frequencies of fat and water decreases with the field strength of the magnet, the chemical saturation technique is more difficult to

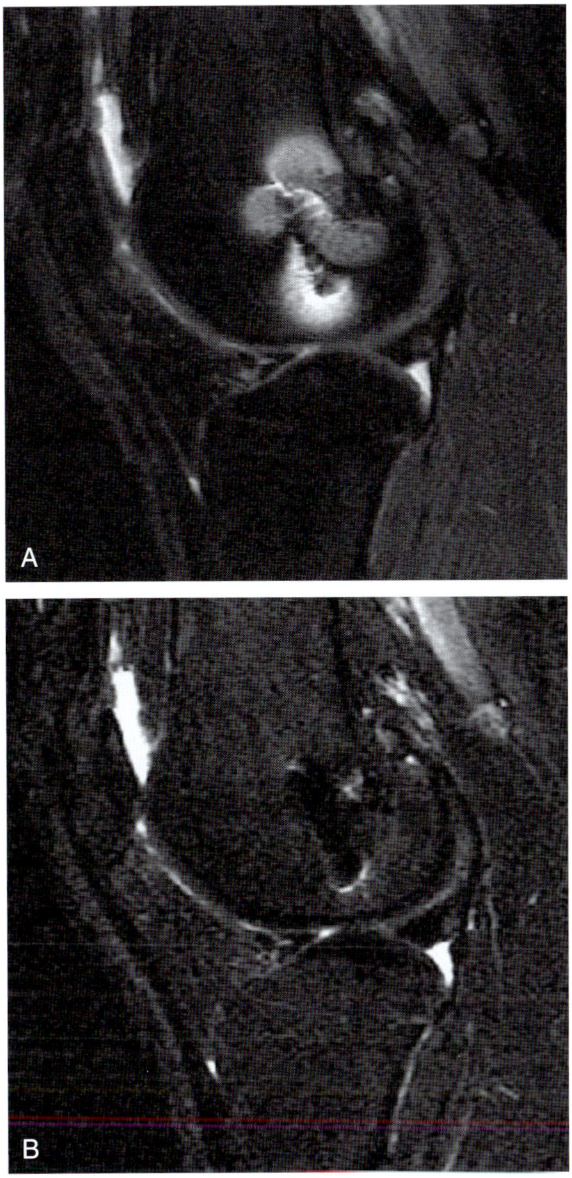

FIGURE 1-13. Examples of inversion recovery imaging. **A,** Sagittal T2-weighted image of the postoperative knee showing metal artifacts. **B,** Fast inversion-recovery image of the same slice showing better fat suppression around the interference screw. The fat suppression here is very homogeneous despite the main field inhomogeneity induced by the metal.

achieve at lower field strengths. Fast STIR techniques, however, are less dependent on field homogeneity and can be used at any field strength.[27] However, the STIR technique is not a fat- or water-specific technique. Any substance with T1 relaxation times similar to fat will have a very low signal on STIR. Thus, STIR should be avoided in conjunction with intravenous or intra-articular administration of a contrast agent.

Another option for suppression signal from fat is spectral-spatial excitation, in which only water spins in a slice are excited.[28] This technique can often provide a more homogeneous low signal from fat than fat saturation (Fig. 1-14). Another technique for images free of fat signal is Dixon-based imaging,[29] in which multiple acquisitions are used to separate fat and water. One variation of this method is called IDEAL (Iterative Decomposition of water and fat with Echo Asymmetry and Least squares estimation).[30,31] This method will be discussed in a later chapter in this book.

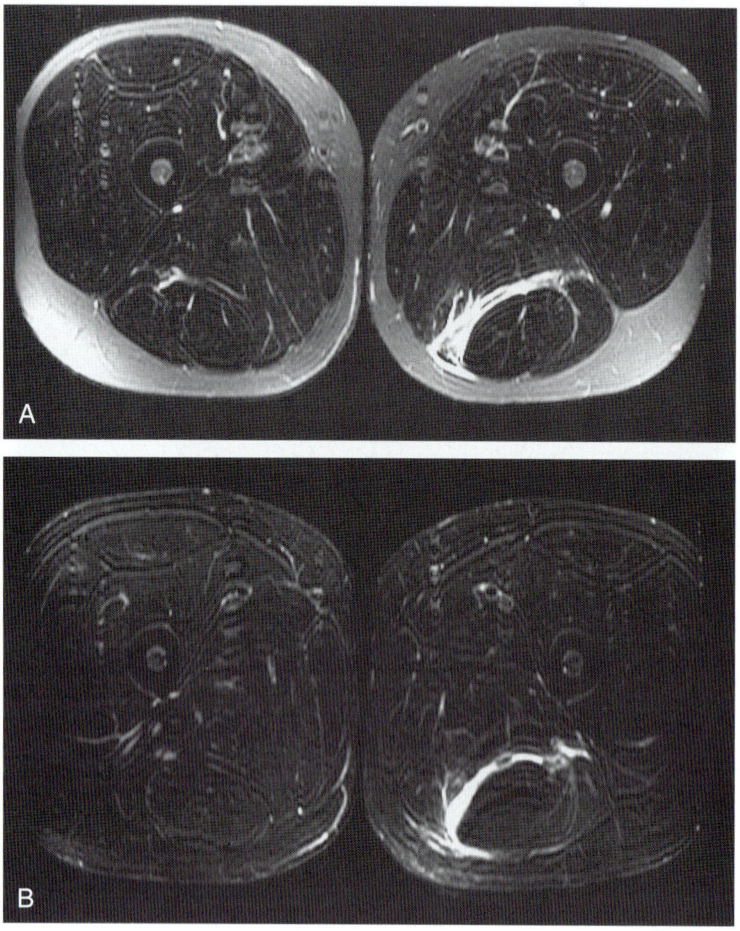

FIGURE 1-14. Images done with conventional fat suppression (**A**) and spectral-spatial excitation (**B**). The image done with spectral-spatial excitation shows uniform excitation of water spins without signal from the subcutaneous fat.

Gradient-Recalled-Echo Imaging

Gradient-echo techniques can provide T1, spin density, or T2* weighting and can be combined with fat suppression (Fig. 1-15) to provide compelling images of articular cartilage.[32] In the wrist, for example, a 3D gradient-echo sequence can be used to obtain high-resolution coronal images of the triangular fibrocartilage and intrinsic carpal ligaments.[21] Metal fragments too small to demonstrate on conventional radiographs are often present in the joint after surgical therapy. These fragments may cause artifacts on gradient-recalled-echo imaging, limiting the utility in some cases. The increased chemical shift at 3.0T means chemical fat suppression pulses may be shorter, resulting in a shorter TR on fat-suppressed 3D gradient-echo examinations and more slices on fat-suppressed 2D multi-slice acquisitions.

STANDARD MRI PROTOCOLS OF ARTHRITIS

In general, protocols should be designed to allow comparison of T1- or PD-weighted images with fat-suppressed or T2-weighted images at the same slice location. The images can be viewed side by side. The high-resolution T1- or PD-weighted images are used for anatomic detail, and the fat-suppressed T2-weighted images are used for delineation of fluid.

Intravenous contrast injections have increased our capabilities to diagnose many features of arthropathy, including soft tissue inflammatory processes such as pannus

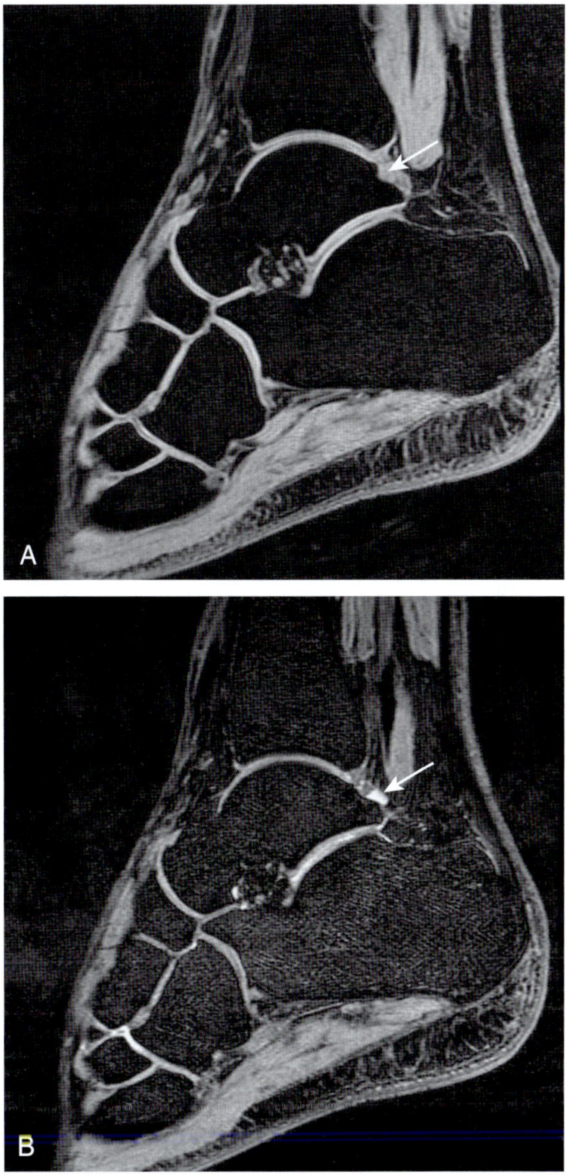

FIGURE 1-15. Gradient-recalled-echo images of the ankle at 3.0T. These images were done with IDEAL (Iterative Decomposition of water and fat with Echo Asymmetry and Least squares estimation) fat/water separation. **A,** IDEAL spoiled gradient-recalled-echo image showing dark fluid (*arrow*) and relative T1 weighting. **B,** IDEAL gradient-recalled-echo image showing relative bright fluid and T2/T1 contrast.

formation and synovitis (Fig. 1-16). In general, techniques that utilize gadolinium as a contrast medium take advantage of the high spatial resolution of fat-suppressed T1-weighted images in multiple planes. Another option for contrast-enhanced imaging is spoiled gradient-echo imaging using a high flip angle and chemical fat suppression.

SUMMARY

High-quality musculoskeletal MRI of arthritis is possible at several field strengths and with several types of MR scanners. Choice of the proper imaging coil for the application is important. Knowledge of the anatomy and pathologic conditions being imaged is also essential. Finally, knowledge of the tradeoffs among image resolution, contrast, and scan time are also important to design an efficient and high-quality imaging protocol.

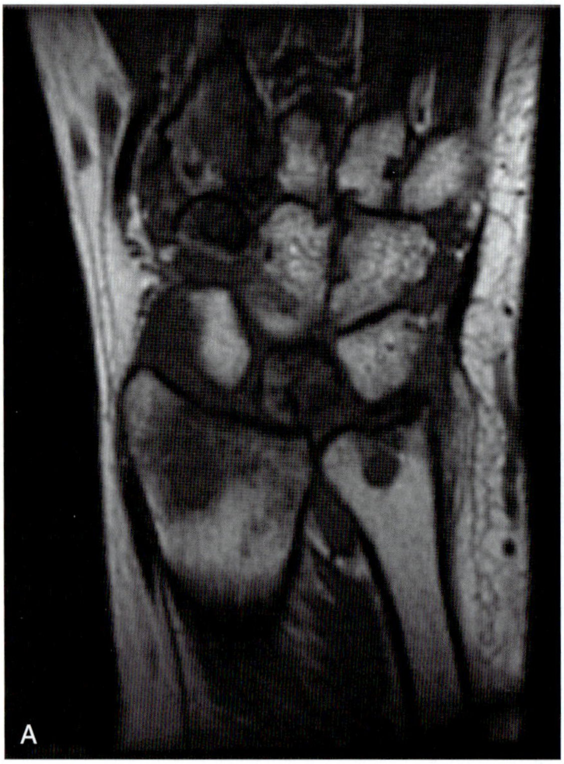

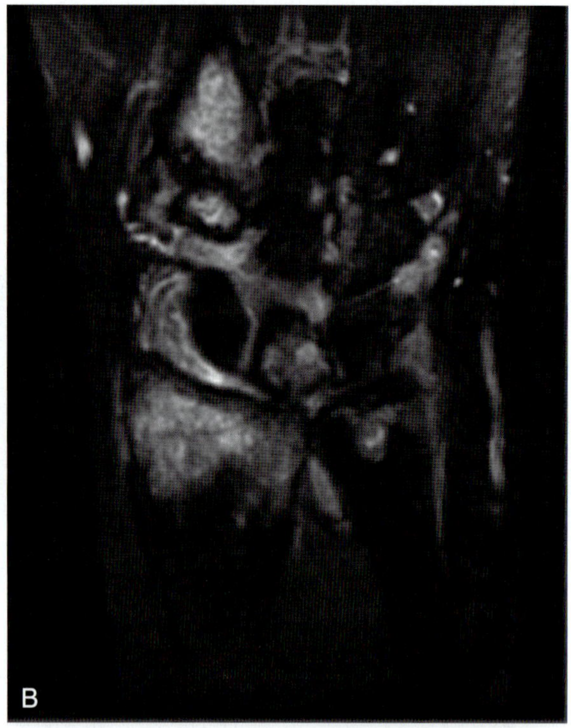

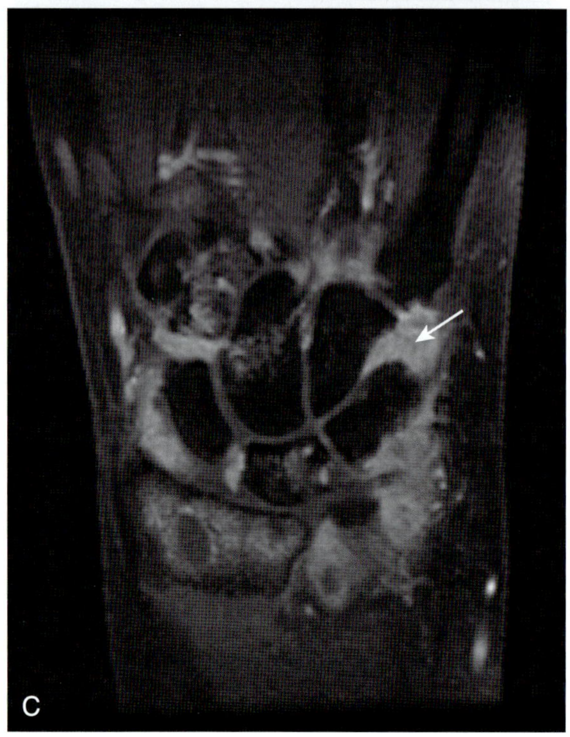

FIGURE 1-16. MR images of the wrist in a patient with rheumatoid arthritis. **A,** Coronal T1-weighted spin-echo image. **B,** Coronal T2-weighted fast spin-echo image with chemical fat suppression. **C,** Coronal T1-weighted spin-echo image with fat suppression after intravenous administration of gadolinium. This image shows enhancing pannus and synovium (*arrow*), which is typical of this inflammatory arthropathy.

References

1. Gold GE, Thedens DR, Pauly JM, et al. MR imaging of articular cartilage of the knee: new methods using ultrashort TEs. AJR Am J Roentgenol 1998; 170:1223-1226.
2. Gold GE, Pauly JM, Macovski A, Herfkens RJ. MR spectroscopic imaging of collagen: tendons and knee menisci. Magn Reson Med 1995; 34:647-654.
3. Maurer J, Requardt H, Sander B, et al. Applications of specialized coils for high-resolution MRI on a whole-body scanner. Magma 1996; 4:27-33.
4. Zlatkin MB. Techniques for MR imaging of joints in sports medicine. Neuroimaging Clin North Am 1999; 7:1-22.
5. Hayes CE, Tsuruda JS, Mathis CM, et al. Brachial plexus: MR imaging with a dedicated phased array of surface coils. Radiology 1997; 203:286-289.
6. Hayes CE, Hattes N, Roemer PB. Volume imaging with MR phased arrays. Magn Reson Med 1991; 18:309-319.
7. Roemer PB, Edelstein WA, Hayes CE, et al. The NMR phased array. Magn Reson Med 1990; 16:192-225.
8. Niitsu M, Mishima H, Miyakawa S, Itai Y. High resolution MR imaging of the bilateral hips with dual phased-array coil. J Magn Reson Imaging 1996; 6:950-953.
9. Kwok WE, Lo KK, Seo G, Totterman SM. A volume adjustable four-coil phased array for high resolution MR imaging of the hip. Magma 1999; 9:59-64.
10. Alley MT, Grist TM, Swan JS. Development of a phased-array coil for the lower extremities. Magn Reson Med 1995; 34:260-267.
11. Lucas P, Kaplan P, Dussault R, Hurwitz S. MRI of the foot and ankle. Curr Probl Diagn Radiol 1997; 26:209-266.
12. Kocharian A, Adkins MC, Amrami KK, et al. Wrist: improved MR imaging with optimized transmit-receive coil design. Radiology 2002; 223:870-876.
13. Escobedo EM, Hunter JC, Zink-Brody GC, et al. Usefulness of turbo spin-echo MR imaging in the evaluation of meniscal tears: comparison with a conventional spin-echo sequence. AJR Am J Roentgenol 1996; 167:1223-1227.
14. Anderson MW, Raghavan N, Seidenwurm DJ, et al. Evaluation of meniscal tears: fast spin-echo versus conventional spin-echo magnetic resonance imaging. Acad Radiol 1995; 2:209-214.
15. Cheung LP, Li KC, Hollett MD, et al. Meniscal tears of the knee: accuracy of detection with fast spin-echo MR imaging and arthroscopic correlation in 293 patients. Radiology 1997; 203:508-512.
16. Ha TP, Li KC, Beaulieu CF, et al. Anterior cruciate ligament injury: fast spin-echo MR imaging with arthroscopic correlation in 217 examinations. AJR Am J Roentgenol 1998; 170:1215-1219.
17. Bredella MA, Tirman PF, Peterfy CG, et al. Accuracy of T2-weighted fast spin-echo MR imaging with fat saturation in detecting cartilage defects in the knee: comparison with arthroscopy in 130 patients. AJR Am J Roentgenol 1999; 172:1073-1080.
18. Goodwin DW, Dunn JF. High-resolution magnetic resonance imaging of articular cartilage: correlation with histology and pathology. Top Magn Reson Imaging 1998; 9:337-347.
19. Kato H, Nakamura R, Shionoya K, et al. Does high-resolution MR imaging have better accuracy than standard MR imaging for evaluation of the triangular fibrocartilage complex? J Hand Surg [Br] 2000; 25:487-491.
20. Link TM, Majumdar S, Peterfy C, et al. High resolution MRI of small joints: impact of spatial resolution on diagnostic performance and SNR. Magn Reson Imaging 1998; 16: 147-155.
21. Potter HG, Asnis-Ernberg L, Weiland AJ, et al. The utility of high-resolution magnetic resonance imaging in the evaluation of the triangular fibrocartilage complex of the wrist. J Bone Joint Surg Am 1997; 79:1675-1684.
22. Rubenstein JD, Li JG, Majumdar S, Henkelman RM. Image resolution and signal-to-noise ratio requirements for MR imaging of degenerative cartilage. AJR Am J Roentgenol 1997; 169:1089-1096.
23. Gold GE, Han E, Stainsby J, et al. Musculoskeletal MRI at 3.0 T: relaxation times and image contrast. AJR Am J Roentgenol 2004; 183:343-351.
24. Henkelman RM, Hardy PA, Bishop JE, et al. Why fat is bright in RARE and fast spin-echo imaging. J Magn Reson Imaging 1992; 2:533-540.
25. Miller TT, Randolph DA Jr, Staron RB, et al. Fat-suppressed MRI of musculoskeletal infection: fast T2-weighted techniques versus gadolinium-enhanced T1-weighted images. Skeletal Radiol 1997; 26:654-658.
26. Sofka CM, Potter HG. Magnetic resonance imaging of the wrist. Semin Musculoskelet Radiol 2001; 5:217-226.
27. Ahn JM, Kwak SM, Kang HS, et al. Evaluation of patellar cartilage in cadavers with a low-field-strength extremity-only magnet: comparison of MR imaging sequences, with macroscopic findings as the standard. Radiology 1998; 208:57-62.
28. Meyer CH, Pauly JM, Macovski A, Nishimura DG. Simultaneous spatial and spectral selective excitation. Magn Reson Med 1990; 15:287-304.

29. Glover GH, Schneider E. Three-point Dixon technique for true water/fat decomposition with B0 inhomogeneity correction. Magn Reson Med 1991; 18:371-383.
30. Reeder SB, Pelc NJ, Alley MT, Gold GE. Rapid MR imaging of articular cartilage with steady-state free precession and multipoint fat-water separation. AJR Am J Roentgenol 2003; 180:357-362.
31. Reeder SB, Pineda AR, Wen Z, et al. Iterative decomposition of water and fat with echo asymmetry and least-squares estimation (IDEAL): Application with fast spin-echo imaging. Magn Reson Med 2005; 54:636-644.
32. Disler DG, McCauley TR. Clinical magnetic resonance imaging of articular cartilage. Top Magn Reson Imaging 1998; 9:360-376.

Chapter 2

FUNCTIONAL ANATOMY AND STRUCTURE OF THE "OSTEOCHONDRAL UNIT"

Timothy J. Mosher

The primary function of articular cartilage is to provide a smooth transfer of force across joints. As such it is useful to consider the cartilage and the underlying subchondral bone as a functional osteochondral unit that must withstand a combination of compressive, tensile, and shear stresses. The stresses are not trivial. For example, it is estimated that with deep knee bending the patellar cartilage undergoes compressive loads that are greater than 6 times body weight.[1] With certain athletic activities such as running, jumping, or weight lifting the forces applied to the joints can reach 10 to 20 times body weight. When considering that human joints are exposed to forces of this magnitude over millions of cycles it is remarkable that normal joint function can be sustained into old age in many individuals. The resiliency of cartilage is due to the highly organized tissue structure. The first portion of this chapter is an overview of osteochondral anatomy as it relates to tissue biomechanics and joint function. The focus in the second half of the chapter is on the role of cartilage structure on the MRI appearance, with particular emphasis on the effect of collagen structure on cartilage T2-weighted signal intensity.

CARTILAGE COMPOSITION

The biomechanical tissue properties of articular cartilage reflect the composition and organization of the extracellular matrix. Articular cartilage is hypocellular and composed of approximately 4% chondrocytes by wet weight.[2] The extracellular matrix is 65% to 85% water, with water content decreasing slightly with depth from the articular surface. The major solid components of the extracellular matrix are type II collagen, which comprises 10% to 20% of the wet weight of cartilage, and large molecules of aggregating proteoglycans, termed *aggrecan,* that contribute 5% to 10% of the wet weight.[3] Most of the extracellular water is in the solution domain of the aggrecan molecules and is freely exchangeable with synovial fluid; however, a small component is bound in the interfibrillar space of the collagen fibrils.[4,5]

The content and structure of collagen and proteoglycans in the matrix differ substantially from bone to the articular surface and strongly influence the biomaterial properties of cartilage.[3,6] The components of type II collagen, tropocollagen molecules, are polymerized into larger collagen fibrils,[7] which, in turn, are organized into a leaflike architecture.[8] As illustrated in Figure 2-1, the orientation and alignment of the collagen matrix vary with depth from the articular surface as well as regionally within the joint. Collagen fibrils cross the bone/cartilage interface at the tidemark

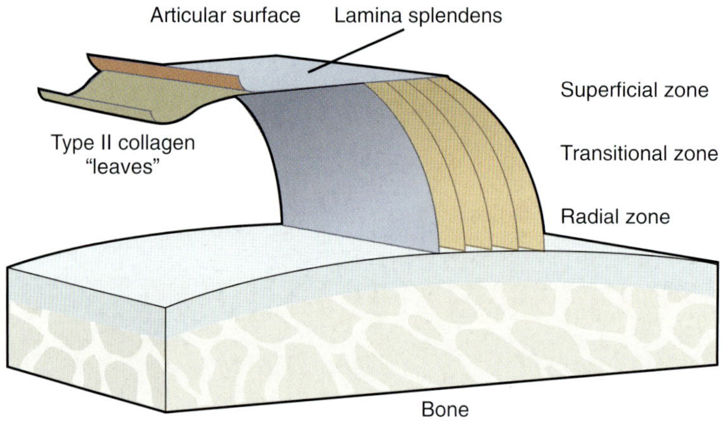

FIGURE 2-1. Structural organization of the type II collagen matrix as a function of depth from the articular surface. The surface of cartilage is covered with a distinct layer termed the *lamina splendens*. Just beneath this layer, collagen fibrils have a preferential orientation parallel to the articular surface. With increasing depth, the collagen matrix assumes a more oblique orientation (transitional zone), ultimately becoming perpendicular to the articular surface in the deep radial zone.

zone and secure cartilage to the subchondral bone.[9] In the deep layer of cartilage near bone, collagen fibrils have a preferential orientation perpendicular to the bone surface. This is frequently termed the *radial zone*, referring to the radial orientation of the collagen matrix[10] as well as the columnar alignment of chondrocytes observed in this layer. Near the surface, the orientation of the collagen matrix curves tangentially in the transitional zone, becoming parallel to the articular surface in the superficial zone.[8,11] Initial studies of the transitional zone suggested a decreased level of orientation of collagen fibrils in this layer; however, more recent studies using MRI[12] and cryofracture scanning electron microscopy[13] demonstrate anisotropy in this layer with a preferential orientation oblique to the articular surface. The thickness of the transitional layer increases near the periphery of the articular surface.[14] The superficial layer is covered with a distinct layer of dense collagen fibers termed the *lamina splendens*.[15] The smooth surface of the lamina splendens, along with the production of unique proteoglycans such as lubricin,[16] surface zone protein, and constituents of synovial fluid greatly reduce friction at the articular surface.[17]

In addition to the zonal variation of the type II collagen matrix, with respect to depth from the articular surface, there are regional differences in composition and organization of collagen within the joint. Regions that are habitually exposed to compressive load, such as the central region of the femoral tibial joint, generally have a thick radial zone and a thinner transitional zone.[18] In addition, habitually loaded regions of cartilage are condensed into thicker fibrils that are spaced at regular intervals.[19] This periodicity is lacking in habitually unloaded cartilage, where collagen fibrils are thinner and have a more random arrangement. Near the periphery of the joint where cartilage experiences primarily shear stress, the transitional zone is thicker and the preferential orientation of the fibers reflects the prevailing direction of shear strain.[14] In addition to regional variation in type II collagen there are also regional differences in expression of nonfibillar collagen proteins responsible for maintaining the organization of the collagen matrix.[20]

Interposed in the meshwork of type II collagen fibrils are large molecules of aggregating proteoglycans consisting of aggrecan.[21] As with collagen and water content, the concentration of proteoglycans also varies within cartilage, with the highest levels found in the middle section and decreasing in concentration near bone and at the articular surface.[22,23] As illustrated in Figure 2-2, aggrecan is composed of a central core fiber filament of hyaluronic acid.[21] Through a linking protein the aggrecan monomers are bound to the hyaluronic acid filament. Aggrecan monomers are composed of a central core protein that binds to large, negatively charged glycosaminoglycan molecules consisting of chondroitin sulfate and keratin sulfate. The ionic groups of the chondroitin sulfate and keratin sulfate confer a net negative fixed charge density to the aggrecan in solution. When these molecules are hydrated, the

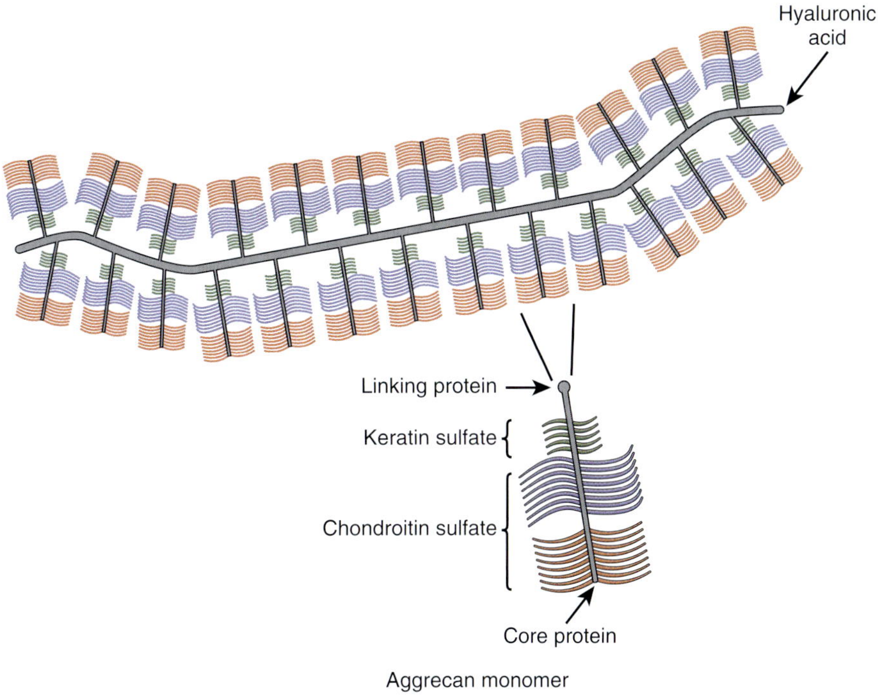

FIGURE 2-2. Structure of the aggrecan. The predominant noncollagen molecule in cartilage is the large aggregating proteoglycans called aggrecan. Each aggrecan monomer consists of a central core protein that serves as the attachment sites for a large number of negatively charged glycosaminoglycans (GAGs): keratin sulfate and chondroitin sulfate. The aggrecan monomers form large aggregates of up to 100 aggrecan monomers by attaching to a central filament of hyaluronic acid. The high concentration of GAG in aggrecan produces a large net negative charge density that binds cations, primarily sodium, leading to high osmotic pressure and swelling of the molecule when hydrated.

high density of negative charges on the proteoglycans binds sodium and draws water into cartilage through osmotic pressure, causing the proteoglycans to swell.[24] Swelling of proteoglycans is constrained by the surrounding collagen meshwork, producing an interstitial fluid pressure of approximately 9 MPa.[25] This pressurization contributes to the compressive stiffness of cartilage, an essential feature for normal cartilage function.

Also critical to the normal cartilage function is the interface with subchondral bone. The subchondral plate illustrated in Figure 2-3 consists of the tidemark zone representing the junction of calcified and uncalcified cartilage, the zone of calcified cartilage, lamellar subchondral cortical bone, and the underlying trabeculae. Collagen fibers in the radial zone extend through the tidemark zone into calcified cartilage but have not been demonstrated to pass into the underlying cortex.[26] The osteochondral junction represents a potential cleavage plane in response to shear stress.[27] The thickness of the subchondral plate varies with respect to the biomechanical force applied to it and thus will vary depending on joint geometry, loading conditions, and factors such as age, weight, and exercise.[28] The subchondral plate can remodel in response to altered biomechanics that may occur as a result of joint injury and damage to overlying cartilage.[29]

CARTILAGE BIOMECHANICS

In activities of daily living, such as walking, the contact region of one articular surface quickly passes over the opposing surface. During this instant the contact pressure at

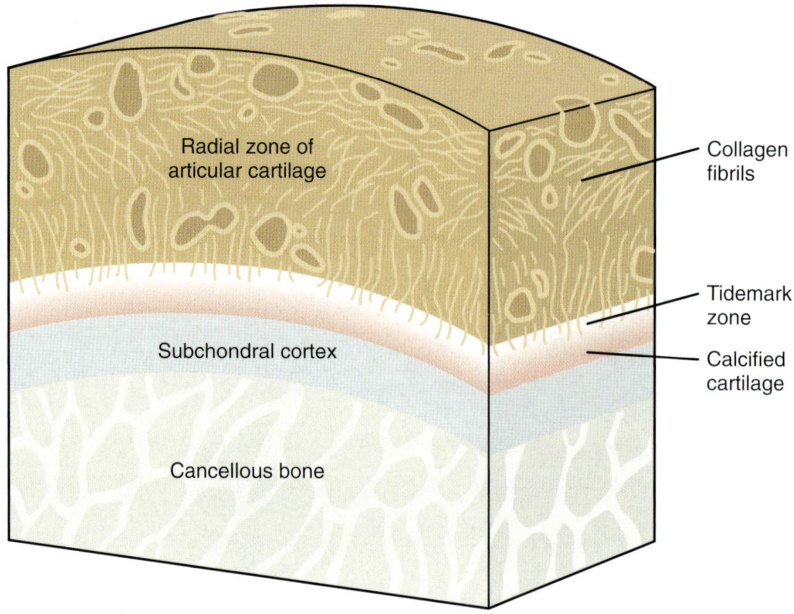

FIGURE 2-3. Structure of the subchondral plate. Type II collagen fibrils oriented perpendicular to the articular surface pass through the tidemark zone, terminating in the zone of calcified cartilage. There is a potential cleavage plane between the zone of calcified cartilage and subchondral cortex of bone. The underlying cortex is supported by trabecular bone that can remodel in response to changes in biomechanical loads.

any one point will rapidly rise in a fraction of a second. When this occurs, cartilage deforms, thereby increasing the local joint congruity and contact area. The intensity of the force imparted onto the articular surface per unit area is termed *stress.* The deformation of the tissue in response to the applied stress is the *tissue strain.* When cartilage is loaded, different forms of strain are generated within the tissue. Portions of the tissue are compressed while others are stretched, placing the tissue under tension. In many biologic tissues, such as cartilage, the strain that develops within the tissue in response to the applied stress will vary over time. These tissues are said to demonstrate viscoelastic properties, which in cartilage are a function of the interaction of the three principal components: water, type II collagen matrix, and aggrecan.[30]

Compression

As cartilage is compressed it deforms, producing bulk flow of water through the extracellular matrix.[31] As the cartilage deforms, fluid is exuded into the synovial space. Because of the viscoelastic properties of cartilage the stiffness of the tissue is a function of the rate at which the compressive force is applied.[32] Cartilage is stiffer when the force is applied rapidly and demonstrates less compressive stiffness when the force is applied slowly. The ability of cartilage to resist compression is a result of the ability of the extracellular matrix to limit water permeability.[33] In healthy cartilage, the frictional drag forces of water flow dissipate the vast majority of energy imparted into the tissue during compression. As water movement becomes less restricted, more of the energy is imparted to the collagen and aggrecan matrix, leading to tissue degradation. Resistance to water flow is a function of the high osmolarity, viscosity, and interstitial pressure of the extracellular matrix.

An important function of cartilage is to transfer the compressive force to the underlying bone, which is substantially stiffer. Cartilage demonstrates a depth-

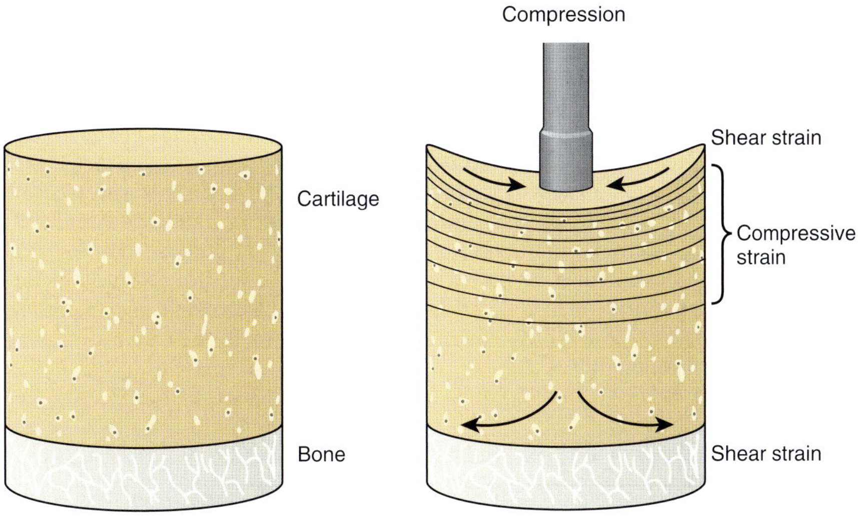

FIGURE 2-4. Depth-dependent response of cartilage to compression. Compression of cartilage produces high tissue deformation and shear strain near the articular surface. With increasing depth from the surface there is less tissue deformation and flow of water through the extracellular matrix. High compressive loads transmitted to the deeper layer of cartilage produce high shear strain in the tidemark zone at the cartilage/bone interface. Shear strain that exceeds the material properties of the tissue can result in cartilage delamination from the subchondral plate.

dependent difference in compressibility, becoming progressively stiffer toward bone.[34] During physiologic loads most of the tissue deformation occurs in the superficial layer of cartilage, with very little compression occurring in the radial zone near the cartilage/bone interface. The depth-dependent response of cartilage to compressive load is illustrated in Figure 2-4.

Tension

As the contour of cartilage is perturbed a portion of the tissue is placed under tension. The ability of cartilage to withstand tensile strain is primarily a function of the fibrillar type II collagen meshwork that is anchored to the calcified tidemark zone of cartilage. The hydrated aggrecan contributes to the tensile stiffness of cartilage by buttressing the collagen meshwork.[35]

Shear

Shear stress occurs when a force is applied tangentially to the surface of a material. In the case of cartilage, shear stress occurs primarily at the articular surface as one cartilage surface passes over the other, and at the bone/cartilage interface, where differences in compressive stiffness of these tissues can produce shear strain during high compressive loads.

For normal cartilage the articular surface has a coefficient of friction that is several orders of magnitude less than man-made materials.[36] This is in part due to the smooth surface of the lamina splendens. Specialized molecules in the surface layer of cartilage such as superficial zone protein and lubricin provide important boundary lubrication. In addition, the extrusion of fluid from the cartilage surface as it is transiently compressed provides a fluid gliding layer that reduces shear strain. In the tangential zone the type II collagen fibrils have a preferential alignment along the direction of habitual shear strain within the joint. As shear strain develops in the surface layer of cartilage, this strain is transferred as tensile strain to the underlying collagen meshwork. Excessive tensile strain can produce fractures within the collagen matrix, leading to cartilage fissures along the collagen "leaves" or flap-type tears at the junction of the transitional and radial cartilage zones.

Differences in biomaterial properties of cartilage and bone can lead to high shear strain at the tidemark zone.[9] As illustrated in Figure 2-4, compressive forces transmitted to the deep layers of cartilage from the articular surface are transferred into shear force as they reach the cartilage/bone interface. This can lead to cleavage of the radial fibers at the tidemark zone, resulting in cartilage delamination.[37] As described previously, the radial collagen fibrils of the radial zone pass through the tidemark, terminating in the zone of calcified cartilage. Because the fibers do not pass into the subchondral cortex there is the potential for cleavage between the calcified cartilage and subchondral bone.

MRI PROPERTIES OF NORMAL CARTILAGE

The MRI relaxation properties of articular cartilage and the appearance of cartilage with standard clinical MRI techniques are strongly influenced by the composition and structure of the extracellular matrix. As a result of this sensitivity, MRI has the potential to function as a noninvasive image marker of structural properties of the extracellular matrix and underlying bone. Because these observations can be made noninvasively in human joints, MRI is a valuable clinical research technique, providing unique information regarding the natural history of cartilage development, physiology, and in-situ biomechanics.

The influence of cartilage structure and composition on MRI signal intensity is most evident on T2-weighted images. As illustrated in Figure 2-5, the signal intensity of cartilage varies with location in the joint as well as with depth from the articular surface. This is primarily a function of regional and zonal differences of the type II collagen matrix, which influences T2 relaxation of cartilage, as well as variation in water content. Within the radial zone the high content and anisotropic orientation of collagen fibrils provide efficient T2 relaxation, leading to low signal intensity on proton-density (PD)- or T2-weighted images. With very high resolution images, the darker radial zone has a striated appearance with alternating fine bands of high and

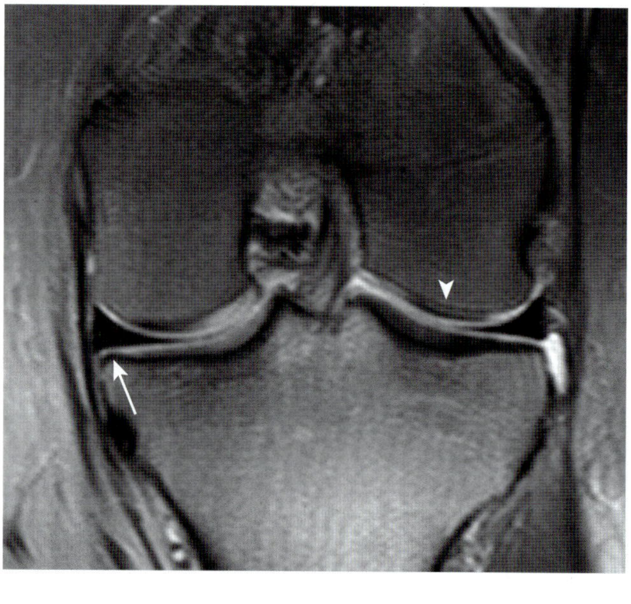

FIGURE 2-5. Normal cartilage. A coronal, 3.0T, T2-weighted, turbo spin-echo (TR/TE: 3200/28 ms) MR image of the femoral tibial joint demonstrates regional variation in the signal intensity of cartilage that reflects structural variation in the architecture of the type II collagen matrix. Central portions of the joint habitually exposed to high compressive loads (*arrowhead*) have a thick radial zone and demonstrate a large hypointense deeper layer of cartilage. Toward the periphery of the joint greater shear stress leads to a smaller radial zone and thicker transitional cartilage zone, reflected in the higher signal intensity of cartilage (*arrow*).

low signal intensity radiating from the bone/cartilage interface. In lower-resolution images, individual striations are not resolved and, instead, this layer is characterized by low signal intensity. Closer to the articular surface, less fibril anisotropy and oblique orientation of the collagen matrix lead to a gradual increase in T2 relaxation time and thus a relative increase in signal intensity on T2-weighted images. At the articular surface, collagen fibers are oriented parallel to the articular surface. The superficial tangential layer and the lamina splendens is approximately 200 μm thick and can be identified on MR microscopy images of excised cartilage specimens as a thin hypointense layer; however, it is too thin to resolve on routine clinical MR images.

The organization and orientation of collagen within the cartilage matrix have a strong influence on the MRI appearance of cartilage. In connective tissues such as tendons, ligaments, and articular cartilage, the highly ordered arrangement of collagen fibers produces residual quadripolar coupling with mobile protons, an efficient mechanism for T2 relaxation.[38,39] For these tissues with a highly preferred or anisotropic organization of collagen fibrils, T2 relaxation is dependent on the relative orientation of the collagen fibers with applied static magnetic field (B0). Tissues containing fibers oriented parallel or perpendicular to B0 have efficient T2 relaxation and low signal intensity on T2-weighted images. However, when fibers are oriented 54 degrees relative to B0 there is averaging of the residual quadripolar coupling, which minimizes this contribution to T2 relaxation and leads to an increase in signal intensity. Because of this effect, 54 degrees is called the "magic angle," derived from the technique of magic angle spinning used to increase the T2 relaxation of crystalline samples in solid-state nuclear magnetic resonance spectroscopy.

The high concentration of collagen in the radial zone also decreases signal intensity through magnetization transfer.[40,41] As suggested by the name, magnetization transfer is a process in which magnetization from a proton located on collagen is transferred to the mobile proton pool that gives rise to the MR signal.[42,43] Magnetization transfer effects are most pronounced for techniques that use a large number of radiofrequency pulses such as multi-slice fast spin-echo (FSE) or turbo spin-echo (TSE) techniques.[44] The rapid application of off-resonance radiofrequency energy quickly saturates protons bound to the collagen molecules but does not saturate the mobile pool in the surrounding water. This saturated magnetization is then transferred either through chemical exchange or exchange of magnetization to nearby water protons in the mobile pool. Types I and II collagen demonstrate substantial magnetization transfer with FSE techniques. The effect of magnetization transfer is to decrease signal intensity of tissues rich in collagen on the MR image. For tissues such as cartilage, incidental magnetization transfer reduces signal intensity by 15% to 20% as the number of slices, and thus the amount of off-resonance irradiation, increases.[44] Because gradient-echo techniques use significantly less radiofrequency energy, there is less incidental magnetization transfer with gradient-echo techniques compared with spin-echo and FSE techniques. As a result of less magnetization transfer and T2 weighting, cartilage has relatively uniform high signal intensity on T1-weighted, fat-suppressed, gradient-echo images. The lack of sensitivity of gradient-echo images to structural changes in the collagen matrix limits detection of cartilage damage that occurs deep to the articular surface, particularly at the bone/cartilage interface.

Recognizing the normal heterogeneity of cartilage is important to avoid erroneously interpreting nonuniform signal as disease on T2-weighted images. As discussed previously, the signal intensity of cartilage normally increases toward the surface.[45] In addition to variation in signal intensity with respect to depth from the articular surface, there are differences with respect to location in the joint and relative orientation of cartilage to the applied magnetic field.[46,47] This variation in signal intensity closely follows variations in histologic and biomechanical properties of cartilage.[48-50] For example, cartilage consistently exposed to high compressive load such as tibial cartilage not covered by meniscus has a thin superficial layer of high signal intensity, corresponding to the thin transitional layer. The more peripheral portion of tibial cartilage covered by the meniscus has a thicker layer of superficial hyperintensity.

Goodwin and associates have correlated this regional variation in signal intensity with obliquity of the collagen matrix cleavage planes on freeze fracture specimens, indicating that the relative orientation of the cartilage matrix to the applied magnetic field is a major factor.[51]

Regional differences in cartilage T2 relaxation are most pronounced in the femoral condyle.[52] This is a result of two processes. First, there are substantial differences in the organization of extracellular matrix and chondrocytes between the central femoral surface and posterior femoral condyles, which are not habitually exposed to a high compressive load but experience shear forces during knee flexion. Whereas type II collagen in the central femoral condyle has a high degree of anisotropy, results from electron microscopy and x-ray diffraction studies indicate the collagen matrix in the posterior femoral condyle has less anisotropy and has a fine fibrillar organization.[19] This region of cartilage lacks the regular bands of condensed collagen seen in the central femoral condyle. Second, the oblique orientation of the collagen matrix in this region with respect to the direction of B0 is close to the magic angle of 54 degrees. As a result of differences in organization and orientation of the type II collagen matrix, cartilage in the posterior femoral condyle demonstrates uniformly high signal intensity compared with the layered pattern of signal intensity observed in the central femoral condyle. Although regional variation in the MRI appearance of cartilage has been extensively studied for the knee, similar variation is observed in other joints with MR images of sufficient resolution. Xia and colleagues have performed high-resolution correlations of cartilage T2 and fibril anisotropy measured with polarized light microscopy in canine humeral head samples.[53] These studies confirmed the high degree of structural variation of the cartilage tissue with respect to location of the joint and the sensitivity of cartilage T2 relaxation to the tissue architecture.

In summary, articular cartilage is relatively acellular. The viscoelastic biomaterial properties of the tissue are a function of three main components—water, type II collagen, and aggrecan—that form a fiber-reinforced composite extracellular matrix. This matrix demonstrates a high level of structural organization with respect to depth from the articular surface, as well as spatial diversity with respect to location in the joint and the prevailing biomechanical forces applied to the tissue. Because the anisotropic arrangement of the type II collagen fibrils provides an efficient pathway for T2 relaxation of interstitial water, T2-weighted MR images are highly sensitive to structural properties of cartilage. Detection of early cartilage injury through identification of changes in cartilage T2-weighted signal intensity is discussed in Chapter 3.

References

1. Huberti HH, Hayes WC. Patellofemoral contact pressures: the influence of q-angle and tendofemoral contact. J Bone Joint Surg Am 1984; 66:715-724.
2. Brandt KD, Doherty M, Lohmander S. Osteoarthritis. New York, Oxford University Press, 2003.
3. Venn M, Maroudas A. Chemical composition and swelling of normal and osteoarthrotic femoral head cartilage. I. Chemical composition. Ann Rheum Dis 1977; 36:121-129.
4. Torzilli PA. Influence of cartilage conformation on its equilibrium water partition. J Orthop Res 1985; 3:473-483.
5. Maroudas A, Schneiderman R. "Free" and "exchangeable" or "trapped" and "non-exchangeable" water in cartilage. J Orthop Res 1987; 5:133-138.
6. Guilak F, Meyer BC, Ratcliffe A, Mow VC. The effects of matrix compression on proteoglycan metabolism in articular cartilage explants. Osteoarthritis Cartilage 1994; 2:91-101.
7. Buehler MJ. Nature designs tough collagen: explaining the nanostructure of collagen fibrils. Proc Natl Acad Sci U S A 2006; 103:12285-12290.
8. Clark JM. The organization of collagen fibrils in the superficial zones of articular cartilage. J Anat 1990; 171:117-130.
9. Redler I, Mow VC, Zimny ML, Mansell J. The ultrastructure and biomechanical significance of the tidemark of articular cartilage. Clin Orthop Relat Res 1975; 112:357-362.
10. Clark JM. Variation of collagen fiber alignment in a joint surface: a scanning electron microscope study of the tibial plateau in dog, rabbit, and man. J Orthop Res 1991; 9:246-257.

11. Speer DP, Dahners L. The collagenous architecture of articular cartilage: correlation of scanning electron microscopy and polarized light microscopy observations. Clin Orthop Relat Res 1979; 139:267-275.
12. Xia Y, Moody JB, Burton-Wurster N, Lust G. Quantitative in situ correlation between microscopic MRI and polarized light microscopy studies of articular cartilage. Osteoarthritis Cartilage 2001; 9:393-406.
13. Clark JM. The organization of collagen in cryofractured rabbit articular cartilage: a scanning electron microscopic study. J Orthop Res 1985; 3:17-29.
14. Thompson AM, Stockwell RA. An ultrastructural study of the marginal transitional zone in the rabbit knee joint. J Anat 1983; 136:701-713.
15. Jeffery AK, Blunn GW, Archer CW, Bentley G. Three-dimensional collagen architecture in bovine articular cartilage. J Bone Joint Surg Br 1991; 73:795-801.
16. Jay GD, Torres JR, Warman ML, et al. The role of lubricin in the mechanical behavior of synovial fluid. Proc Natl Acad Sci U S A 2007; 104:6194-6199.
17. Schmidt TA, Gastelum NS, Nguyen QT, et al. Boundary lubrication of articular cartilage: role of synovial fluid constituents. Arthritis Rheum 2007; 56:882-891.
18. Moger CJ, Barrett R, Bleuet P, et al. Regional variations of collagen orientation in normal and diseased articular cartilage and subchondral bone determined using small angle X-ray scattering (SAXS). Osteoarthritis Cartilage 2007; 15:682-687.
19. Gomez S, Toffanin R, Bernstorff S, et al. Collagen fibrils are differently organized in weight-bearing and not-weight-bearing regions of pig articular cartilage. J Exp Zool 2000; 287:346-352.
20. Julkunen P, Kiviranta P, Wilson W, et al. Characterization of articular cartilage by combining microscopic analysis with a fibril-reinforced finite-element model. J Biomech 2007; 40:1862-1870.
21. Roughley PJ. The structure and function of cartilage proteoglycans. Eur Cell Mater 2006; 12:92-101.
22. Franzen A, Inerot S, Hejderup SO, Heinegard D. Variations in the composition of bovine hip articular cartilage with distance from the articular surface. Biochem J 1981; 195:535-543.
23. Bayliss MT, Venn M, Maroudas A, Ali SY. Structure of proteoglycans from different layers of human articular cartilage. Biochem J 1983; 209:387-400.
24. Maroudas AI, Ziv I, Weisman N, Venn M. Studies of hydration and swelling pressure in normal and osteoarthritic cartilage. Biorheology 1985; 22:159-169.
25. Maroudas AI. Balance between swelling pressure and collagen tension in normal and degenerate cartilage. Nature 1976; 260:808-809.
26. Clark JM, Huber JD. The structure of the human subchondral plate. J Bone Joint Surg Br 1990; 72:866-873.
27. Otterness IG, Chang M, Burkhardt JE, et al. Histology and tissue chemistry of tidemark separation in hamsters. Vet Pathol 1999; 36:138-145.
28. Doube M, Firth EC, Boyde A. Variations in articular calcified cartilage by site and exercise in the 18-month-old equine distal metacarpal condyle. Osteoarthritis Cartilage 2007; 15:1283-1292.
29. Inoue H. Alterations in the collagen framework of osteoarthritic cartilage and subchondral bone. Int Orthop 1981; 5:47-52.
30. Mow VC, Huiskes R. Basic Orthopaedic Biomechanics & Mechano-biology. Philadelphia, Lippincott Williams & Wilkins, 2005.
31. Lu XL, Mow VC. Biomechanics of articular cartilage and determination of material properties. Med Sci Sports Exerc 2008; 40:193-199.
32. Mow VC, Holmes MH, Lai WM. Fluid transport and mechanical properties of articular cartilage: a review. J Biomech 1984; 17:377-394.
33. Armstrong CG, Mow VC. Variations in the intrinsic mechanical properties of human articular cartilage with age, degeneration, and water content. J Bone Joint Surg Am 1982; 64:88-94.
34. Wong M, Carter DR. Articular cartilage functional histomorphology and mechanobiology: a research perspective. Bone 2003; 33:1-13.
35. Schmidt MB, Mow VC, Chun LE, Eyre DR. Effects of proteoglycan extraction on the tensile behavior of articular cartilage. J Orthop Res 1990; 8:353-363.
36. Chen AC, Klisch SM, Bae WC, et al. Mechanical characterization of native and tissue-engineered cartilage. Methods Mol Med 2004; 101:157-190.
37. Levy AS, Lohnes J, Sculley S, et al. Chondral delamination of the knee in soccer players. Am J Sports Med 1996; 24:634-639.
38. Xia Y. Magic-angle effect in magnetic resonance imaging of articular cartilage: a review. Invest Radiol 2000; 35:602-621.
39. Bydder M, Rahal A, Fullerton GD, Bydder GM. The magic angle effect: a source of artifact, determinant of image contrast, and technique for imaging. J Magn Reson Imaging 2007; 25:290-300.
40. Wolff SD, Chesnick S, Frank JA, et al. Magnetization transfer contrast: MR imaging of the knee. Radiology 1991; 179:623-628.
41. Regatte RR, Akella SV, Reddy R. Depth-dependent proton magnetization transfer in articular cartilage. J Magn Reson Imaging 2005; 22:318-323.
42. Kim DK, Ceckler TL, Hascall VC, et al. Analysis of water-macromolecule proton magnetization transfer in articular cartilage. Magn Reson Med 1993; 29:211-215.

43. Lattanzio PJ, Marshall KW, Damyanovich AZ, Peemoeller H. Macromolecule and water magnetization exchange modeling in articular cartilage. Magn Reson Med 2000; 44:840-851.
44. Yao L, Gentili A, Thomas A. Incidental magnetization transfer contrast in fast spin-echo imaging of cartilage. J Magn Reson Imaging 1996; 6:180-184.
45. Xia Y, Farquhar T, Burton-Wurster N, Lust G. Origin of cartilage laminae in MRI. J Magn Reson Imaging 1997; 7:887-894.
46. Xia Y. Heterogeneity of cartilage laminae in MR imaging. J Magn Reson Imaging 2000; 11:686-693.
47. Goodwin DW. Visualization of the macroscopic structure of hyaline cartilage with MR imaging. Semin Musculoskelet Radiol 2001; 5:305-312.
48. Kurkijarvi JE, Nissi MJ, Kiviranta I, et al. Delayed gadolinium-enhanced MRI of cartilage (dGEMRIC) and T2 characteristics of human knee articular cartilage: topographical variation and relationships to mechanical properties. Magn Reson Med 2004; 52:41-46.
49. Nieminen MT, Rieppo J, Toyras J, et al. T2 relaxation reveals spatial collagen architecture in articular cartilage: a comparative quantitative MRI and polarized light microscopic study. Magn Reson Med 2001; 46:487-493.
50. Goodwin DW, Zhu H, Dunn JF. In vitro MR imaging of hyaline cartilage: correlation with scanning electron microscopy. AJR Am J Roentgenol 2000; 174:405-409.
51. Goodwin DW, Dunn JF. High-resolution magnetic resonance imaging of articular cartilage: correlation with histology and pathology. Top Magn Reson Imaging 1998; 9:337-347.
52. Mosher TJ, Smith H, Dardzinski BJ, et al. MR imaging and T2 mapping of femoral cartilage: in vivo determination of the magic angle effect. AJR Am J Roentgenol 2001; 177:665-669.
53. Xia Y, Moody JB, Alhadlaq H, et al. Characteristics of topographical heterogeneity of articular cartilage over the joint surface of a humeral head. Osteoarthritis Cartilage 2002; 10:370-380.

Chapter 3

Clinical MRI of Osteoarthritis and Osteochondral Injury

Timothy J. Mosher

As discussed in Chapter 2, the structural integrity and function of cartilage and underlying bone are intimately coupled. Chondral injury leads to increased stress on subchondral bone, and, conversely, failure of the subchondral osseous plate undermines integrity of overlying cartilage. Although unique imaging findings are observed within cartilage, bone, and the cartilage/bone interface, it is reasonable to consider these as injuries of the osteochondral unit. It can be difficult to visualize directly chondral injury in joints such as the ankle, hip, and shoulder where cartilage is thin and covering a curved surface. Often, altered signal intensity in subchondral bone marrow is the most conspicuous finding to indicate there has been an osteochondral injury. Certain features in combination with the clinical history may provide clues as to the type and duration of injury. Recognizing the pattern of injury can assist in focusing attention to specific areas of the articular surface that are likely to have been exposed to trauma. This information may suggest an underlying mechanism and time course of the injury. The contour of the chondral margins and marrow abnormalities may help differentiate acute traumatic insult from chronic degeneration. Pooling information gathered from evaluation of the entire joint will lead to greater confidence in the diagnosis of osteochondral injury.

CLINICAL MRI OF OSTEOARTHRITIS

Although MRI is a potentially valuable clinical research tool for longitudinal studies of osteoarthritis (OA),[1-4] it plays a very limited role in the clinical evaluation of patients with established radiographic findings. There are occasions, such as when there is discrepancy between severity of clinical and radiographic findings, that MRI is a valuable clinical problem-solving tool.[5] This most often occurs in patellofemoral and hip OA when radiographic evaluation of joint space narrowing can be unreliable and underestimate the degree of articular damage. MRI may exclude confounding pathologic processes such as meniscal tears that can mimic symptoms of OA and require different therapy. As illustrated in the case presented in Figure 3-1, there is a role for MRI in OA patients who have acute worsening of pain that may indicate a new pathologic process that may impact patient management, such as an insufficiency fracture of subchondral bone.

Many factors, including biomechanics, genetics, and inflammation, affect the heterogeneous condition of OA.[6] The combination of these factors contributes to patient symptoms of pain, stiffness, and joint dysfunction. An active area of clinical MRI

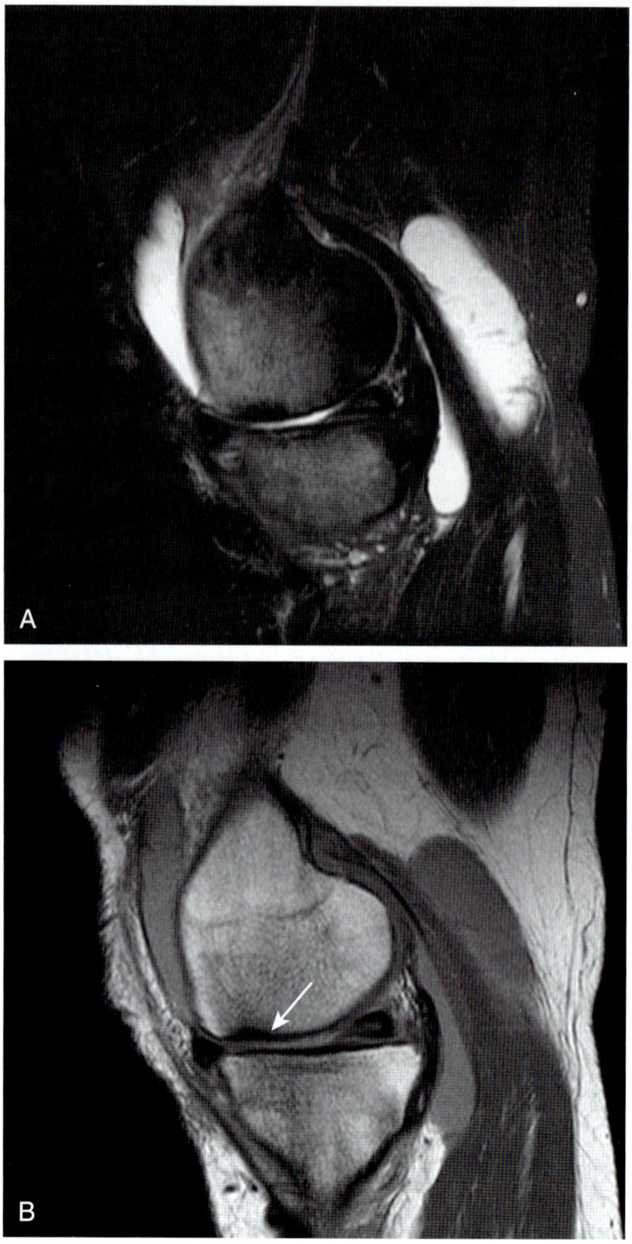

FIGURE 3-1. Insufficiency fracture in a 55-year-old man with acute exacerbation of knee pain. **A,** Sagittal, fat-suppressed, T2-weighted, turbo spin-echo (TR/TE: 4350/70 ms) image demonstrates extensive marrow "edema" in the medial femoral condyle. **B,** Sagittal, PD-weighted, turbo spin-echo (TR/TE: 1600/20 ms) image demonstrates subchondral crescentic region of low signal intensity (*arrow*) consistent with insufficiency fractures in a patient with a medial meniscal tear and advanced osteoarthritis of the medial femoral tibial compartment.

research in the management of patients with OA is identifying sources of pain based on objective imaging findings.[7-10] In the future, MRI may provide differentiation that could help guide and target treatment.[11] For example, the presence of joint effusion and synovitis may indicate patients for whom the inflammatory component of OA is a primary source of symptoms. Such a patient may benefit from treatment with anti-inflammatory medications, in contrast to patients with focal subchondral marrow changes in whom dysfunctional biomechanics may be a more important factor.[12] Another research goal in MRI is identification of imaging features that may identify patients at risk for rapid disease progression who would benefit from more aggressive intervention or alteration in lifestyle. Preliminary studies have identified subchondral bone marrow degenerative signal[13] and focal osteochondral defects[14-16] as two risk factors for knee OA progression.

OSTEOCHONDRAL INJURY

There is growing recognition that focal osteochondral injury represents a substantial risk factor for the development of OA (Fig. 3-2).[17,18] Particularly in the younger patient, MRI plays an important clinical role in the diagnosis of pre-radiographic OA and focal osteochondral injury. Increased awareness of osteochondral injuries, development of cartilage repair techniques, and advances in MRI technology have increased the diagnostic frequency of these lesions.[19] The historical dependence on radiography has emphasized the osseous component of osteochondral injuries. Although radiography continues to be the first-line imaging modality in evaluation

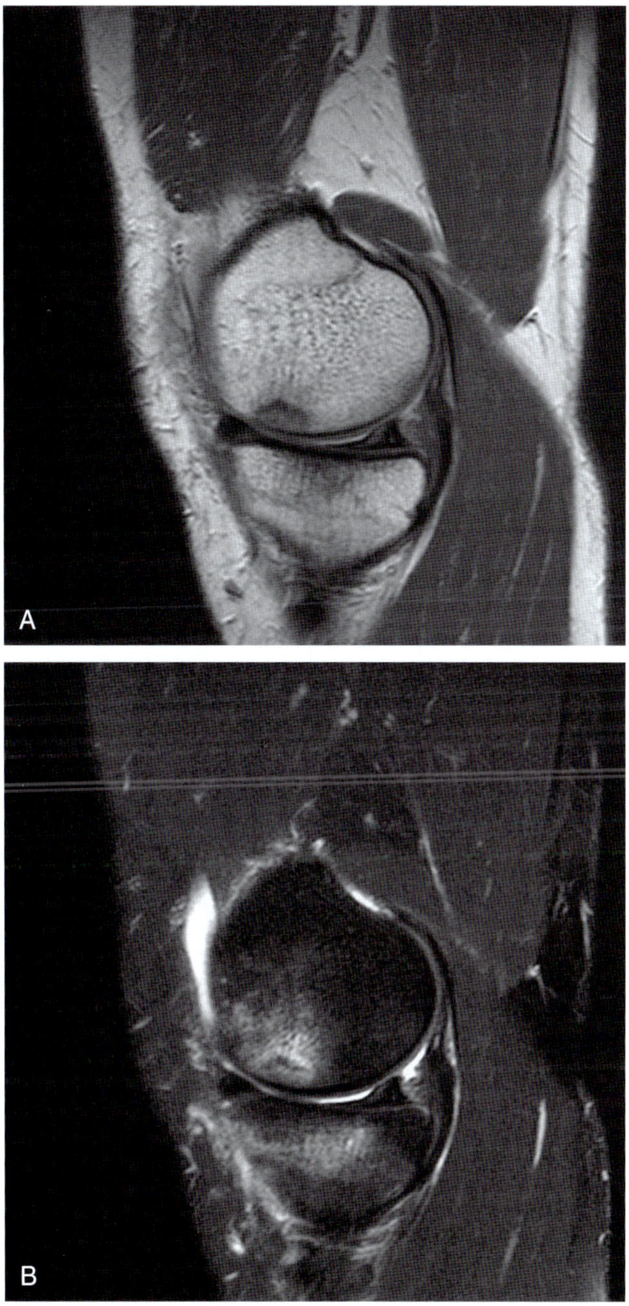

FIGURE 3-2. Osteochondral fracture. Sagittal PD-weighted (**A**) and T2-weighted turbo spin-echo (**B**) images demonstrate a nondisplaced osteochondral fracture of the medial femoral condyle. Follow-up sagittal PD-weighted (**C**) and T2-weighted turbo spin-echo (**D**) images 4 years later demonstrate complete loss of cartilage in the medial femoral tibial compartment, a meniscal tear, and a large unstable osteochondral fracture of the femoral condyle.

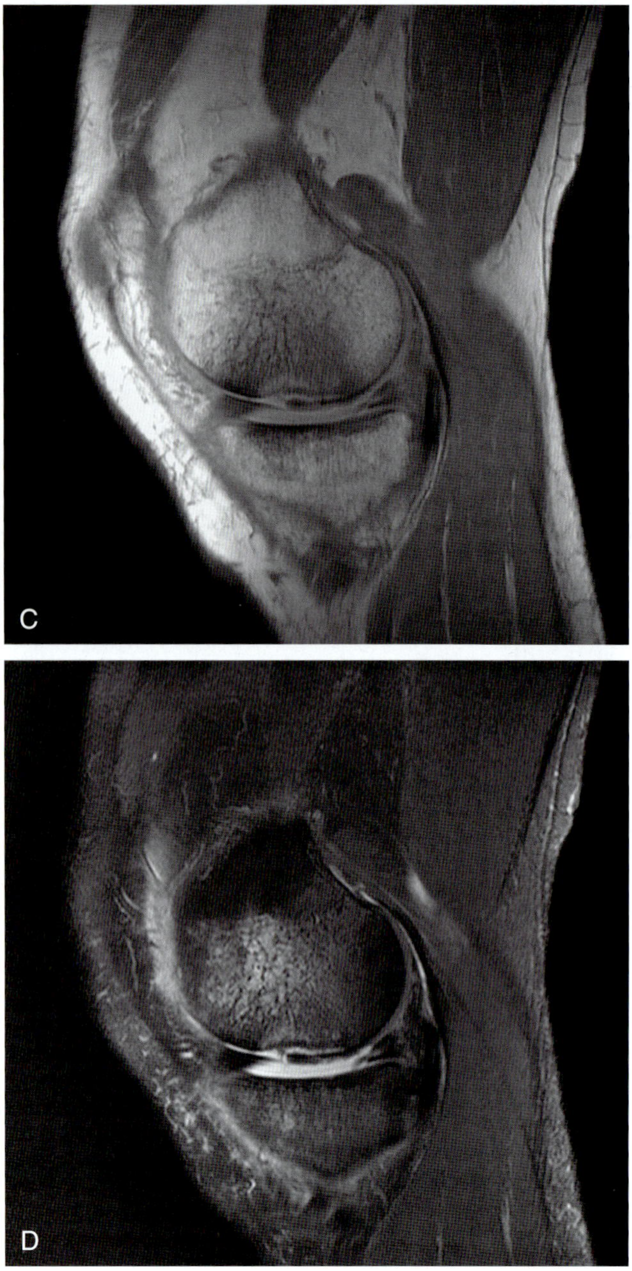

FIGURE 3-2, cont'd

of articular injuries, it is insensitive to isolated cartilage injury.[20,21] MRI has become a standard diagnostic tool in evaluation of osteochondral injuries[22,23] because it is the only noninvasive imaging technique that provides direct assessment of articular cartilage and associated subchondral marrow pathologic processes.

The thin, curved contour of articular cartilage places high technical demands on MRI. Compared with evaluation of meniscal or ligamentous injury, the accuracy and the sensitivity of MRI for cartilage injury are substantially lower and quite variable and depend on technique and experience.[24-26] Over recent years, advances in MRI hardware and acquisition techniques have improved the abilities to visualize and quantitatively monitor morphologic changes in small cartilage lesions. In addition to clinical methods focused on changes in cartilage morphology there has been development of physiologic MRI techniques that are sensitive to changes in cartilage composition and organization of the extracellular matrix that precede loss of tissue.[27,28] These techniques have the potential to provide novel information on the natural history of early cartilage injury, in-vivo cartilage biomechanics, and longitudinal evaluation of cartilage repair.[29,30]

Osteochondral injuries represent a spectrum of articular conditions ranging from acute cartilage tears to chronic osteochondral defects, including osteochondritis dissecans (OCD). Although there is ongoing debate regarding the pathogenesis of OCD, there is a consensus supporting a traumatic/mechanical theory of injury to the osteochondral unit. The imaging appearance of chondral/osteochondral injury differs based on severity and acuity of the trauma and the reparative response of the tissue. A single episode of high-impact trauma may result in a chondral or osteochondral fracture. In certain locations with appropriate mechanisms of injury, the forces applied to the bone/cartilage unit result in a de-bonding or delamination of the cartilage from the underlying bone. In cases in which acute trauma does not produce a structural defect it may alter the biomechanical properties of the osteochondral unit, leading to progressive loss of articular cartilage and degenerative change in subchondral bone. In the absence of an acute traumatic insult, chronic repetitive microtrauma, such as overuse injuries, can produce focal microfracture, necrosis, and healing response of subchondral bone with localized degenerative changes in the overlying cartilage.

MRI Assessment of Chondral Injury

Current MRI grading systems of focal articular cartilage damage are based on modifications of the Outerbridge classification originally described for surgical grading of patellar lesions.[31] The original surgical Outerbridge classification is based on size of surface fragmentation and fissuring. The MRI modification of the Outerbridge classification incorporates depth of the lesion from the articular surface. In addition, several MRI classifications have been proposed for grading osteochondral lesions.[32,33]

Grade 0: Normal Cartilage

By definition, grade 0 cartilage has both normal morphology and signal intensity; however, signal intensity of normal cartilage varies with depth from the articular surface,[34] location in the joint,[35] age of the patient,[36] and the particular pulse sequence used to acquire the image. The appearance of normal cartilage was discussed in Chapter 2.

Grade I Lesions: Isolated Change in Cartilage Signal Intensity

In the surgical form of the Outerbridge classification, grade I lesions are identified by a subjective determination of cartilage softening or discoloration with an intact articular surface. Because there is no direct MRI finding that corresponds to cartilage softening, this has been modified to reflect isolated MRI signal changes without disruption of the articular surface. Early studies found poor correlation between grade I MRI lesions and arthroscopy,[37,38] as well as low sensitivity in MRI detection of patellar cartilage softening found at arthroscopy.[39] Recent studies indicate diagnostic accuracy is improved with 3.0T MRI technology.[40]

With the lack of findings at arthroscopy there is a tendency to discount MRI findings of early cartilage injury. Studies performed on excised cartilage specimens suggest that poor correlation reflects inherent differences in the properties of cartilage evaluated with MRI and arthroscopy. It has been postulated that elevation in cartilage signal intensity on T2-weighted sequences is a result of alterations in the organization of the collagen matrix that reduce collagen fibril anisotropy and increase cartilage water content.[41] In studies of enzymatically treated cartilage specimens, degradation of the type II collagen matrix was strongly correlated with elevation in cartilage T2, whereas removal of proteoglycans using either trypsin or interleukin-2 had minimal effect.[41] Similarly, it has been shown that although removal of proteoglycan significantly decreases cartilage stiffness, degradation of the collagen matrix associated with elevation in cartilage T2 correlated poorly with Young's modulus.[42,43] Based on results of ex-vivo studies, it is likely that focal elevation in T2-weighted signal intensity reflects structural changes of the collagen matrix that do not substantially alter the visible appearance or compressibility of cartilage. Although such damage may not have an immediate impact on tissue biomechanics, because of the inability of cartilage to repair or replace type II collagen, it places cartilage at risk for further degeneration. Preliminary studies have shown grade I lesions frequently progress to higher grades.[44] Long-term natural history trials such as the National Institutes of Health–funded Osteoarthritis Initiative (OAI) are needed to determine the clinical significance of these lesions.

An early manifestation of OA is failure of the type II collagen matrix. This may occur as a result of a single traumatic insult in which tensile strain in the collagen network exceeds the biomaterial properties or through repetitive stress that can lead to fatigue fracture. Age is an important factor in modifying the material properties of the collagen matrix. Because of the slow rate of turnover of type II collagen in cartilage there is accumulation of advanced glycation end products and crosslinking of collagen.[45,46] These age-related factors increase the stiffness and friability of collagen, making it more brittle and prone to fracture.

As originally describe by Maroudas and colleagues, fragmentation of the collagen network may be one of the earliest manifestations of osteochondral injuries leading to OA.[47] As illustrated in Figure 3-3, fractures in the collagen network prevent constraint on the hydrated aggrecan, allowing the tissue to swell. As the tissue swells there is a measurable increase in water content and loss of the normally high interstitial swelling pressure. This reduces the ability of cartilage to restrict the flow of water through the tissue as it undergoes compression. With loss of restricted water movement, more energy deposited in the tissue from compressive force is transferred

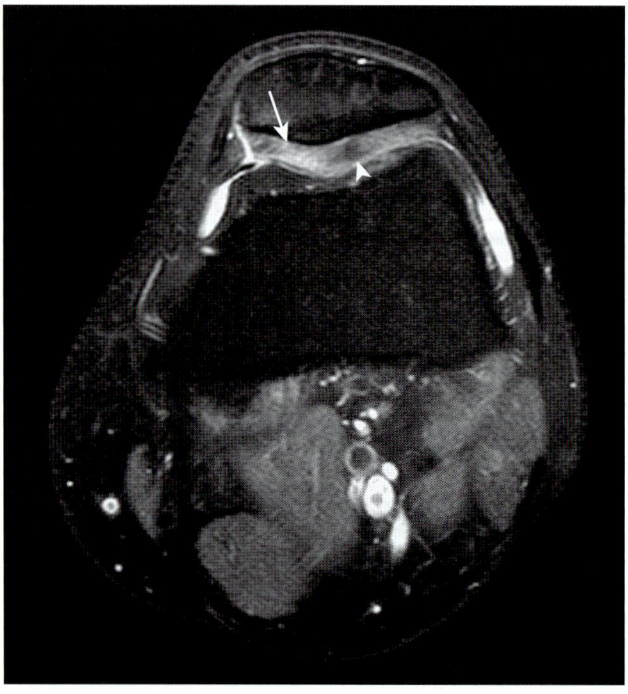

FIGURE 3-3. Structural changes of the cartilage matrix with early osteoarthritis produce an increase in cartilage T2-weighted signal intensity (*arrow*). Fractures within the type II collagen matrix allow unconstrained swelling of the hydrated aggrecan and loss of collagen fibril anisotropy. As the aggrecan swells there is an increase in the content and mobility of interstitial cartilage water, which, along with decreased tissue anisotropy, results in longer cartilage T2 values. Adjacent regions of T2-weighted hypointense signal are frequently observed in the subacute and chronic settings (*arrowhead*).

to the solid extracellular matrix. This leads to progressive degradation and fragmentation of the extracellular matrix. Concurrently, high magnitude compressive strain in cartilage leads to chondrocyte injury and apoptosis, limiting ability to synthesize new proteoglycan. This results in a mismatch where degradation from excessive biomechanical loads exceeds the biomaterial properties of the tissue. With time, this imbalance results in visible cartilage damage and, ultimately, loss of tissue.

Many of these earliest changes in cartilage injury increase the T2 relaxation time of cartilage water and produce changes in MRI signal intensity that can be visualized with standard T2-weighted, turbo spin-echo MRI techniques. Breaks in the collagen matrix, particularly those occurring in regions of high structural anisotropy such as the radial zone, reduce the residual dipolar coupling with water, leading to prolongation of the cartilage T2 relaxation time. The concurrent elevation in cartilage water content and increased mobility of water are also factors that lead to longer T2 relaxation in early cartilage injury.

Focal areas of T2 hyperintensity are frequently found in patients without a discrete cartilage defect. Although the clinical significance of this finding is unknown, as illustrated in Figure 3-4, these lesions often progress to sites of morphologic damage.[44] A more diffuse heterogeneous pattern of high T2-weighted signal can be observed after acute trauma, frequently in association with hyperintensity in the adjacent subchondral bone marrow. Isolated areas of T2 hyperintensity may be observed in the cartilage of patients with no reported history of trauma. As demonstrated in Figure 3-4, this can be associated with a focal blister or smooth contour abnormality of the overlying articular surface. Similar findings of focal swelling and alterations in the fibril density in the superficial zone of patellar cartilage have been reported in the electron microscopy literature,[48,49] supporting the hypothesis that these lesions represent structural reorganization/degeneration of the collagen matrix.

In addition to T2 hyperintensity, which is frequently present in the acute setting, focal areas of decreased T2-weighted cartilage signal are frequently observed adjacent to sites of cartilage injury. Decreased T2-weighted signal is generally not observed immediately after trauma but, as demonstrated by the case illustrated in Figure 3-5, is observed with subacute and chronic osteochondral injuries. The etiology of the decreased T2 signal intensity has not been determined but may reflect fragmentation of collagen fibrils leading to a greater number of exposed water-binding sites. In addition to providing more efficient T2 relaxation, collagen fragmentation may decrease overall signal intensity through magnetization transfer between collagen fragments and cartilage water. Alternatively, T2 hypointensity can result from formation of fibrocartilage repair tissue. Areas of low T2-weighted signal intensity are also observed with sites of chondrocalcinosis, particularly with gradient-echo techniques[50] or with high magnetic field strengths.[51]

GRADE II/III LESIONS: PARTIAL-THICKNESS CARTILAGE INJURY

Grade II lesions represent fissures, erosion, ulceration, or fibrillation involving the superficial 50% of cartilage thickness. In the modified Outerbridge classification, lesions that extend to the deep 50% of cartilage are considered grade III. These injuries can occur in the setting of acute trauma or chronic cartilage wear; however, imaging features are different. Acute osteochondral injuries are suggested by the presence of adjacent soft tissue edema, joint effusion, and subchondral bone marrow T2 hyperintensity with ill-defined margins. The presence of well-demarcated or cystic lesions in subchondral bone is suggestive of chronicity. As discussed previously, chronic lesions are frequently heterogeneous, with areas of increased and decreased signal intensity in cartilage on proton density (PD)–weighted or T2-weighted fast spin-echo sequences.

There is no consensus in the MRI literature regarding terminology used to describe morphology of focal cartilage lesions. Fissures represent linear clefts of the articular surface (Fig. 3-6). They are most frequently observed acutely after joint trauma, particularly in patellar cartilage. These clefts frequently follow the preferential ori-

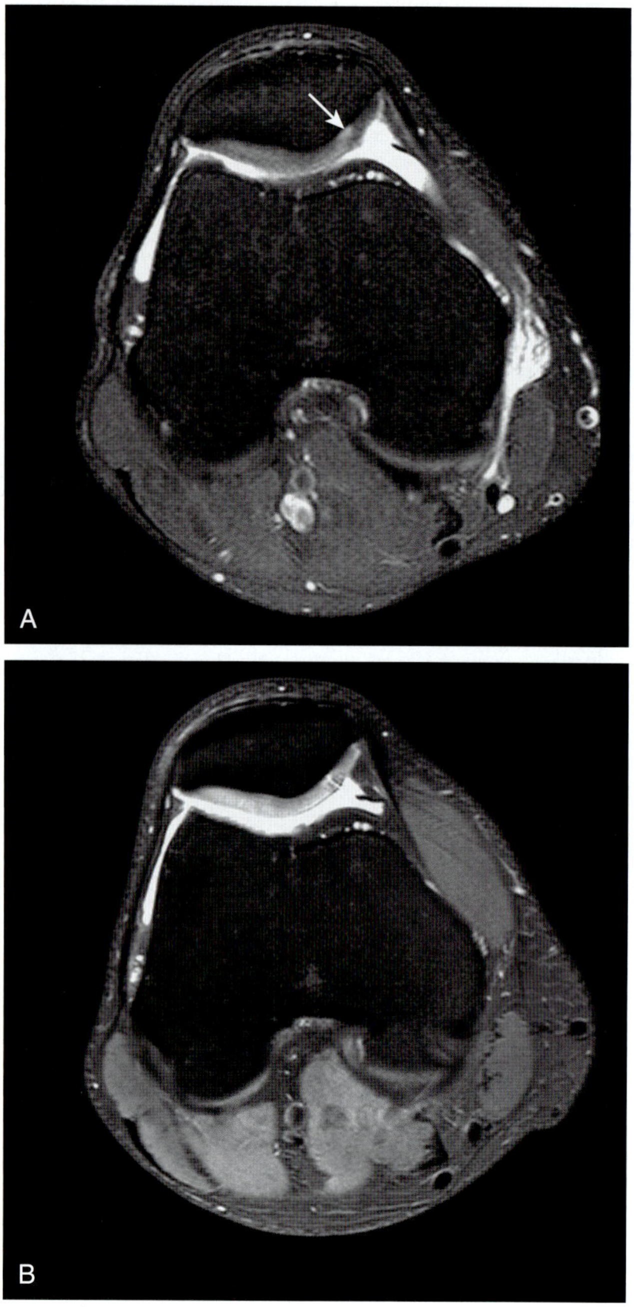

FIGURE 3-4. Chondral delamination and basal cystic degeneration produce focal T2 elevation in cartilage signal intensity in the deep radial zone and a smooth "blister" of the patellar articular surface of a 27-year-old professional hockey player with knee pain secondary to sprain of the medial collateral ligament (not shown). **A,** Axial, 1.5T, PD-weighted turbo spin-echo (TR/TE: 2000/40 ms) image demonstrates focal T2 hyperintensity of the deep radial zone of the medial facet (*arrow*). **B,** Axial, 3.0T, PD-weighted turbo spin-echo (TR/TE: 1785/30 ms) image obtained 1 year later demonstrates interval progression to grade III lesion with a full-thickness fissure extending to the articular surface.

entation of the collagen matrix. The rate and magnitude of loading of cartilage influence the location of injury. When shear force is applied at high speed but with low energy, cracks are produced along the articular cartilage surface. At low speed and low energy, splits initially occur in the deeper layers.[52]

As seen in Figure 3-7, obliquely oriented fissures or flap tears can be seen as linear defects extending from the articular surface. Such tears may result from excessive shear strain, resulting in failure of the collagen network at the junction of the transitional and radial zones. Because chondral flap tears may produce symptoms of locking, patients can present with clinical symptoms mimicking a meniscal tear.

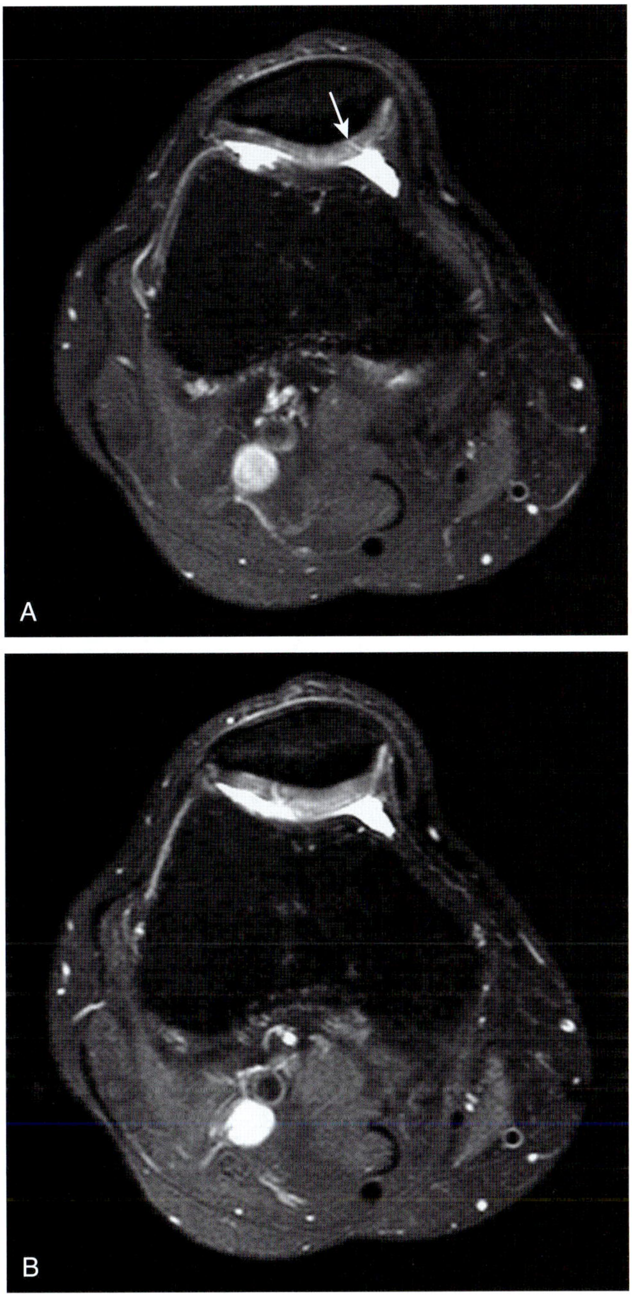

FIGURE 3-5. Focal T2 hypointensity in a 36-year-old man with chronic knee pain and locking symptoms. **A,** Axial, turbo spin-echo, fat-suppressed, PD-weighted image (TR/TE: 3000/30 ms) demonstrates medial patellar cartilage fissuring (*arrow*). **B,** Focal chondral hypointensity adjacent to the chondral fissure of the lateral patellar facet suggests a subacute/chronic chondral injury.

Ulceration of superficial cartilage blisters results in a small focal irregular crater. Erosion refers to a smoothly marginated area of thinned cartilage and is frequently seen in older patients. Cartilage erosion is often identified in the posterior tibial plateau and femoral condyle, particularly in patients with chronic tears of the anterior cruciate ligament (Fig. 3-8). Fibrillation or fraying of the articular surface appears visually as a fine velvety surface and is a common finding in subjects with OA and in asymptomatic older individuals. MRI has insufficient spatial resolution to resolve the individual fibrillations[53] and generally appears as an indistinct articular margin. Although MRI has poor correlation with arthroscopy for Outerbridge grade I lesions, sensitivity and specificity are greater than 85% for grade II lesions and higher.[54]

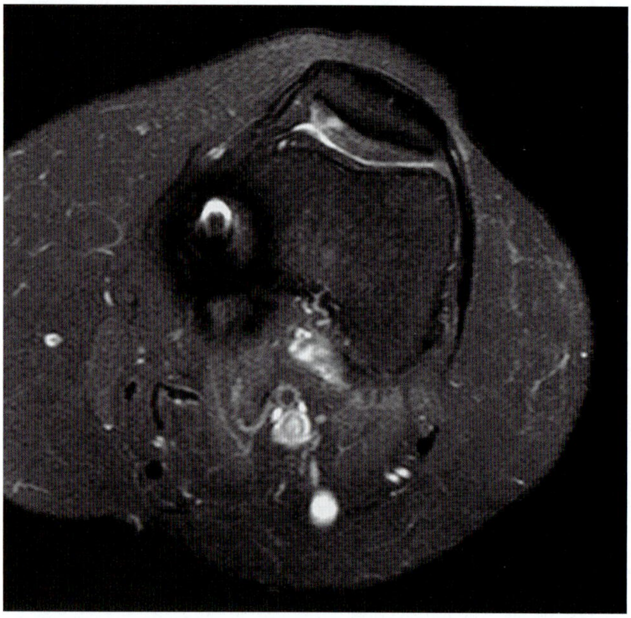

FIGURE 3-6. Grade III chondral injury in a 24-year-old woman status post anterior cruciate ligament reconstruction with persistent pain. Axial, PD-weighted, fat-suppressed, turbo spin-echo (TR/TE: 1600/33 ms) image shows a superficial fissure extending to a large area of hyperintense signal in the deep radial zone of the medial patellar facet consistent with a grade III chondral lesion. A 2.5-cm region of chondral delamination was identified at arthroscopy.

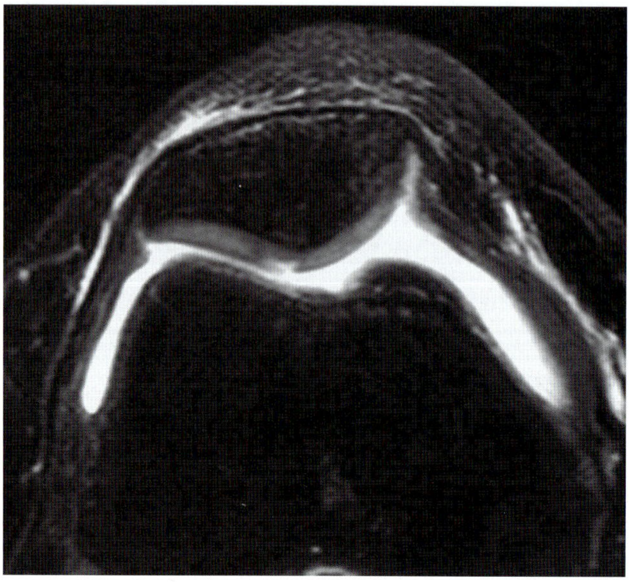

FIGURE 3-7. Grade II chondral injury in a 38-year-old woman with intermittent locking of the knee and suspected meniscal tear. Axial, PD-weighted, fat-suppressed, turbo spin-echo image (TR/TE: 4400/30 ms) demonstrates a superficial flap tear of the articular surface. Note subtle areas of decreased signal intensity in adjacent cartilage suggestive of a subacute/chronic injury.

GRADE IV LESIONS: FULL-THICKNESS CARTILAGE LESIONS

Full-thickness lesions with exposure of the underlying subchondral bone are classified as grade IV lesions. The margin of the lesion can suggest the mechanism of cartilage injury. As shown in Figure 3-9, sharply marginated borders are characteristic of traumatic cartilage injuries, whereas shallow or irregular margins are features more characteristic of chronic degeneration. Abnormal signal from the underlying bone marrow and central osteophytes is frequently associated with grade IV lesions[55] but is also observed in lower-grade chondral lesions. MRI has demonstrated high specificity and sensitivity for detection of grade IV defects.

MRI Findings in Injury of the Cartilage/Bone Interface

Excessive shear forces to the cartilage/bone interface can injure the tidemark zone and disrupt collagen fibers that bind cartilage to subchondral bone. In addition to shear force applied directly to the articular surface, high shear strain at the bone/cartilage interface develops with axial compression.[56] Cleavage of collagen fibers leads to delamination or de-bonding of cartilage from the underlying bone. As illustrated in Figure 3-10, this can result in a displaced chondral fragment. In less severe cases, cartilage delamination may not be readily apparent at arthroscopy, because the

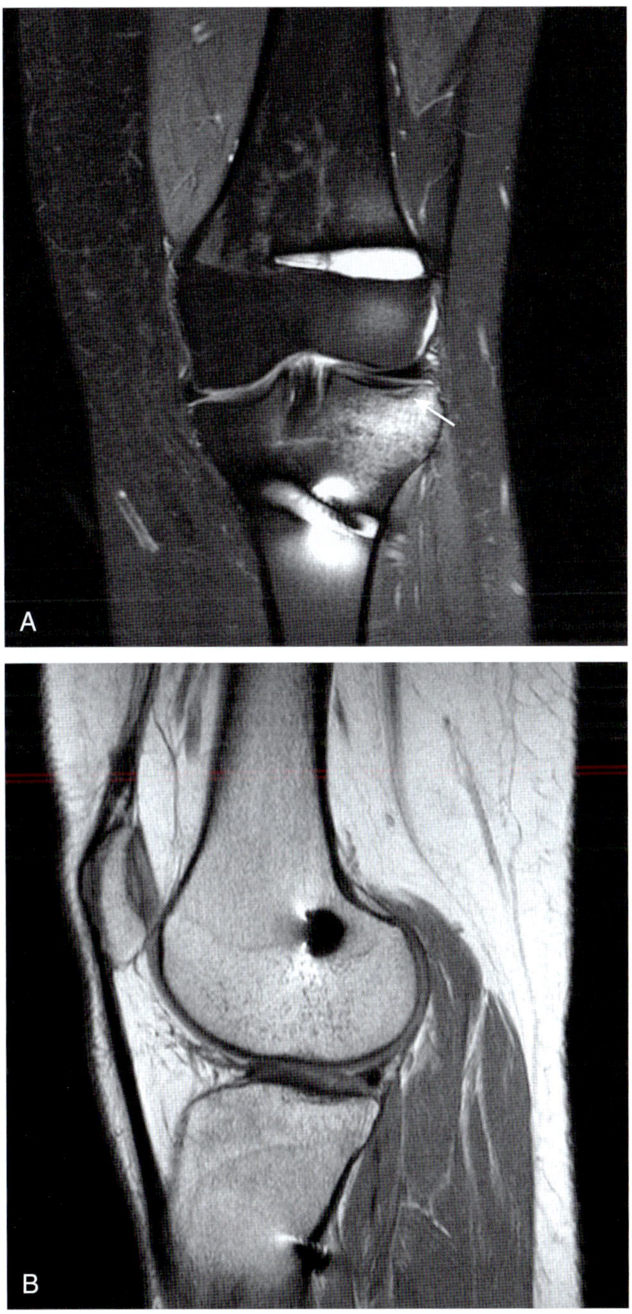

FIGURE 3-8. A 23-year-old woman presented 6 years after anterior cruciate ligament (ACL) reconstruction with acute exacerbation of knee pain. **A,** Coronal, fat-suppressed, PD-weighted, turbo spin-echo (TR/TE: 3000/30 ms) image demonstrates a nondisplaced fracture (*arrow*) of the lateral tibial plateau with surrounding marrow edema consistent with an acute injury. Sagittal, PD-weighted (TR/TE: 2000/15 ms) (**B**) and fat-suppressed T2-weighted (TR/TE: 2500 ms/70 ms) turbo spin-echo (**C**) images demonstrate diffusely increased T2 hyperintensity in the cartilage of the posterior lateral tibial plateau and anterior translation of the tibia consistent with ACL graft insufficiency and degenerative wear of tibial cartilage.

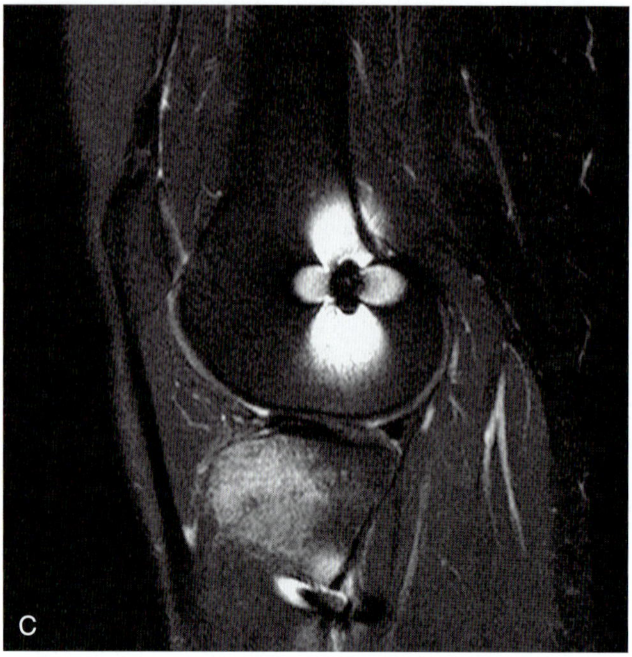

FIGURE 3-8, cont'd

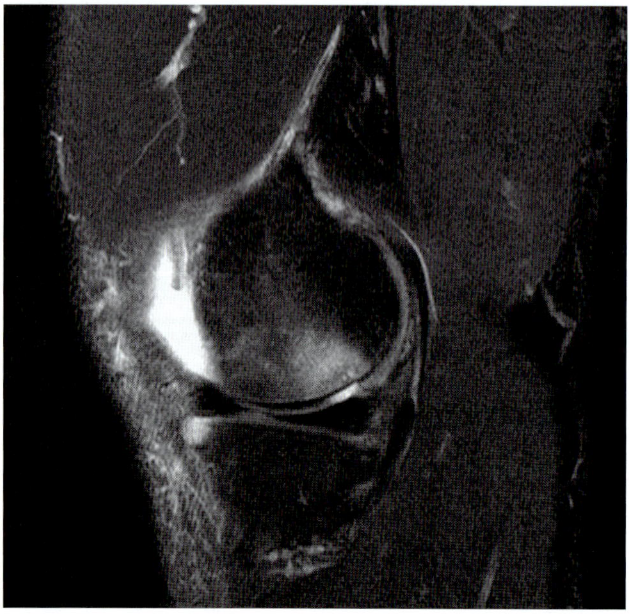

FIGURE 3-9. Acute grade IV chondral injury in a 44-year-old man 16 days after a twisting injury of the knee, resulting in an acute anterior cruciate ligament tear (not shown). Sagittal, T2-weighted, fat-suppressed, turbo spin-echo (TR/TE: 2500/70 ms) image shows a full-thickness chondral lesion of the posterior medial femoral condyle with sharp chondral margins characteristic of an acute injury. Note the large amount of subchondral marrow hyperintensity and flattening of the subchondral cortex consistent with a fracture of the subchondral plate.

articular surface is often intact.[57] In addition to biomechanical factors, recent evidence demonstrates that genetic factors influence the risk of cartilage delamination.[58]

MRI findings of cartilage delamination consist of linear T2 elevation at the bone/cartilage interface.[59] This is likely due to focal elevation in water content as well as loss of collagen fiber anisotropy in the radial zone, which occurs when cartilage is cleaved from bone.[60] In the knee, delamination injuries may be seen in the femoral condyle, frequently in cartilage adjacent to the posterior horn of the meniscus. In the setting of patellar dislocation, shearing injury can lead to delamination injuries

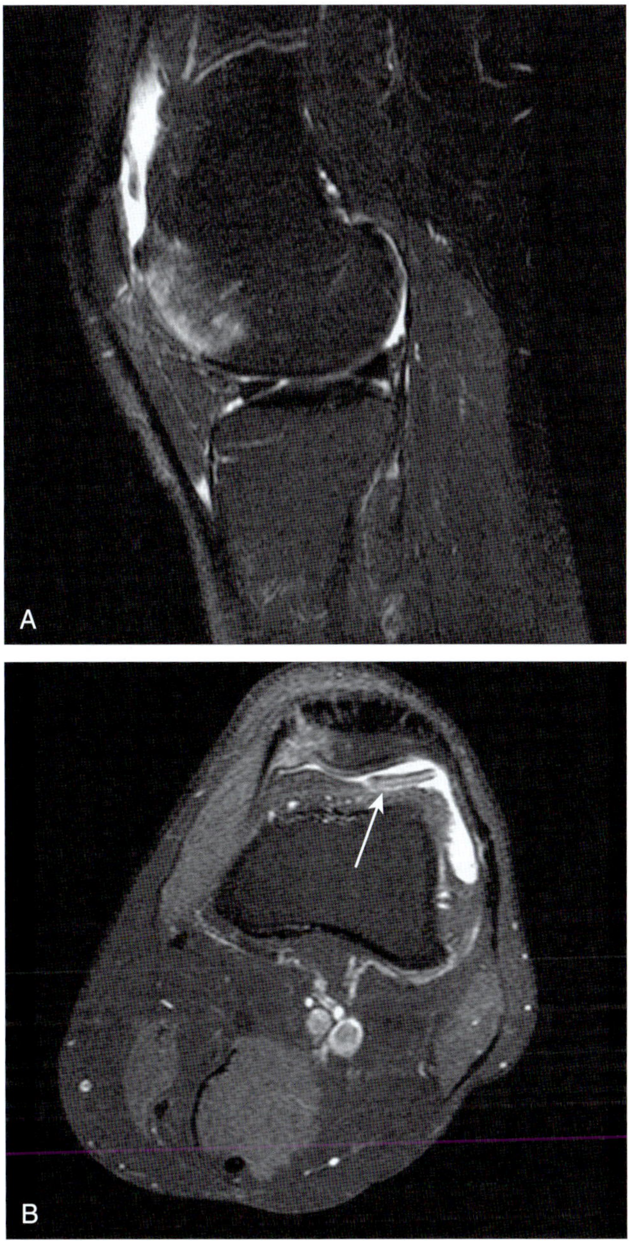

FIGURE 3-10. Cartilage delamination of the knee in a 55-year-old man with a suspected meniscal tear. **A,** Sagittal, fat-suppressed, T2-weighted, turbo spin-echo (TR/TE: 2500/70 ms) image shows a large chondral defect of the lateral femoral trochlea and subchondral signal hyperintensity. **B,** Axial, fat-suppressed, PD-weighted, turbo spin-echo (TR/TE: 1500/33 ms) image shows a large delaminated chondral fragment in the lateral suprapatellar recess (*arrow*).

of the median patellar ridge and may be associated with full-thickness cartilage fissures or flap tears. Delamination injuries are also frequently observed in the femoral trochlea after blunt anterior knee trauma, frequently in association with patellar cartilage injury.

Delamination of cartilage from the anterosuperior acetabulum is a frequent finding in the cam pattern of femoral acetabular impingement.[61,62] It is hypothesized that the aspherical femoral head produces high shear stress on acetabular cartilage at this site during hip flexion and internal rotation. Because of thin acetabular cartilage and high degree of joint congruity that presses delaminated cartilage against the acetabulum, detection of chondral delamination in the hip is a diagnostic challenge. As illustrated in Figure 3-11, MR arthrography can be helpful in detection. With this

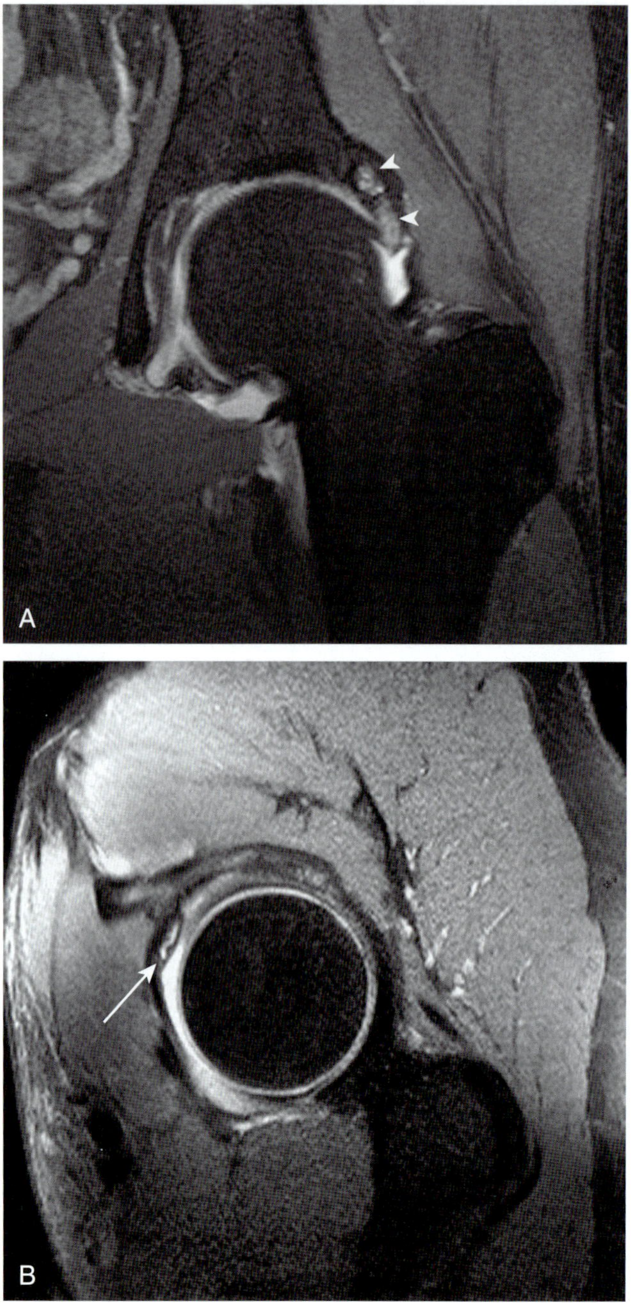

FIGURE 3-11. Acetabular cartilage delamination in a 40-year-old runner with clinical diagnosis of femoral acetabular impingement. **A,** A 3.0T, coronal, fat-suppressed, PD-weighted, turbo spin-echo (TR/TE: 2600/30 ms) image from a hip MR arthrogram shows large anterosuperior intralabral and paralabral cysts (*arrowheads*) with chondrosis of the acetabular cartilage. **B,** Sagittal, fat-suppressed, PD-weighted, turbo spin-echo (TR/TE: 5100/15 ms) image aligned perpendicular to the osteochondral junction demonstrates focal chondral delamination of the anterosuperior acetabulum (*arrow*).

technique, cartilage delamination is indicated by the presence of high signal on T1-weighted, fat-suppressed images between bone and cartilage.[63]

Careful attention to MRI acquisition parameters is needed to diagnose injuries of the deeper layer of cartilage and cartilage/bone interface. These injuries are best seen on PD-weighted, turbo spin-echo images with fat saturation. Because the T2 relaxation time of water in the deep radial cartilage zone is in the range of 10 to 15 ms,[64] the echo time values for turbo spin-echo imaging of cartilage should be in the range of 25 to 35 ms to provide sufficient signal to visualize injuries of the cartilage/bone interface while generating adequate contrast of the articular surface. Although longer echo time values increase bulk fluid/cartilage at the articular surface, they may limit detection of deep chondral injuries where T2 values are substantially shorter. The addition of fat suppression increases the dynamic range of cartilage signal intensity and improves conspicuity of internal cartilage lesions. Fat suppression also reduces the effects of chemical shift artifact from subchondral bone marrow that may obscure the cartilage/bone interface. As a general guideline, the receiver bandwidth should be optimized such that the chemical shift is less than 50% the thickness of bone. If the receiver bandwith is set too low, fat signal can obscure the cartilage/bone interface. Setting the receiver bandwidth too high will reduce image signal to noise. The application of driven equilibrium can improve contrast resolution of cartilage while allowing the use of shorter repetition time values to decrease image acquisition time.

MRI Findings in Subchondral Bone Associated with Osteochondral Injuries

BONE MARROW "EDEMA" SIGNAL

Increased T2-weighted signal from subchondral bone marrow is a frequent finding in acute traumatic osteochondral injury[65] as well as chronic osteochondral injury, or OA.[66-68] Similar alteration in bone marrow signal intensity is observed after high-intensity exercise or with altered joint biomechanics.[69,70] It is a nonspecific MRI finding but can be associated with pain[67] and with internal derangement in the knee.[70,71]

Characteristics of the MRI signal abnormality in the marrow are similar to water, which is dark on short echo time sequences and bright on fluid-sensitive sequences such as fat-saturated, PD-weighted or T2-weighted, spin-echo, turbo spin-echo, or short tau inversion recovery (STIR) images.[72] Because the abnormal signal closely follows water, this finding has been erroneously termed bone marrow *edema*.[73] Correlation studies with histology indicate a mixture of tissue types contribute to the abnormal marrow signal. In the setting of acute trauma, areas of fluid-like signal are associated with regions of trabecular microfracture, hemorrhage, necrosis, and edema.[74] In this clinical setting the marrow findings represent a bone marrow contusion. Follow-up studies have shown abnormal marrow signal can persist for several months after resolution of symptoms and are infrequently associated with long-term sequelae.[75,76] In contrast to lesions with an ill-defined reticular border, bone marrow contusions that have a well-demarcated margin that extends to the subchondral plate have a 50% likelihood of progressing to localized cartilage loss.[77]

In the presence of OA or chronic focal osteochondral injury, the region of abnormal marrow signal has a heterogeneous histology consisting of necrosis, fibrosis, subchondral cysts, edema, hemorrhage, and granulation tissue.[73,78,79] The presence of elevated T2-weighted signal in bone marrow may be a secondary indication of an overlying full-thickness articular cartilage defect.[80] In correlation with arthroscopic grading of focal cartilage defects, prevalence of subchondral marrow hyperintense T2-weighted signal is 1% for arthroscopically normal cartilage, 10% for partial-thickness defects, and 53% for full-thickness articular cartilage defects.[80]

Although more common in the hip,[81] transient bone marrow edema in the absence of trauma has been observed in the knee. For the hip, this condition is most frequently observed in middle-aged males.[82,83] As illustrated in Figure 3-1, a diffuse pattern of marrow edema is frequently seen in association with subchondral insufficiency fractures. This is most frequently encountered in the medial femoral condyle of middle-aged and elderly females, often in association with meniscal tears or meniscal dysfunction, as indicated by meniscal extrusion.[84] Although this lesion has been referred to as spontaneous osteonecrosis of the knee, more recent studies suggest this entity is likely a result of increased loading forces resulting in fracture of the subchondral plate.[70,85] The risk of fracture and development of stress-related marrow abnormality in the subchondral marrow is likely influenced by osteoporosis. In a study of over 800 postmenopausal women there was a significantly lower prevalence of subchondral bone marrow edema-like lesions in women receiving alendronate and estrogen compared with women not receiving anti-resorptive therapy.[86]

Subchondral Marrow Findings in Osteochondritis Dissecans

Whereas the bone marrow "edema" pattern can be seen with chronic articular conditions such as OA, the classic OCD pattern exhibits a well-demarcated crescent or oval lesion that is low signal on T1-weighted images and heterogeneous on T2-weighted images, as illustrated in Figure 3-12. These lesions undergo varying degrees

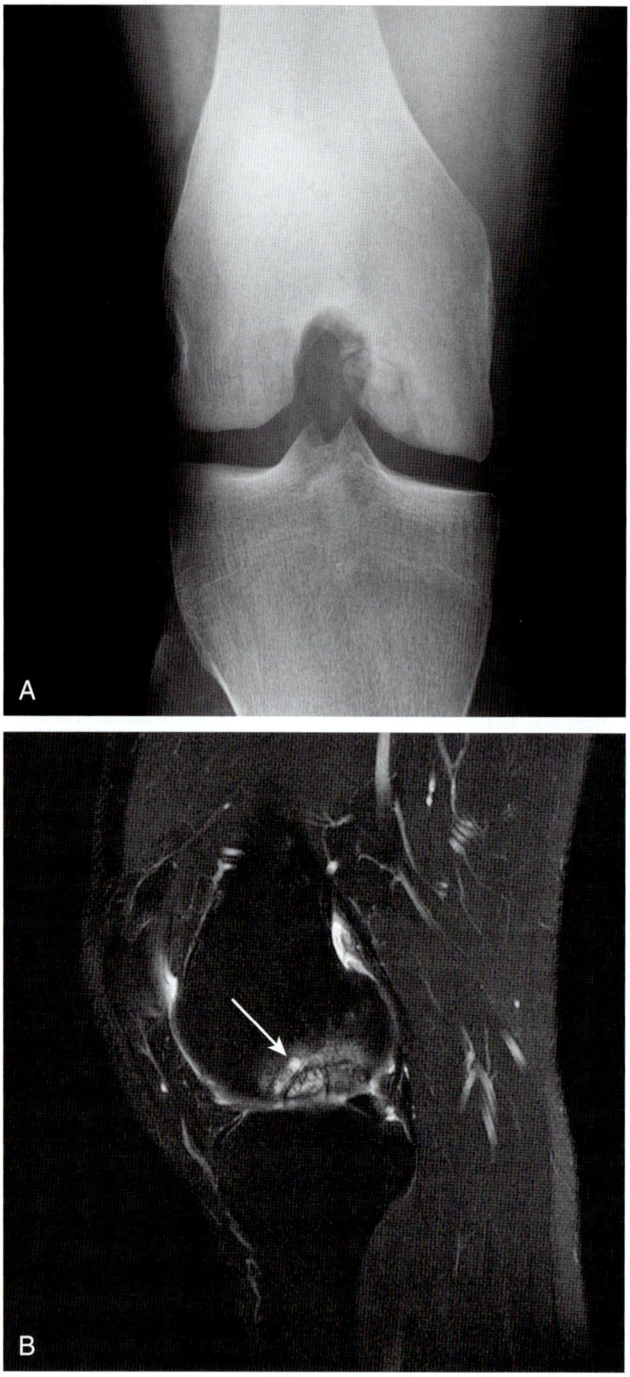

FIGURE 3-12. Unstable osteochondritis dissecans (OCD). **A,** Anteroposterior tunnel view of OCD of the medial femoral condyle in a 25-year-old man with knee pain. **B,** Sagittal, fat-suppressed, T2-weighted (TR/TE: 2500/70 ms) MR image demonstrates a 5-mm subchondral cyst (*arrow*) of the subchondral bone. **C,** Coronal, fat-suppressed, PD-weighted, turbo spin-echo (TR/TE: 1750/30 ms) MR image demonstrates linear T2 hyperintensity at the osseous interface of the OCD suggestive of instability, which was confirmed at surgery.

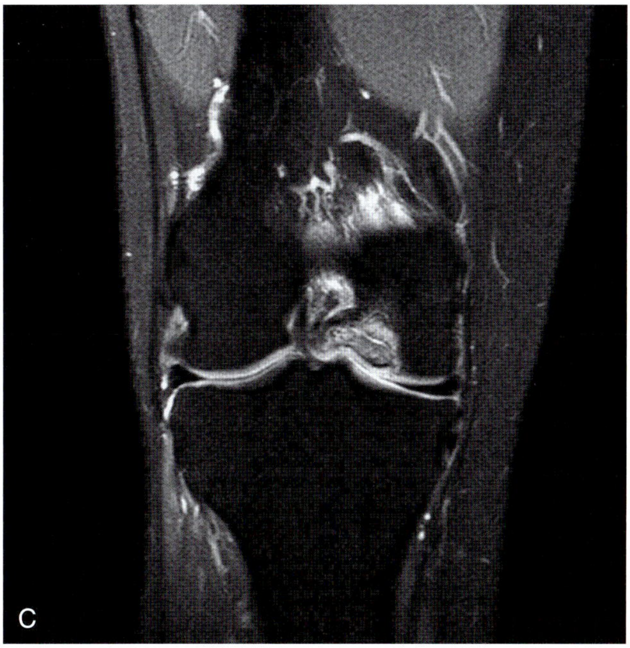

FIGURE 3-12, cont'd

of enhancement that indicate an active reparative process. The demarcation zone between the subchondral lesion and healthy marrow is frequently bright on T2-weighted images and can represent granulation tissue or fluid communicating with the articular surface. Low signal at the demarcation zone on T2-weighted images is ascribed to healing and suggests stability of the lesion. This is an important differentiator because treatment is dependent on stability of the osteochondral fragment. MRI findings of fragment instability include (1) a high signal intensity line on T2-weighted images of the demarcation zone measuring greater than 5 mm in length or circumferentially surrounding the osteochondral fragment; (2) a round, homogeneously bright area on T2-weighted images measuring at least 5 mm in diameter in the subchondral bone; or (3) a focal cartilage defect of greater than 5 mm.[87] The most common sign of instability is high T2-weighted signal at the demarcation zone between healthy marrow and the osteochondral fragment (see Fig. 3-12). The reported accuracy of this finding in the literature has been variable,[87-89] primarily because of the difficulty differentiating fluid from high T2-weighted signal intensity of granulation tissue. Specificity for identifying an unstable osteochondral fragment is improved if the hypertense demarcation zone is accompanied by a chondral defect.[90] To improve specificity in diagnosis of an unstable fragment, intra-articular injection of gadolinium contrast has been used to demonstrate communication of the demarcation zone with the articular surface.[89] After intravenous administration of gadolinium, enhancement of the demarcation zone is indicative of reparative granulation tissue.[91] Although in an animal model this finding was associated with unstable fragments,[91] other authors have interpreted this finding as a sign of stability and healing.[32]

The presence of subchondral cysts greater than 5 mm is less common but is indicative of unstable lesions. At surgery, cystic lesions in the talus contained loose granulation tissue rather than fluid.[88] For knee examinations, current MRI techniques generally have sufficient contrast resolution to identify overlying cartilage defects; however, this finding can be equivocal in thinner cartilage of the talar dome. In follow-up studies, the presence of an overlying chondral defect was predictive of a poor outcome.[92] Skeletally mature patients with fused growth plates also are more likely to have poor outcomes. Several recent studies have highlighted the importance of skeletal maturity when assessing the specificity of MRI findings as a marker of osteochondral stability and long-term prognosis.

Patterns of Osteochondral Injuries

In the setting of acute trauma, identifying the pattern of marrow abnormality is helpful in directing the search for potential sites of cartilage injury. From these patterns it is possible to infer instability patterns related to the principal mechanisms of injury.[93] Sanders and colleagues have described five basic patterns in the knee that are associated with soft tissue injury.[94] These consist of the pivot shift injury, dashboard injury, hyperextension injury, clip injury, and lateral patellar dislocation. This patterned approach in diagnosis is also helpful in the evaluation of osteochondral injury.

The pivot shift injury pattern is characterized by marrow hyperintensity in the posterior lateral tibial plateau and the central portion of the lateral femoral condyle near the terminal sulcus. This injury pattern is a result of a valgus load applied to the flexed knee combined with internal rotation of the femur or with external rotation of the tibia and is associated with disruption of the anterior cruciate ligament. Impaction of the lateral femoral condyle on the tibial plateau can result in osteochondral fractures or delamination injuries of cartilage in the terminal sulcus of the lateral femoral condyle (deep sulcus sign) or posterior lateral tibial plateau.

The term *dashboard injury* reflects the common mechanism of injury in which the flexed knee of a front seat passenger strikes against the dashboard in a head-on motor vehicle collision. When the force is applied to the superior tibia, this can produce posterior translation of the tibia, leading to disruption of the posterior cruciate ligament and posterior joint capsule. Blunt trauma applied more superiorly to the patella of a flexed knee may result in osteochondral fractures of the patellofemoral joint.[95] Lower velocity loading of the patellofemoral joint, such as from a fall on a flexed knee, can produce acute chondral injuries of the patella and trochlea in a "kissing" pattern reflecting the contact points at the time of injury. Patellar chondral injuries are generally best seen on axial views and consist of fissures often associated with high signal in the deep radial zone of cartilage. Injuries of trochlear cartilage are better evaluated on sagittal images. Delamination injuries are also encountered with this mechanism and can be recognized by linear signal at the bone/cartilage interface on fat-suppressed PD- or T2-weighted images. With this mechanism of injury, the femoral cartilage is frequently injured at the inferior margin of the trochlear groove and is best visualized on sagittal images.

Hyperextension injuries resulting in marrow contusions in the anterior femoral condyle and tibial plateau can produce anterior cruciate ligament, posterior cruciate ligament, and meniscal injuries. When combined with a varus force, the marrow contusions are located medially and are associated with injuries of the posterolateral corner. As illustrated in Figure 3-13, the hyperextension mechanism can be associated with shear injuries or osteochondral fractures of the anterior femoral condyle, best seen on coronal or sagittal images.

Clip injuries of the knee result from a direct valgus force applied to a partially flexed or extended knee, producing compressive loading of the lateral compartment and tensile stress of the medial stabilizers. Soft tissue injuries consist of sprain injuries of the medial collateral and anterior cruciate ligaments, as well as meniscal tears. Compressive loading of the lateral compartment can result in impaction injuries of the central femoral and tibial surfaces.[96] Avulsion osteochondral fractures can result medially.

Transient lateral dislocation of the patella can be recognized by focal marrow edema of the inferomedial patella and anterolateral margin of the lateral femoral condyle. In athletes, transient patella dislocation typically occurs in adolescents and young adults as a result of a twisting motion while the knee is in 10 to 20 degrees of flexion with the foot planted. Patellar dislocations are associated with injuries of the medial retinaculum; these include sprain injuries and avulsion fractures of the medial patellofemoral ligament, either from the adductor tubercle or medial patella, or strain injuries of the vastus medialis obliquus muscle. Suspicion of a transient patellar dislocation should lead to careful evaluation of the patellofemoral articular surfaces for evidence of cartilage injury or osteochondral fracture, which at arthroscopy is present in more than 66% of cases.[97] The prevalence of osteochondral injury identified on MRI studies obtained after patellar dislocation is similar, ranging from 58% to 78%.[98-101] Osteochondral injuries are particularly prevalent in the inferomedial patella and adjacent to the median ridge. In a review of 81 patients with lateral

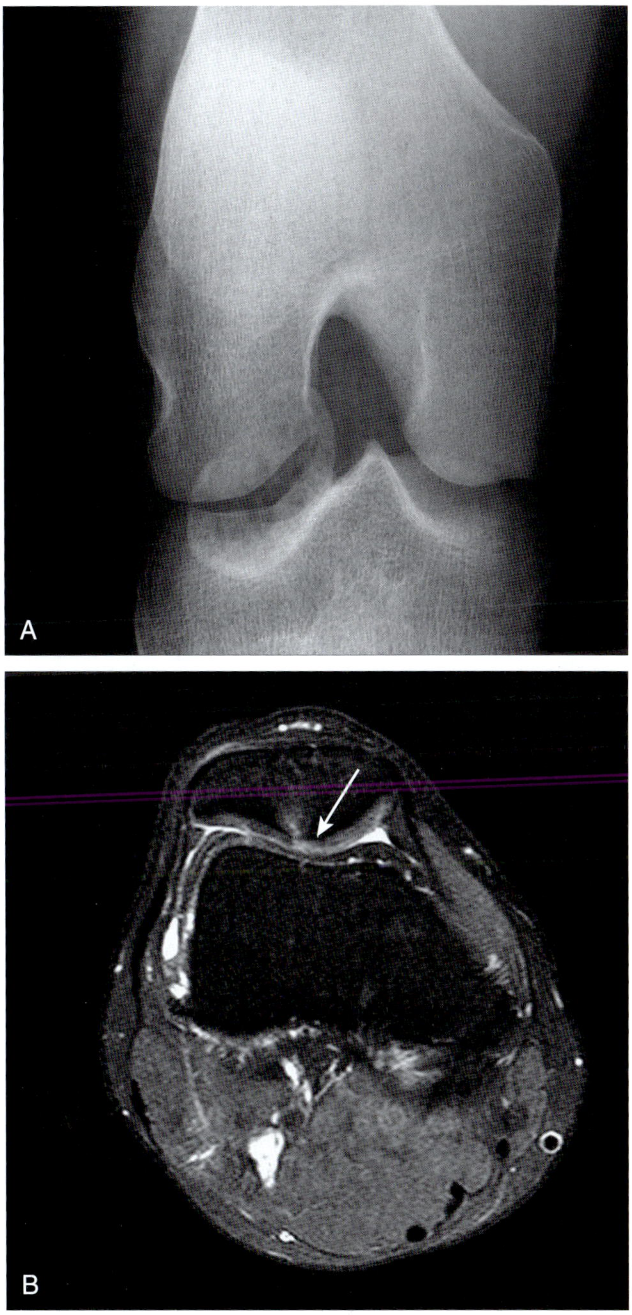

FIGURE 3-13. Chronic osteochondral fracture. **A,** Anteroposterior tunnel view demonstrates a calcified osteochondral body in a 20-year-old male patient with chronic knee pain 6 years after a hyperextension injury of the right knee. The pattern of injury suggests a chronic transient patellar dislocation with a large chronic osteochondral fracture of the lateral femoral trochlea. **B,** Grade III chondral injury of the median patellar ridge (*arrow*). Note the lack of marrow change on sagittal PD-weighted (**C**) and T2-weighted (**D**) images at the site of osteochondral fracture (*arrows*).

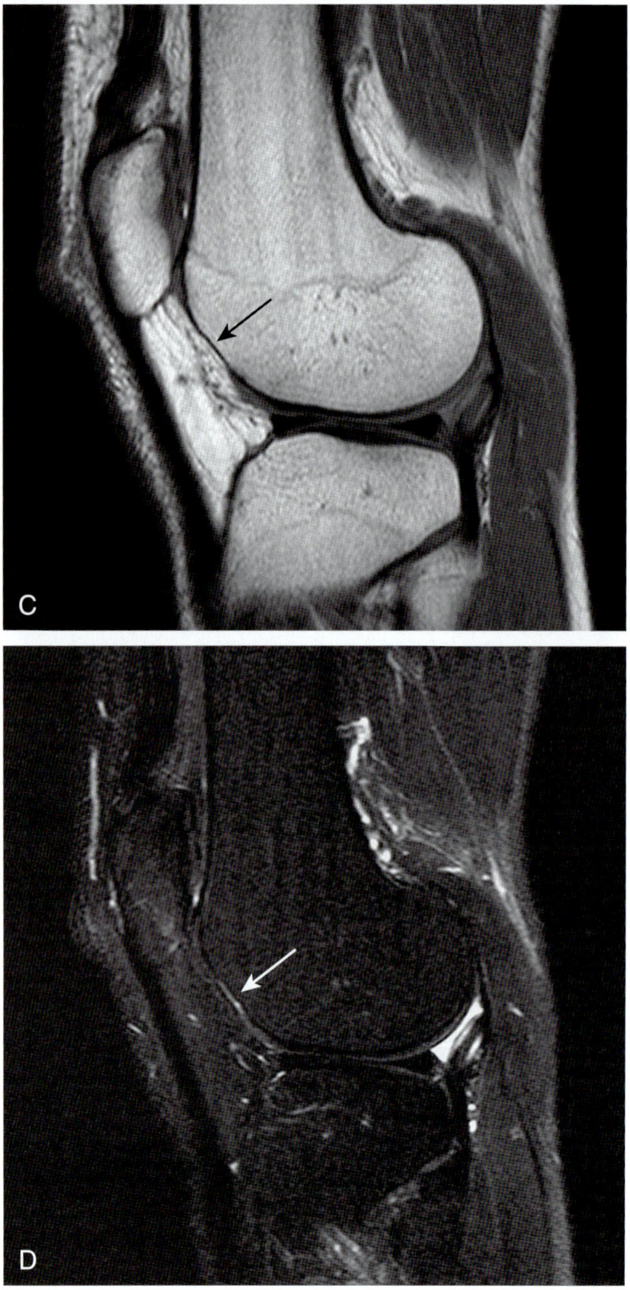

FIGURE 3-13, cont'd

patellar dislocation, Elias and colleagues observed osteochondral injuries on MRI in the inferomedial patella of 70% of subjects and the anterolateral femoral condyle in 5% of subjects.[98] This study demonstrated a concave deformity of the inferomedial patellar surface consistent with an osteochondral impaction fracture in 44% of subjects. Shear forces applied to the cartilage of the median ridge can result in oblique flap tears or delamination injuries that appear as linear hyperintensities on fat-suppressed, PD-weighted, fast spin-echo images (see Fig. 3-7).

After transient patellar dislocation, many young athletes have persistent retropatellar pain or evidence of patellofemoral instability.[102] It appears that individuals with a single episode of patellar dislocation are at greater risk of developing patellofemoral

OA than individuals with a recurrent pattern of dislocation.[103] This may be a result of greater force needed to dislocate a stable patella and a higher potential for osteochondral injury.

The knee is the most common joint for OCD, but the pattern of involvement differs from osteochondral injuries typically observed after acute trauma. The lateral margin of the medial femoral condyle is the most common site of involvement (85%), followed by the inferocentral portion of the lateral femoral condyle (13%) and the anterior lateral femoral condyle (2%).[104] Less frequently, OCD can involve the patellofemoral joint[105,106] and can be a source of persistent anterior knee pain in the young athlete.[107,108] Radiographs are relatively insensitive to osteochondral lesions of the patella, which are likely under-recognized as a cause of anterior knee pain. OCD usually occurs in the distal half of the patella and is frequently associated with a history of anterior knee trauma.[109] On the femoral trochlea, the lesion is most often observed on the anterior lateral femoral condyle close to midline[110] in adolescent athletes with repetitive flexion extension related to running or jumping activities.[111]

SUMMARY

Osteoarthritis and osteochondral injuries are frequent sources of symptoms that may mimic other causes of articular pathology, such as a meniscal tear in the knee. There is growing appreciation that focal osteochondral injury represents a significant risk factor for OA and can lead to persistent symptoms and long-term disability. With the ability to directly demonstrate articular cartilage, MRI is the most sensitive noninvasive technique for identifying osteochondral injuries but requires careful attention to image acquisition techniques, understanding of the MRI appearance of normal and injured cartilage, and a targeted examination of the joint based on patterns of soft tissue injury.

References

1. Peterfy CG, Gold G, Eckstein F, et al. MRI protocols for whole-organ assessment of the knee in osteoarthritis. Osteoarthritis Cartilage 2006; 14(Suppl A):A95-A111.
2. Hunter DJ, Niu J, Zhang Y, et al. Change in cartilage morphometry: a sample of the progression cohort of the Osteoarthritis Initiative. Ann Rheum Dis 2008; Apr 13 [Epub ahead of print].
3. Eckstein F, Mosher T, Hunter D. Imaging of knee osteoarthritis: data beyond the beauty. Curr Opin Rheumatol 2007; 19:435-443.
4. Amin S, LaValley MP, Guermazi A, et al. The relationship between cartilage loss on magnetic resonance imaging and radiographic progression in men and women with knee osteoarthritis. Arthritis Rheum 2005; 52:3152-3159.
5. Conaghan P. Is MRI useful in osteoarthritis? Best Pract Res Clin Rheumatol 2006; 20:57-68.
6. Felson DT, Zhang Y. An update on the epidemiology of knee and hip osteoarthritis with a view to prevention. Arthritis Rheum 1998; 41:1343-1355.
7. Hunter DJ, Lo GH, Gale D, et al. The reliability of a new scoring system for knee osteoarthritis MRI and the validity of bone marrow lesion assessment: BLOKS (Boston Leeds Osteoarthritis Knee Score). Ann Rheum Dis 2008; 67:206-211.
8. Torres L, Dunlop DD, Peterfy C, et al. The relationship between specific tissue lesions and pain severity in persons with knee osteoarthritis. Osteoarthritis Cartilage 2006; 14:1033-1040.
9. Zhai G, Cicuttini F, Ding C, et al. Correlates of knee pain in younger subjects. Clin Rheumatol 2007; 26:75-80.
10. Felson DT, Chaisson CE, Hill CL, et al. The association of bone marrow lesions with pain in knee osteoarthritis. Ann Intern Med 2001; 134:541-549.
11. Conaghan PG, Felson D, Gold G, et al. MRI and non-cartilaginous structures in knee osteoarthritis. Osteoarthritis Cartilage 2006; 14(Suppl A):A87-A94.
12. Pessis E, Drape JL, Ravaud P, et al. Assessment of progression in knee osteoarthritis: results of a 1 year study comparing arthroscopy and MRI. Osteoarthritis Cartilage 2003; 11:361-369.
13. Felson DT, McLaughlin S, Goggins J, et al. Bone marrow edema and its relation to progression of knee osteoarthritis. Ann Intern Med 2003; 139:330-336.
14. Davies-Tuck ML, Wluka AE, Wang Y, et al. The natural history of cartilage defects in people with knee osteoarthritis. Osteoarthritis Cartilage 2008; 16:337-342.

15. Ding C, Cicuttini F, Scott F, et al. Association of prevalent and incident knee cartilage defects with loss of tibial and patellar cartilage: a longitudinal study. Arthritis Rheum 2005; 52:3918-3927.
16. Wang Y, Ding C, Wluka AE, et al. Factors affecting progression of knee cartilage defects in normal subjects over 2 years. Rheumatology (Oxford) 2006; 45:79-84.
17. Wluka AE, Ding C, Jones G, et al. The clinical correlates of articular cartilage defects in symptomatic knee osteoarthritis: a prospective study. Rheumatology (Oxford) 2005; 44:1311-1316.
18. Larsen E, Jensen PK, Jensen PR. Long-term outcome of knee and ankle injuries in elite football. Scand J Med Sci Sports 1999; 9:285-289.
19. Loomer R, Fisher C, Lloyd-Smith R, et al. Osteochondral lesions of the talus. Am J Sports Med 1993; 21:13-19.
20. Wright RW, Boyce RH, Michener T, et al. Radiographs are not useful in detecting arthroscopically confirmed mild chondral damage. Clin Orthop Relat Res 2006; 442:245-251.
21. Anderson IF, Crichton KJ, Grattan-Smith T, et al. Osteochondral fractures of the dome of the talus. J Bone Joint Surg Am 1989; 71:1143-1152.
22. Loredo R, Sanders TG. Imaging of osteochondral injuries. Clin Sports Med 2001; 20:249-278.
23. Schachter AK, Chen AL, Reddy PD, Tejwani NC. Osteochondral lesions of the talus. J Am Acad Orthop Surg 2005; 13:152-158.
24. Vaz CE, Camargo OP, Santana PJ, Valezi AC. Accuracy of magnetic resonance in identifying traumatic intra-articular knee lesions. Clinics 2005; 60:445-450.
25. Riel KA, Reinisch M, Kersting-Sommerhoff B, et al. 0.2-Tesla magnetic resonance imaging of internal lesions of the knee joint: a prospective arthroscopically controlled clinical study. Knee Surg Sports Traumatol Arthrosc 1999; 7:37-41.
26. Yoon YS, Rah JH, Park HJ. A prospective study of the accuracy of clinical examination evaluated by arthroscopy of the knee. Int Orthop 1997; 21:223-227.
27. Mosher TJ, Dardzinski BJ. Cartilage MRI T2 relaxation time mapping: overview and applications. Semin Musculoskelet Radiol 2004; 8:355-368.
28. Burstein D, Gray M. New MRI techniques for imaging cartilage. J Bone Joint Surg Am 2003; 85(Suppl 2):70-77.
29. Potter HG, Foo LF. Magnetic resonance imaging of articular cartilage: trauma, degeneration, and repair. Am J Sports Med 2006; 34:661-677.
30. Lang P, Noorbakhsh F, Yoshioka H. MR imaging of articular cartilage: current state and recent developments. Radiol Clin North Am 2005; 43:629-639, vii.
31. Outerbridge RE. The etiology of chondromalacia patellae. J Bone Joint Surg Br 1961; 43:752-757.
32. Bohndorf K. Osteochondritis (osteochondrosis) dissecans: a review and new MRI classification. Eur Radiol 1998; 8:103-112.
33. Mintz DN, Tashjian GS, Connell DA, et al. Osteochondral lesions of the talus: a new magnetic resonance grading system with arthroscopic correlation. Arthroscopy 2003; 19:353-359.
34. Modl JM, Sether LA, Haughton VM, Kneeland JB. Articular cartilage: correlation of histologic zones with signal intensity at MR imaging. Radiology 1991; 181:853-855.
35. Goodwin DW, Wadghiri YZ, Zhu H, et al. Macroscopic structure of articular cartilage of the tibial plateau: influence of a characteristic matrix architecture on MRI appearance. AJR Am J Roentgenol 2004; 182:311-318.
36. Chung T, Jaramillo D. Normal maturing distal tibia and fibula: changes with age at MR imaging. Radiology 1995; 194:227-232.
37. Gagliardi JA, Chung EM, Chandnani VP, et al. Detection and staging of chondromalacia patellae: relative efficacies of conventional MR imaging, MR arthrography, and CT arthrography. AJR Am J Roentgenol 1994; 163:629-636.
38. van Leersum M, Schweitzer ME, Gannon F, et al. Chondromalacia patellae: an in vitro study. Comparison of MR criteria with histologic and macroscopic findings. Skeletal Radiol 1996; 25:727-732.
39. De Smet AA, Monu JU, Fisher DR, et al. Signs of patellar chondromalacia on sagittal T2-weighted magnetic resonance imaging. Skeletal Radiol 1992; 21:103-105.
40. von Engelhardt LV, Kraft CN, Pennekamp PH, et al. The evaluation of articular cartilage lesions of the knee with a 3-Tesla magnet. Arthroscopy 2007; 23:496-502.
41. Nieminen MT, Toyras J, Rieppo J, et al. Quantitative MR microscopy of enzymatically degraded articular cartilage. Magn Reson Med 2000; 43:676-681.
42. Nissi MJ, Toyras J, Laasanen MS, et al. Proteoglycan and collagen sensitive MRI evaluation of normal and degenerated articular cartilage. J Orthop Res 2004; 22:557-564.
43. Kurkijarvi JE, Nissi MJ, Kiviranta I, et al. Delayed gadolinium-enhanced MRI of cartilage (dGEMRIC) and T2 characteristics of human knee articular cartilage: topographical variation and relationships to mechanical properties. Magn Reson Med 2004; 52:41-46.
44. Biswal S, Hastie T, Andriacchi TP, et al. Risk factors for progressive cartilage loss in the knee: a longitudinal magnetic resonance imaging study in forty-three patients. Arthritis Rheum 2002; 46:2884-2892.

45. Verzijl N, DeGroot J, Ben ZC, et al. Crosslinking by advanced glycation end products increases the stiffness of the collagen network in human articular cartilage: a possible mechanism through which age is a risk factor for osteoarthritis. Arthritis Rheum 2002; 46:114-123.
46. Bank RA, Bayliss MT, Lafeber FP, et al. Ageing and zonal variation in post-translational modification of collagen in normal human articular cartilage: the age-related increase in non-enzymatic glycation affects biomechanical properties of cartilage. Biochem J 1998; 330(Pt 1):345-351.
47. Maroudas AI. Balance between swelling pressure and collagen tension in normal and degenerate cartilage. Nature 1976; 260:808-809.
48. Hwang WS, Li B, Jin LH, et al. Collagen fibril structure of normal, aging, and osteoarthritic cartilage. J Pathol 1992; 167:425-433.
49. Mori Y, Kubo M, Okumo H, Kuroki Y. A scanning electron microscopic study of the degenerative cartilage in patellar chondropathy. Arthroscopy 1993; 9:247-264.
50. Beltran J, Marty-Delfaut E, Bencardino J, et al. Chondrocalcinosis of the hyaline cartilage of the knee: MRI manifestations. Skeletal Radiol 1998; 27:369-374.
51. Suan JC, Chhem RK, Gati JS, et al. 4 T MRI of chondrocalcinosis in combination with three-dimensional CT, radiography, and arthroscopy: a report of three cases. Skeletal Radiol 2005; 34:714-721.
52. Tomatsu T, Imai N, Takeuchi N, et al. Experimentally produced fractures of articular cartilage and bone: the effects of shear forces on the pig knee. J Bone Joint Surg Br 1992; 74:457-462.
53. Rubenstein JD, Li JG, Majumdar S, Henkelman RM. Image resolution and signal-to-noise ratio requirements for MR imaging of degenerative cartilage. AJR Am J Roentgenol 1997; 169:1089-1096.
54. Nakanishi K, Inoue M, Harada K, et al. Subluxation of the patella: evaluation of patellar articular cartilage with MR imaging. Br J Radiol 1992; 65:662-667.
55. Kijowski R, Stanton P, Fine J, De Smet A. Subchondral bone marrow edema in patients with degeneration of the articular cartilage of the knee joint. Radiology 2006; 238:943-949.
56. Wong M, Carter DR. Articular cartilage functional histomorphology and mechanobiology: a research perspective. Bone 2003; 33:1-13.
57. Levy AS, Lohnes J, Sculley S, et al. Chondral delamination of the knee in soccer players. Am J Sports Med 1996; 24:634-639.
58. Holderbaum D, Malvitz T, Ciesielski CJ, et al. A newly described hereditary cartilage debonding syndrome. Arthritis Rheum 2005; 52:3300-3304.
59. Kendell SD, Helms CA, Rampton JW, et al. MRI appearance of chondral delamination injuries of the knee. AJR Am J Roentgenol 2005; 184:1486-1489.
60. Keinan-Adamsky K, Shinar H, Navon G. The effect of detachment of the articular cartilage from its calcified zone on the cartilage microstructure, assessed by 2H-spectroscopic double quantum filtered MRI. J Orthop Res 2005. 23:109-117.
61. Kassarjian A, Yoon LS, Belzile E, et al. Triad of MR arthrographic findings in patients with cam-type femoroacetabular impingement. Radiology 2005; 236:588-592.
62. Pfirrmann CW, Mengiardi B, Dora C, et al. Cam and pincer femoroacetabular impingement: characteristic MR arthrographic findings in 50 patients. Radiology 2006; 240:778-785.
63. Beaule PE, Zaragoza E, Copelan N. Magnetic resonance imaging with gadolinium arthrography to assess acetabular cartilage delamination: a report of four cases. J Bone Joint Surg Am 2004; 86:2294-2298.
64. Freeman DM, Bergman G, Glover G. Short TE MR microscopy: accurate measurement and zonal differentiation of normal hyaline cartilage. Magn Reson Med 1997; 38:72-81.
65. Sanders RK, Crim JR. Osteochondral injuries. Semin Ultrasound CT MR 2001; 22:352-370.
66. Felson DT. An update on the pathogenesis and epidemiology of osteoarthritis. Radiol Clin North Am 2004; 42:1-9, v.
67. Hofmann S, Kramer J, Vakil-Adli A, et al. Painful bone marrow edema of the knee: differential diagnosis and therapeutic concepts. Orthop Clin North Am 2004; 35:321-333, ix.
68. Mandalia V, Fogg AJ, Chari R, et al. Bone bruising of the knee. Clin Radiol 2005; 60:627-636.
69. Lazzarini KM, Troiano RN, Smith RC. Can running cause the appearance of marrow edema on MR images of the foot and ankle? Radiology 1997; 202:540-542.
70. Yao L, Stanczak J, Boutin RD. Presumptive subarticular stress reactions of the knee: MRI detection and association with meniscal tear patterns. Skeletal Radiol 2004; 33:260-264.
71. Zanetti M, Pfirrmann CW, Schmid MR, et al. Patients with suspected meniscal tears: prevalence of abnormalities seen on MRI of 100 symptomatic and 100 contralateral asymptomatic knees. AJR Am J Roentgenol 2003; 181:635-641.
72. Arndt WF 3rd, Truax AL, Barnett FM, et al. MR diagnosis of bone contusions of the knee: comparison of coronal T2-weighted fast spin-echo with fat saturation and fast spin-echo STIR images with conventional STIR images. AJR Am J Roentgenol 1996; 166:119-124.
73. Zanetti M, Bruder E, Romero J, Hodler J. Bone marrow edema pattern in osteoarthritic knees: correlation between MR imaging and histologic findings. Radiology 2000; 215:835-840.
74. Rangger C, Kathrein A, Freund MC, et al. Bone bruise of the knee: histology and cryosections in 5 cases. Acta Orthop Scand 1998; 69:291-294.

75. Roemer FW, Bohndorf K. Long-term osseous sequelae after acute trauma of the knee joint evaluated by MRI. Skeletal Radiol 2002; 31:615-623.
76. Boks SS, Vroegindeweij D, Koes BW, et al. Follow-up of occult bone lesions detected at MR imaging: systematic review. Radiology 2006; 238:863-871.
77. Vellet AD, Marks PH, Fowler PJ, Munro TG. Occult posttraumatic osteochondral lesions of the knee: prevalence, classification, and short-term sequelae evaluated with MR imaging. Radiology 1991; 178:271-276.
78. Bergman AG, Willen HK, Lindstrand AL, Pettersson HT. Osteoarthritis of the knee: correlation of subchondral MR signal abnormalities with histopathologic and radiographic features. Skeletal Radiol 1994; 23:445-448.
79. Nolte-Ernsting CC, Adam G, Buhne M, et al. MRI of degenerative bone marrow lesions in experimental osteoarthritis of canine knee joints. Skeletal Radiol 1996; 25:413-420.
80. Kijowski R, Stanton P, Fine J, De Smet A. Subchondral bone marrow edema in patients with degeneration of the articular cartilage of the knee joint. Radiology 2006; 238:943-949.
81. Watson RM, Roach NA, Dalinka MK. Avascular necrosis and bone marrow edema syndrome. Radiol Clin North Am 2004; 42:207-219.
82. Moosikasuwan JB, Miller TT, Math K, Schultz E. Shifting bone marrow edema of the knee. Skeletal Radiol 2004; 33:380-385.
83. Arjonilla A, Calvo E, Alvarez L, Fernandez Yruegas D. Transient bone marrow oedema of the knee. Knee 2005; 12:267-269.
84. Uetani M, Hashmi R, Ito M, et al. Subchondral insufficiency fracture of the femoral head: magnetic resonance imaging findings correlated with micro-computed tomography and histopathology. J Comput Assist Tomogr 2003; 27:189-193.
85. Ramnath RR, Kattapuram SV. MR appearance of SONK-like subchondral abnormalities in the adult knee: SONK redefined. Skeletal Radiol 2004; 33:575-581.
86. Carbone LD, Nevitt MC, Wildy K, et al. The relationship of antiresorptive drug use to structural findings and symptoms of knee osteoarthritis. Arthritis Rheum 2004; 50:3516-3525.
87. De Smet AA, Ilahi OA, Graf BK. Reassessment of the MR criteria for stability of osteochondritis dissecans in the knee and ankle. Skeletal Radiol 1996; 25:159-163.
88. De Smet AA, Fisher DR, Graf BK, Lange RH. Osteochondritis dissecans of the knee: value of MR imaging in determining lesion stability and the presence of articular cartilage defects. AJR Am J Roentgenol 1990; 155:549-553.
89. Kramer J, Stiglbauer R, Engel A, et al. MR contrast arthrography (MRA) in osteochondrosis dissecans. J Comput Assist Tomogr 1992; 16:254-260.
90. O'Connor MA, Palaniappan M, Khan N, Bruce CE. Osteochondritis dissecans of the knee in children: a comparison of MRI and arthroscopic findings. J Bone Joint Surg Br 2002; 84:258-262.
91. Adam G, Buhne M, Prescher A, et al. Stability of osteochondral fragments of the femoral condyle: magnetic resonance imaging with histopathologic correlation in an animal model. Skeletal Radiol 1991; 20:601-606.
92. De Smet AA, Ilahi OA, Graf BK. Untreated osteochondritis dissecans of the femoral condyles: prediction of patient outcome using radiographic and MR findings. Skeletal Radiol 1997; 26:463-467.
93. Chung CB, Lektrakul N, Resnick D. Straight and rotational instability patterns of the knee: concepts and magnetic resonance imaging. Radiol Clin North Am 2002; 40:203-216.
94. Sanders TG, Medynski MA, Feller JF, Lawhorn KW. Bone contusion patterns of the knee at MR imaging: footprint of the mechanism of injury. RadioGraphics 2000; 20(Spec No):S135-151.
95. Bealle D, Johnson DL. Subchondral contusion of the knee caused by axial loading from dashboard impact: detection by magnetic resonance imaging. J South Orthop Assoc 2000; 9:13-18.
96. Shelbourne KD, Nitz PA. The O'Donoghue triad revisited: combined knee injuries involving anterior cruciate and medial collateral ligament tears. Am J Sports Med 1991; 19:474-477.
97. Sallay PI, Poggi J, Speer KP, Garrett WE. Acute dislocation of the patella: a correlative pathoanatomic study. Am J Sports Med 1996; 24:52-60.
98. Elias DA, White LM, Fithian DC. Acute lateral patellar dislocation at MR imaging: injury patterns of medial patellar soft-tissue restraints and osteochondral injuries of the inferomedial patella. Radiology 2002; 225:736-743.
99. Kirsch MD, Fitzgerald SW, Friedman H, Rogers LF. Transient lateral patellar dislocation: diagnosis with MR imaging. AJR Am J Roentgenol 1993; 161:109-113.
100. Quinn SF, Brown TR, Demlow TA. MR imaging of patellar retinacular ligament injuries. J Magn Reson Imaging 1993; 3:843-847.
101. Virolainen H, Visuri T, Kuusela T. Acute dislocation of the patella: MR findings. Radiology 1993; 189:243-246.
102. Hinton RY, Sharma KM. Acute and recurrent patellar instability in the young athlete. Orthop Clin North Am 2003; 34:385-396.
103. Maenpaa H, Lehto MU. Patellofemoral osteoarthritis after patellar dislocation. Clin Orthop Relat Res 1997; (339):156-162.
104. Obedian RS, Grelsamer RP. Osteochondritis dissecans of the distal femur and patella. Clin Sports Med 1997; 16:157-174.

105. Edwards DH, Bentley G. Osteochondritis dissecans patellae. J Bone Joint Surg Br 1977; 59:58-63.
106. Peters TA, McLean ID. Osteochondritis dissecans of the patellofemoral joint. Am J Sports Med 2000; 28:63-67.
107. Murray J. Chronic knee pain in the athlete. Pediatr Ann 1984; 13:613-615, 618-619, 621.
108. Mori Y, Kubo M, Shimokoube J, Kuroki Y. Osteochondritis dissecans of the patellofemoral groove in athletes: unusual cases of patellofemoral pain. Knee Surg Sports Traumatol Arthrosc 1994; 2:242-244.
109. Schwarz C, Blazina ME, Sisto DJ, Hirsh LC. The results of operative treatment of osteochondritis dissecans of the patella. Am J Sports Med 1988; 16:522-529.
110. Boutin RD, Januario JA, Newberg AH, et al. MR imaging features of osteochondritis dissecans of the femoral sulcus. AJR Am J Roentgenol 2003; 180:641-645.
111. Smith JB. Osteochondritis dissecans of the trochlea of the femur. Arthroscopy 1990; 6:11-17.

Chapter 4

SURGICAL APPROACHES FOR OSTEOCHONDRAL REPAIR AND POSTOPERATIVE IMAGING CONSIDERATIONS

Lawrence M. White and Michael P. Recht

Articular cartilage is a highly specialized tissue with complex ultrastructure and unique biomechanical properties providing for load distribution and a low-friction weight-bearing surface essential for normal pain-free movement of synovial joints. Traumatic articular cartilage injuries are well-recognized sequelae of acute or repetitive impact or twisting injuries to a joint. The incidence and prevalence of traumatic cartilage injuries have not been fully delineated and are somewhat difficult to gauge clinically. However, arthroscopic studies have highlighted that such injuries are common. In a retrospective study of surgical reports from 19,827 patients undergoing knee arthroscopy, chondral lesions were documented in 63% of cases, with an average of 2.7 lesions per knee.[1] Similar results have been more recently described in a prospective review of 993 knee arthroscopies illustrating cartilage abnormalities in 66% of patients, with full-thickness cartilage lesions (Fig. 4-1) seen in 11% of cases.[2]

Traumatic injuries may manifest as cartilage matrix and cellular injury with morphologically intact articular cartilage surface cover; mechanical disruption of articular cartilage in the forms of partial- or full-thickness cartilage fissures, flap tears, and segmental cartilage defects; or osteochondral injuries involving both articular cartilage and underlying subchondral bone. Injuries involving articular cartilage have a limited capacity for intrinsic repair secondary to insufficient vascularity of the cartilage and the chondrocytes' inability to divide and migrate to repair significant tissue defects. Full-thickness injuries of articular cartilage that extend to involve subchondral bone do cause hemorrhage and fibrin clot formation and initiate an inflammatory response stimulating osseous and articular cover repair. However, although this repair tissue may anatomically fill an osteochondral defect and alleviate symptoms temporarily, this repair tissue rarely replicates the mechanical and biologic properties of normal native articular cartilage.[3-7] Such repair tissue typically illustrates evidence of degeneration, fragmentation, fibrillation, and tissue depletion within 1 year or less after injury.

The majority of cartilage injuries may not result in clinical symptoms or disability; however, some patients may present with complaints of swelling, pain with move-

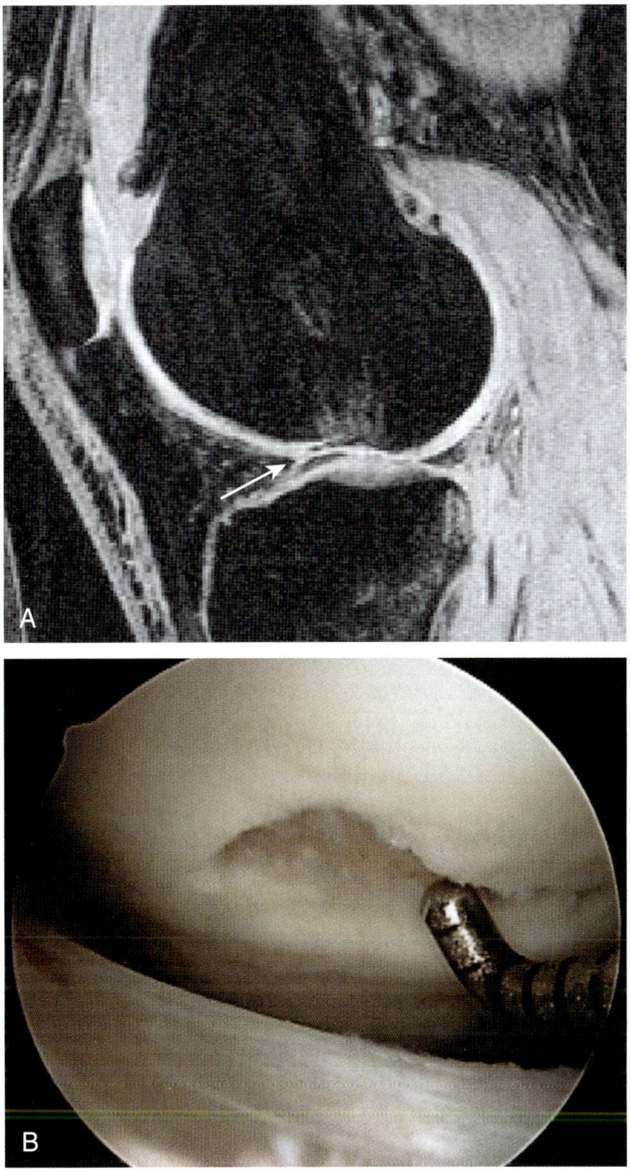

FIGURE 4-1. **A,** Sagittal, 3D, fat-suppressed, T1-weighted, gradient-echo image (TR/TE/FA: 50 ms/11 ms/45°) of a 27-year-old man with an anterior cruciate ligament tear. There is an osteochondral fracture of the lateral femoral condyle (*arrow*) with subjacent bone marrow edema. There is also bone marrow edema in the posterior lateral tibial plateau secondary to an osteochondral impaction injury. **B,** Arthroscopic image demonstrating the acute osteochondral fracture lifted by the surgical probe. (**B** courtesy of Richard Parker, MD.)

ment, or mechanical symptoms of catching, locking, or giving way. Additionally, although the determinant of the true natural history of an articular cartilage lesion is likely multifactorial and somewhat poorly delineated at present, there is evidence to support the concept of lesional progression, degeneration, and, ultimately, the development of osteoarthritic disease.[8]

Increased awareness of the prevalence and significance of articular cartilage lesions coupled with the limited natural capacity of cartilage for effective intrinsic repair have contributed to growing interest in surgical techniques for the treatment of articular cartilage lesions. Such operative techniques have advanced considerably over the past decade, paralleling advances in biologic science and results of experimental models of cartilage regeneration and repair. The most widely employed surgical treatment options for repair of cartilage lesions currently include marrow stimulation, osteochondral transplantation, and chondrocyte transplantation techniques. Success rates for these surgical options vary depending on defect location, size, and depth; status of underlying subchondral bone and adjacent surrounding cartilage; joint stability; biomechanical joint alignment; and clinical factors including patient age, weight, and general health status.

MAGNETIC RESONANCE IMAGING

MRI has been well established as an accurate noninvasive means of assessing articular cartilage, enabling accurate assessment of cartilage morphology and volume and providing insight into its constituent biochemical composition.[9-25] MRI has similarly been well described as a valuable technique in the postoperative evaluation of cartilage repair procedures.[26-32] As in the preoperative setting, critical user-dependent image acquisition factors that affect the MRI assessment of cartilage repair techniques include acquisition pulse sequences that determine image contrast, image spatial resolution, and overall image signal-to-noise ratio.

Although multiple existing and developing MRI pulse sequences have been evaluated in the assessment of articular cartilage, two classes of pulse sequence acquisitions have been found to be most accurate in this regard: 3D spoiled gradient-echo (SPGR) or fast low-angle shot (FLASH) sequences and intermediate-weighted or T2-weighted fast spin-echo (FSE) techniques.

Fat-suppressed 3D SPGR and FLASH acquisitions provide high-resolution contiguous thin-slice images with high contrast between bright cartilage and dark fluid, bone, fat, and muscle. However, such sequences may be limited in their assessment of internal cartilage pathology and small intrasubstance fissures or defects.[28] An additional potential limitation of SPGR and FLASH acquisitions is their relative sensitivity to susceptibility and intravoxel dephasing artifacts, which may be important image quality considerations in a patient after cartilage repair.[31] FSE acquisitions are less prone to postoperative metal-related artifacts originating from metallic debris from prior surgical instrumentation and possible stabilization hardware in the vicinity of the joint. Such metal-related artifacts may compromise image quality, particularly in the setting of prior osteochondral allograft transplants and autologous chondrocyte implantation.[26]

Intermediate- and T2-weighted FSE acquisitions can provide high-resolution, high-contrast imaging of articular cartilage and repair tissue in postoperative patients, with excellent depiction of surface morphology as well as intrinsic signal changes potentially reflective of intrasubstance pathologic processes.

Intra-articular contrast material, either through direct or indirect MR arthrographic techniques, may offer advantages of improved definition of the integrity and integration of repair tissue. Investigators have advocated the use of indirect MR arthrography in the MR evaluation of surface morphology and potential delamination of repair tissue after autologous chondrocyte implantation.[33] In contrast, other investigators have concluded that nonenhanced high-resolution fluid-sensitive imaging acquisitions are sufficient for accurate assessment of tissue integration and delamination without the need for contrast agent administration.[27,29]

Because of the high image spatial resolution and signal-to-noise requisites of MRI assessment of postoperative cartilage repair procedures, imaging studies in such patients should ideally be performed on high field (1.0T or higher) MR scanners. Imaging at 3.0T provides the potential advantage of imaging with relative increased image signal to noise ratio or higher spatial resolution at similar imaging acquisition times, compared with 1.0T or 1.5T imaging (albeit with somewhat increased sensitivity to postoperative metal-related artifacts). In contrast, imaging at low field strength (0.18-0.2T) should generally be avoided in the evaluation of cartilage repair procedures and has been shown to have substantial limitations in visualizing cartilage pathology compared with imaging at 1.5T.[34-36]

In addition to a routine assessment of joint anatomy, a complete MRI evaluation of cartilage repair procedures should include specific assessments of (1) repair tissue: defect fill, surface morphology, and MR signal characteristics; (2) adjacent cartilage and bone: repair tissue integration to native cartilage and subchondral bone and MR signal characteristics of subchondral bone; and (3) the articulation: joint effusion, synovitis, adhesions, and loose bodies.[29]

SURGICAL CARTILAGE REPAIR PROCEDURES

Marrow Stimulation

Marrow stimulation techniques for cartilage repair include subchondral drilling, abrasion arthroplasty, and microfracture. The surgical objectives of marrow stimulation techniques are the introduction of pluripotent repair cells into the site of a cartilage defect via the induction of hemorrhage, facilitated through surgical penetration of the subchondral bone plate. Penetration of subchondral blood vessels and underlying subchondral bone marrow leads to filling of the chondral defect with a fibrin clot, with subsequent migration of undifferentiated mesenchymal cells into the clot. Proliferation and differentiation of these mesenchymal cells result in partial or complete filling of a defect with subchondral new bone formation and overlying fibrocartilaginous repair tissue.[3,37-40]

Microfracture

Of the marrow stimulation methods described in the literature, the most widely employed surgical technique is microfracture. The technique is a commonly employed treatment option for the surgical management of full-thickness defects in the knee and other articulations. Developed and elaborated on by Steadman and coworkers,[41,42] microfracture is a minimally invasive one-stage arthroscopic procedure that is relatively easy to technically perform, is cost effective, and does not preclude repeat surgical intervention if clinically warranted. Ideal candidates for microfracture cartilage repair include patients younger than 45 years of age, with isolated well-contained lesions of less than 4 cm^2 involving the weight-bearing femoral condyles, trochlea, or patella, without concomitant meniscal or ligamentous insufficiency.[40,43-45]

Technically, the procedure involves débridement of a cartilage lesion to stable articular cartilage margins, curettage and removal of the calcified cartilage layer, and creation of multiple perpendicular microperforations of the subchondral bone with arthroscopic awls or picks at 3- to 4-mm intervals throughout the defect (Fig. 4-2). Postoperatively, weight bearing is generally avoided for at least 6 weeks, with gradually advanced weight bearing, physiotherapy, and return to full activity (including high impact sports or professional activities) usually by 6 to 8 months postoperatively.[37,39,40]

Histologic evaluation of repair tissue formed after microfracture or other marrow stimulation techniques in experimental and clinical models typically illustrates partial or complete filling of an articular defect primarily with fibrocartilaginous repair tissue, composed mostly of type I collagen.[6,46-49] This is in contrast to the composition of native hyaline articular cartilage, which is composed primarily of type II collagen produced by chondrocytes.

Clinical results of microfracture surgical repair of focal articular cartilage lesions in the knee have shown the most substantial functional improvements within the first 2 years postoperatively.[43,45,50,51] Optimal outcomes in these investigations were generally observed in younger active patients with a short duration of symptoms, low body mass index, and lesions involving the femoral condyles.[43-45,51] However, despite initial improvements in clinical function, some clinical studies have shown a subsequent deterioration in clinical results beginning at 18 to 24 months postoperatively.[43,44] These observations have been hypothesized to correlate to the histologic and biomechanical properties of fibrocartilage (type I collagen) observed in

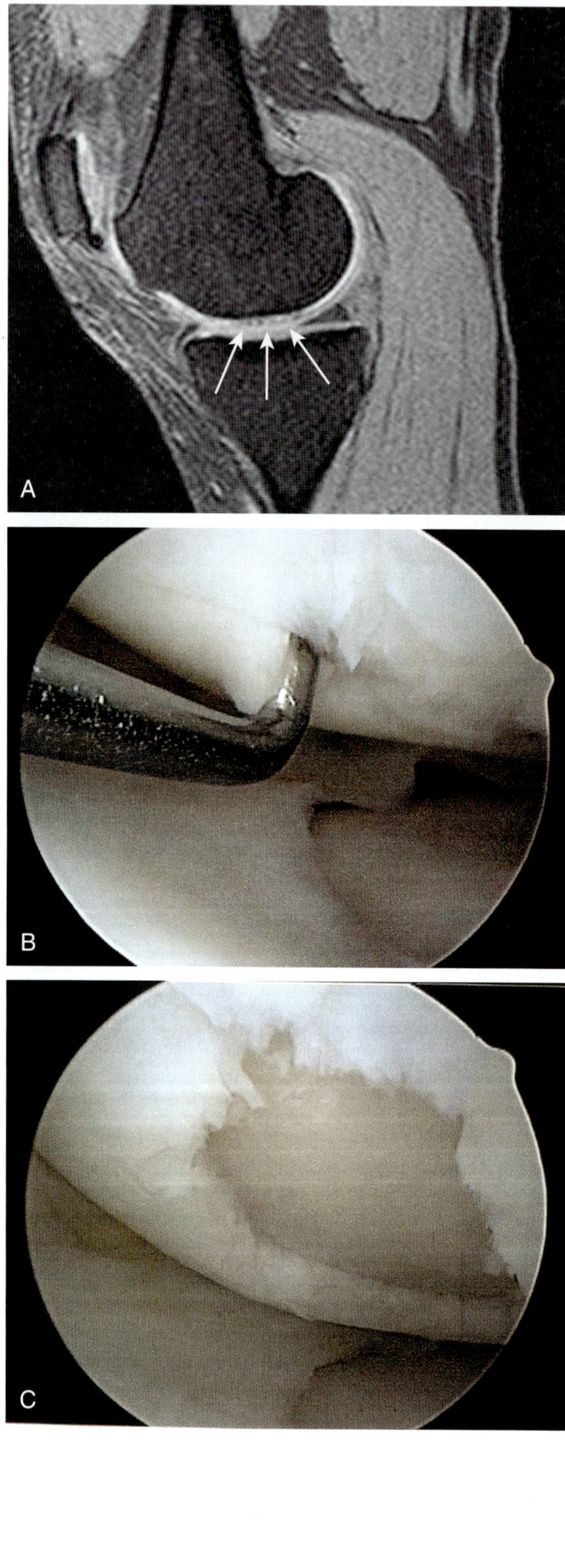

FIGURE 4-2. **A,** Sagittal, 3D, fat-suppressed, T1-weighted, gradient-echo image (TR/TE/FA: 50 ms/11 ms/45°) of a 34-year-old female soccer player. There is surface irregularity and internal signal abnormality (*arrows*) within the articular cartilage of the medial femoral condyle. **B** to **E,** Arthroscopic image demonstrates microfracture of the chondral defect. **B,** Probe demonstrating the surface irregularity of the articular cartilage of the medial femoral condyle. **C,** The defect is débrided, and (**D**) a surgical awl is used to penetrate the subchondral bone (**E**), causing bleeding. (Courtesy of Richard Parker, MD.)

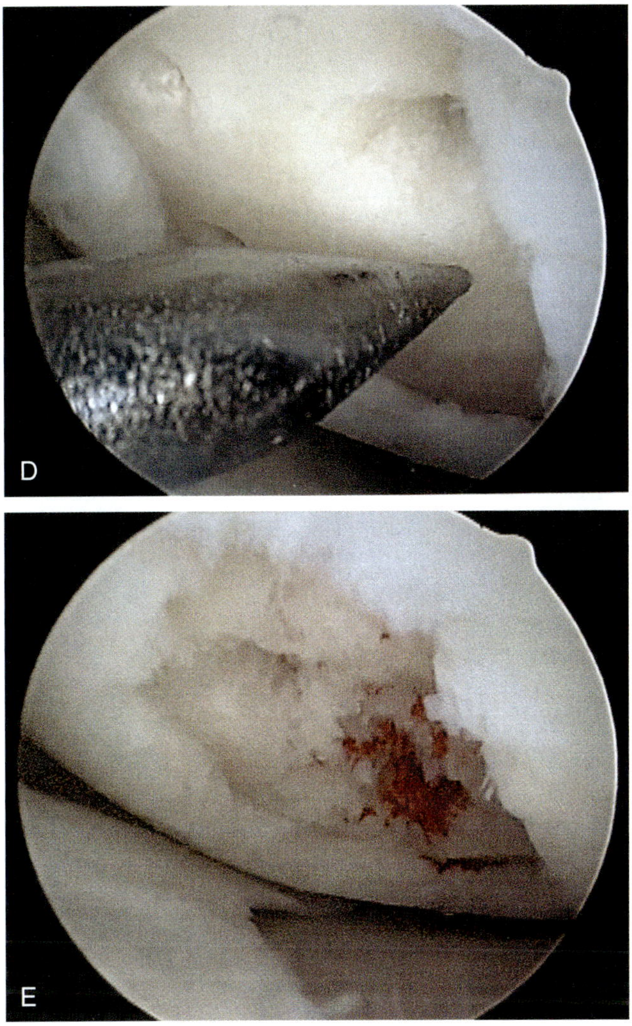

FIGURE 4-2, cont'd

experimental animal models. In such models, fibrocartilaginous repair tissue illustrates degeneration, reduced stiffness, and a predilection for degradation after an initial period of fibrocartilage repair tissue formation and healing.[52-54]

MRI of Microfracture

The MRI appearance of areas of microfracture repair varies over time postoperatively.[26] Within the first few months after surgery, MRI illustrates repair tissue partially or fully filling the articular defect (Fig. 4-3). This repair tissue typically shows increased signal on intermediate or T2-weighted imaging[32,43] compared with native articular cartilage. Over time, within the first year postoperatively, the volume of repair tissue may increase with progressive defect fill (Fig. 4-4).[26,30-32] Despite good defect fill, some MRI investigations have described varying degrees of persistent depression of the repair cartilage's surface morphology, mild persistent increased signal intensity on FSE imaging relative to adjacent native hyaline cartilage, and fissures or gaps between native and repair cartilage in the majority of microfracture cases imaged.[27,43]

Subchondral bone subjacent to sites of microfracture repair may illustrate a less distinct, thin, and irregular appearance relative to adjacent subchondral bone.

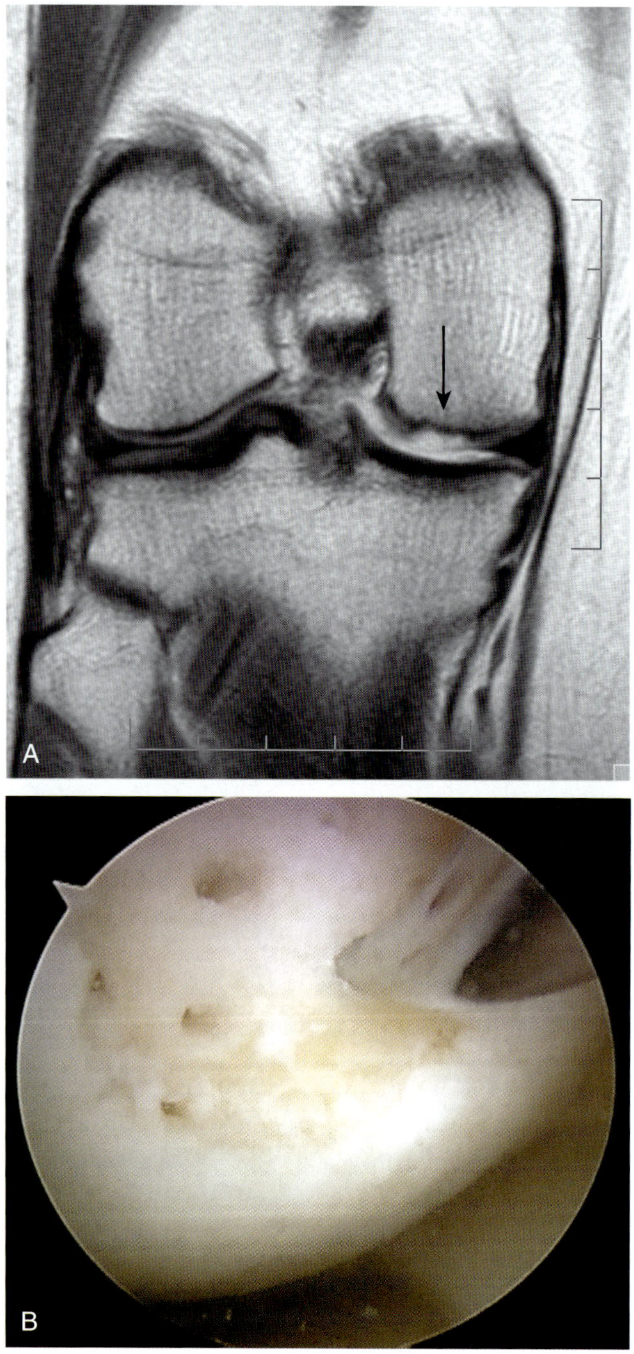

FIGURE 4-3. A 42-year-old woman presented with an anterior cruciate ligament (ACL) tear and post-traumatic cartilage defect of the medial femoral condyle sustained during an alpine ski injury. Preoperative coronal, intermediate-weighted, fast spin-echo (TR/TE: 4000/35 ms) MR image (**A**) shows a full-thickness defect along the weight-bearing aspect of the medial femoral condyle (*arrow*). Intraoperative arthroscopic image (**B**) during microfracture of the débrided articular cartilage defect shows, arthroscopic awl creating perforations of the subchondral bone plate. (**C**) Coronal intermediate-weighted, fast spin-echo (TR/TE: 4000/35 ms) image obtained 6 months postoperatively shows a smooth articular surface contour at the microfracture site with low-to-intermediate–weighted signal repair tissue filling the previously seen articular cartilage defect (*arrow*). Intact ACL reconstruction graft (*arrowheads*) is seen in the intercondylar notch.

Subchondral marrow edema is also frequently seen in the initial postoperative period. Typically, this marrow edema progressively decreases over time, although mild degrees of persistent marrow edema-like signal may be observed in asymptomatic patients at varying time points postoperatively.[26,27] Subchondral osseous overgrowth may also be observed at the microfracture repair site, possibly related to enchondral ossification of repair tissue or hypertrophic osseous healing of the multiple perforations of the subchondral bone plate.[27] Such osseous overgrowth may contribute to overall defect volume fill, with relative thinning of overlying repair tissue, with

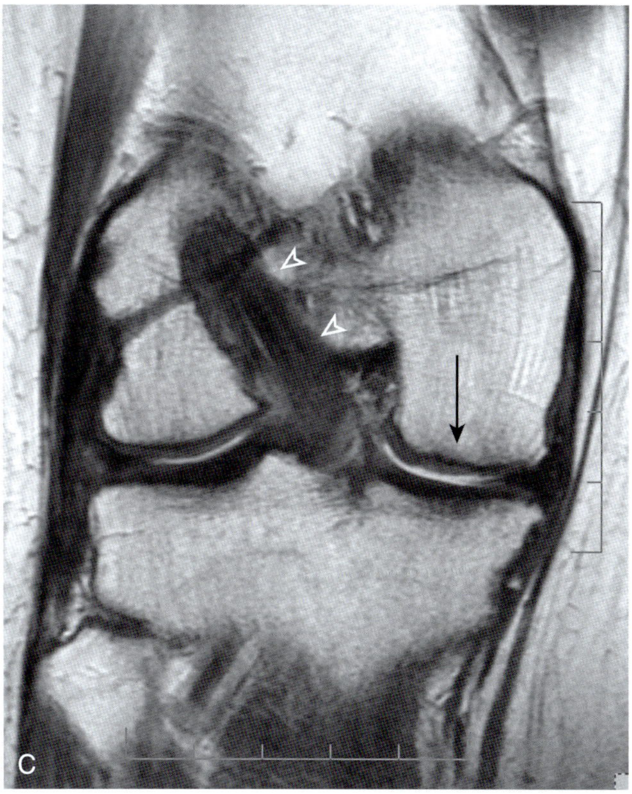

FIGURE 4-3, cont'd

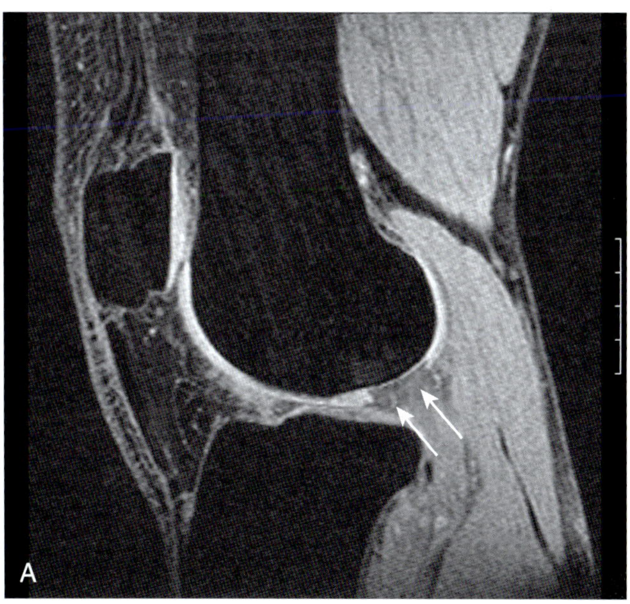

FIGURE 4-4. **A,** Sagittal, fat-suppressed, T1-weighted, gradient-echo image (TR/TE/FA: 30 ms/10 ms/45°) of a 24-year-old professional football player demonstrating a full-thickness chondral defect (*arrows*) of the lateral femoral condyle. **B,** Image 5 months after microfracture shows partial fill (*arrows*) of the defect with repair tissue. **C,** Image 12 months after microfracture shows progressive fill (*arrows*) of the defect. The player was able to resume his professional career.

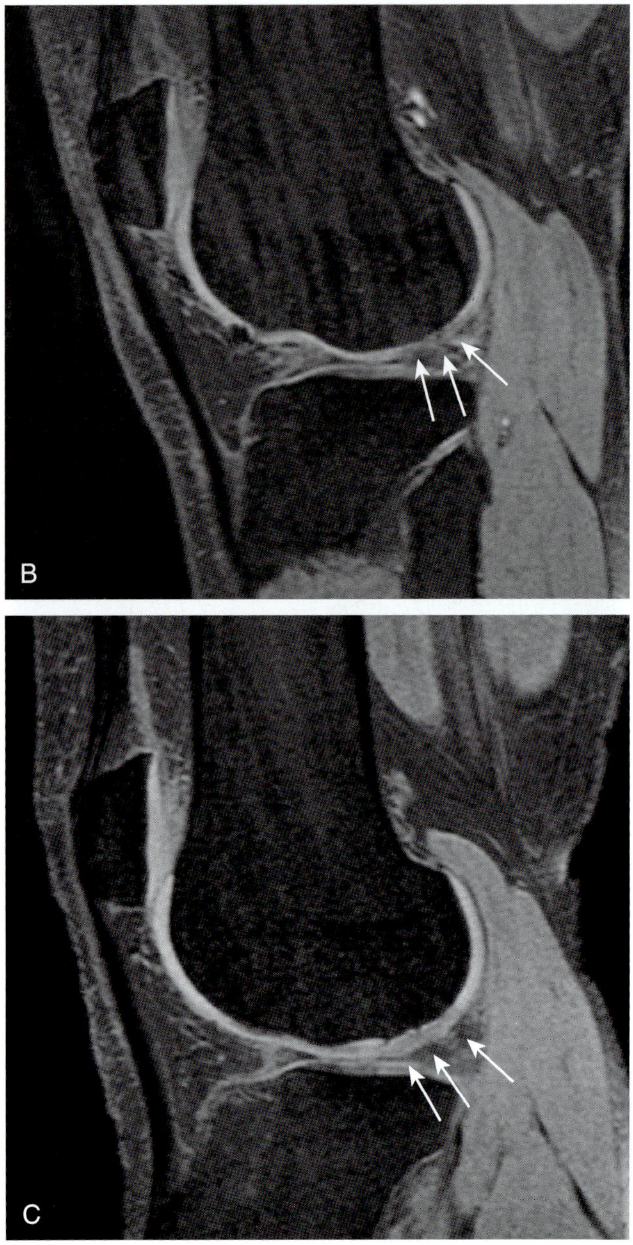

FIGURE 4-4, cont'd

potential implications on function and durability of the repair cartilage over time.[55,56]

Clinical function after microfracture treatment has been correlated to postoperative MRI findings of defect fill.[43] In this study, investigators found a correlation between good repair tissue defect fill and improved clinical knee function postoperatively and an association of limited/poor fill grade (<33% defect fill) and decreasing functional scores 24 months postoperatively.

MRI features of other potential complications or failure of microfracture cartilage repair may include visualization of chondral flaps and fissures, progressive tissue thinning, and defect enlargement suggestive of repair tissue breakdown and degeneration.

Osteochondral Transplantation

Osteochondral transplantation techniques of cartilage repair involve the use of autograft or allograft constructs of bone and overlying articular cartilage for restoration of an articular surface. Such repair techniques provide the theoretical advantage of implanting an articular surface composed of fully formed hyaline articular matrix with viable intrinsic chondrocytes.

OSTEOCHONDRAL AUTOGRAFTS

Autologous osteochondral transplantation (AOT) techniques include a series of similar procedures with varying names based on surgical instrumentation manufacturers: MosaicPlasty (Acuflex, Smith and Nephew), OATS (Osteochondral autograft transfer system, Arthrex), SDS (Soft delivery system, Sulzer Medica), and COR (Mitek). These techniques all involve the transplantation of one or more cylindrical plugs of autologous bone with overlying hyaline cartilage harvested from normal relatively non–weight-bearing aspects of the joint. These plugs are then transplanted into similarly sized holes created within the defect site to restore chondral and subchondral defects of the joint (Fig. 4-5). Graft plugs utilized may vary in overall dimensions from 2.7 to 8.5 mm in diameter and 10 to 25 mm in length.

AOT procedures can be performed arthroscopically or utilizing a small arthrotomy, which may be of added benefit when treating large defects or defects posteriorly located within the joint.[3] AOT procedures are usually done in one stage with multiple transplant plugs used to graft large defects and one or two plugs used to treat small articular defects.

Optimal candidates for osteochondral autograft transplantation are symptomatic young patients younger than 50 years of age with focal chondral or osteochondral defects 1 to 4 cm^2 in size.[57-59] Although larger lesions of up to 8 cm^2 have been treated, donor site graft availability, operative morbidity, and other technical issues limit the absolute size of lesions that can be effectively treated with AOT techniques.[37] AOT is used most commonly in the knee and ankle joints but has also been utilized in the repair of articular defects of other diarthrodial surfaces, including the tibia, humeral capitellum, and femoral head.[60-62] As with other cartilage reparative procedures, malalignment and ligamentous or meniscal insufficiency are relative contraindications and are typically treated simultaneously or as a staged procedure with AOT repair.[37,63]

Technically, AOT procedures involve débridement of a defect's margins back to healthy hyaline cartilage and the base of a defect down to viable subchondral bone. The defect recipient site is then measured to determine the number and size of grafts required for reconstruction of the articular surface. Recipient tunnels are then cut with coring instruments, removing evenly spaced, properly sized bone plugs oriented perpendicular to the articular surface at the defect site. After preparation of the recipient site, an appropriate number of correspondingly sized osteochondral plugs are harvested, perpendicular to the articular surface, using tubular harvesting instruments. Harvested plugs are obtained from relatively non–weight-bearing "donor" aspects of the joint. Typical donor sites in the knee include the margins of the inferior lateral trochlear ridge, intercondylar notch, or supracondylar ridge. The harvested osteochondral graft plug(s) are then transplanted atraumatically into the recipient tunnel(s) using press-fit fixation. The surgical goal of the transplantation is reconstruction of the contour of the articulation, with positioning and orientation of the transplantation plugs flush with the surface of adjacent native cartilage. Graft plug positioning proud or recessed relative to the native articular surface of the joint, either secondary to technical difficulties at surgery or graft subsidence and motion, is associated with worse clinical outcomes likely secondary to excess mechanical stress on the transplant plugs or subjacent cartilage.[64,65]

After AOT, patients are initially kept non–weight bearing postoperatively and then advanced to partial protective weight bearing with weight-bearing exercises and

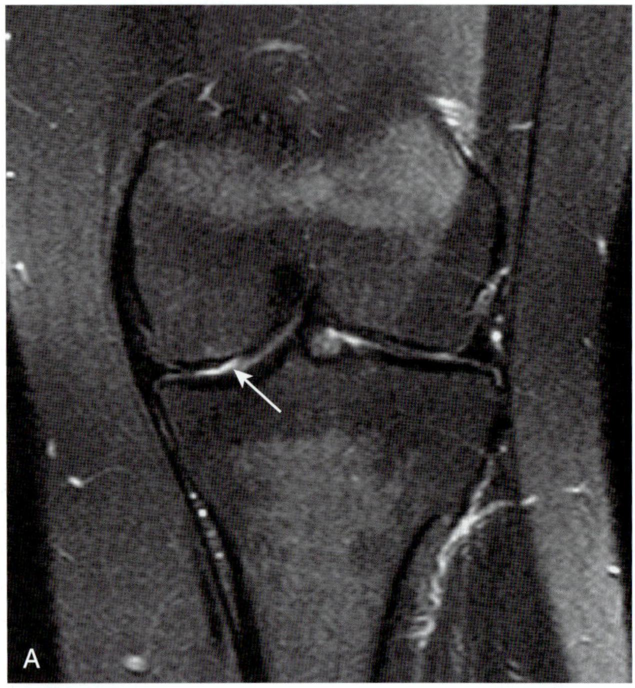

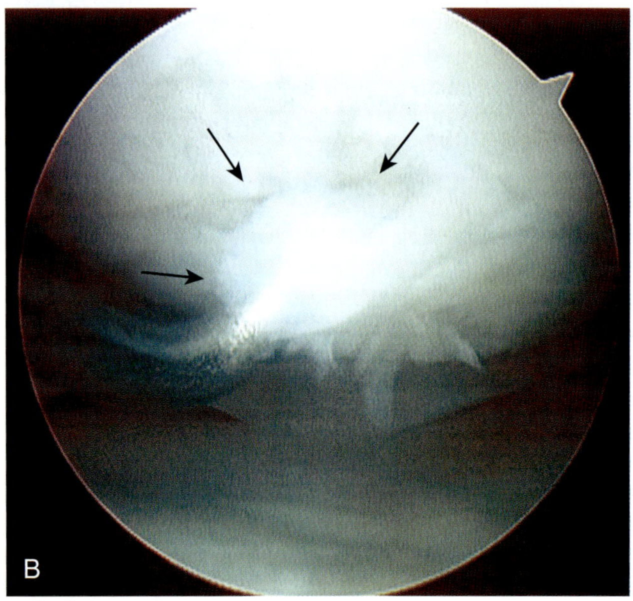

FIGURE 4-5. Autologous chondrocyte transplantation in a 34-year-old woman. **A,** Coronal, fat-suppressed, T2-weighted fast spin-echo image (TR/TE: 3000/80 ms) demonstrating a chondral defect of the medial femoral condyle (*arrow*). Arthroscopic images demonstrate the defect (**B**, *arrows*), débridement of the defect (**C**, *arrows*), four osteochondral plugs filling the defect (**D**), and two donor sites on the medial femoral trochlea (**E**, *arrows*). (Courtesy of Richard Parker, MD.)

subsequent progressive advancement to full weight bearing, This phased and conservative approach to weight bearing postoperatively is employed to avoid early graft damage and to promote early graft osseous incorporation and healing. Timing of the progress of postoperative rehabilitation is dependent on the size of the treated defect, patient age, patient body mass index, and level of anticipated postoperative patient activity.[59]

Second-look arthroscopic and histologic evaluations of autologous osteochondral transplants have shown consistent survival of transplanted hyaline cartilage overlying the osseous transplantation plugs.[57,66,67] Fibrocartilaginous repair tissue has also been documented between transplant graft plug interstices and their junction with native articular cartilage of the joint.[58,68,69]

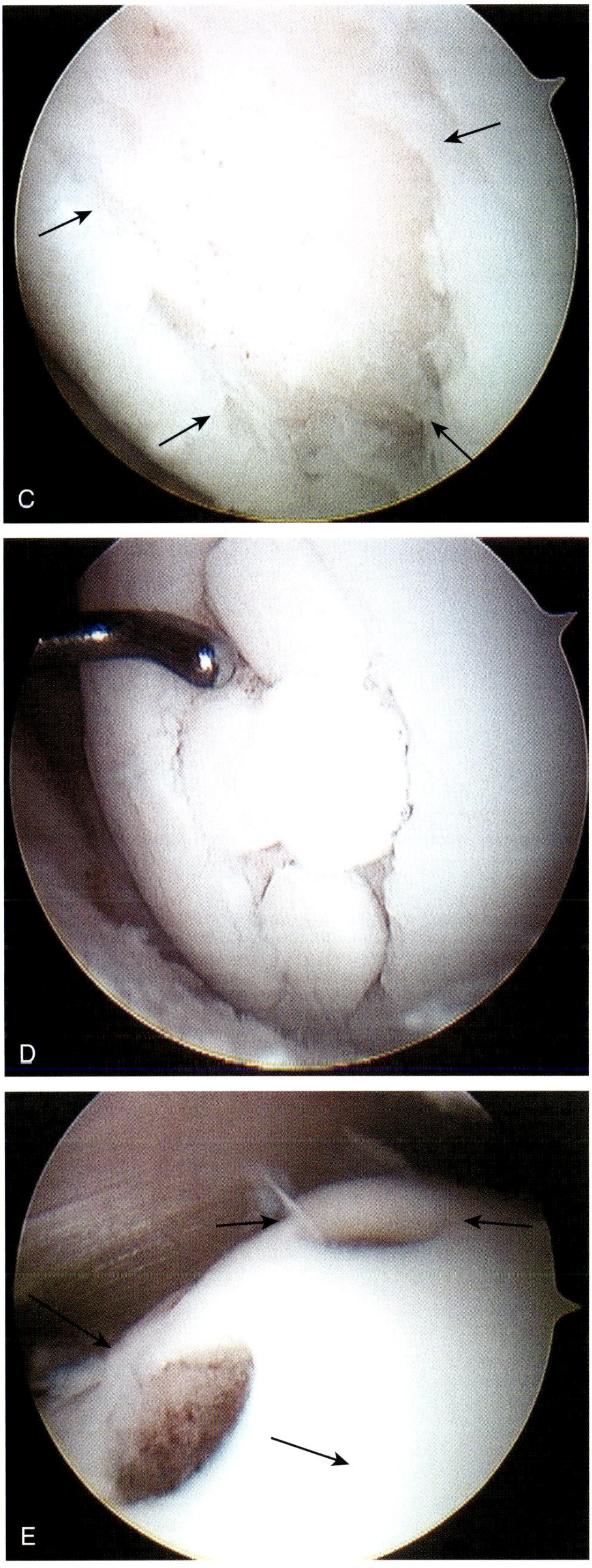

Figure 4-5, cont'd

Clinically, postoperative follow-up studies have reported high rates of symptomatic relief and functional improvement[58,66,70-77] up to 7 years postoperatively.[60,70-72,78-80] However, less favorable outcomes have been reported when defects greater than 4 cm^2 are repaired[81,82] and for repair of defects utilizing a larger number of transplant graft plugs.[78]

Few comparative investigations of AOT relative to other cartilage repair procedures are available in the literature. However, one such study of 413 arthroscopic resurfacing procedures (mosaicplasty, subchondral drilling, abrasion arthroplasty, and microfracture) showed superior long-term clinical outcome results for mosaicplasty relative to the other techniques evaluated.[71] Other randomized clinical trials have shown outcomes after mosaicplasty to be superior to microfracture[83] and comparable with outcome results after autologous chondrocyte implantation for repair of small- to medium-sized defects.[84,85]

MRI after Autologous Osteochondral Transplantation

MRI after AOT procedures can provide information regarding congruity of repair articular surface, graft incorporation, as well as status of the donor site. At the donor sites, tubular regions of low T1 and increased T2 signal intensity are normally seen within the harvest marrow space, with corresponding defects seen in the overlying articular cartilage. These observed subchondral signal changes at the donor sites progressively resolve, returning to normal fatty marrow signal (Fig. 4-6), while the associated articular defects may become less apparent as they progressively fill-in with fibrocartilaginous repair tissue.[57-59,68,69,74]

Congruence of the repair site articular surface after AOT is an important determinant of clinical repair success. Incongruent grafts may be subject to micromotion interfering with incorporation[86] and to accelerated mechanical wear and degeneration.[64,65] Graft incongruity may occur secondary to technical surgical challenges during graft insertion or subsequent subsidence or degradation of transplanted plugs. Postoperatively, MRI should ideally illustrate a smooth congruent cartilage/cartilage interface at the AOT repair site (Fig. 4-7). In the setting of graft incongruity, surface stepoff deformities are seen either between individual transplant plugs or between transplant plugs and the native articular surface of the joint. Such stepoff incongruities and gaps may become less marked over time (Fig. 4-8), with gradual improvement in apparent congruity secondary to fibrocartilaginous repair tissue overgrowth originating from subchondral bone of the repair site and extending through the osteochondral transplant graft interstices.[58]

In contrast to surface incongruities, incongruity of subchondral bone/bone interfaces is a common normal finding reflective of the thinner hyaline cartilage cover of donor osteochondral plugs. The donor osteochondral plugs are harvested from relative non–weight-bearing aspects of the joint where articular cartilage is typically thinner in depth than native articular cartilage at the site of transplantation. Because harvested plugs are inserted to a depth providing for a congruent smooth repair articular surface, the bone/bone interface between transplant plugs and native subchondral bone will often be incongruous (Figs. 4-9 and 4-10).

The signal characteristics of the repair articular cartilage after AOT typically mirror those of adjacent native articular cartilage.[87,88] Signal changes of marrow edema are normally seen within the transplant osseous plugs and surrounding subchondral bone postoperatively (see Fig. 4-10A), with associated intense enhancement after the administration of intravenous contrast material.[88] These changes are believed to correlate to graft revascularization with corresponding perigraft fibrovascular reparative and inflammatory reactive changes observed in animal studies 6 to 14 weeks postoperatively.[89,90] Resolution of such edema-like signal changes are typically observed on MRI 9 to 12 months postoperatively (see Fig. 4-10B) as the transplant grafts become fully incorporated into the surrounding subchondral bone. After osseous incorporation, normal marrow signal is typically seen within and surrounding the osteochondral transplantation plugs; however, in some cases, persistence of a mild

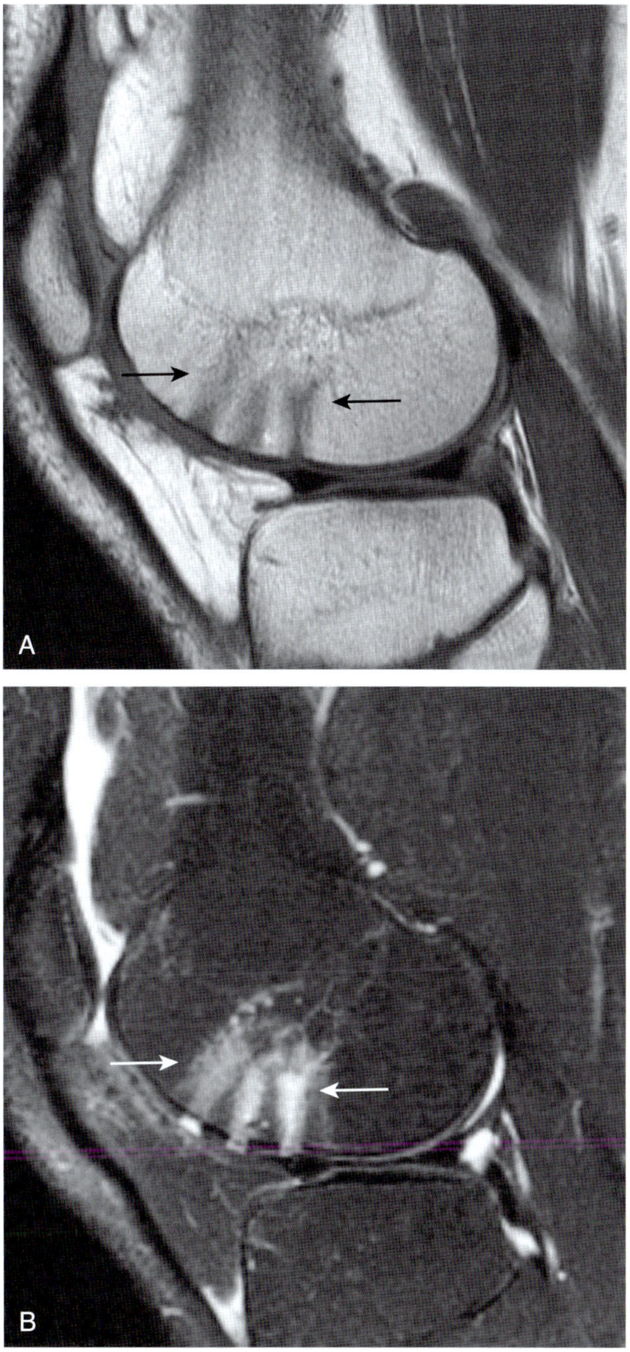

FIGURE 4-6. A 26-year-old man underwent mosaicplasty and autogenic osteochondral transplantation of the medial femoral condyle. Postoperative sagittal, intermediate-weighted (TR/TE: 4000/20 ms) (**A**) and fat-suppressed, T2-weighted (TR/TE: 3500/70 ms) (**B**) fast spin-echo MR images of the lateral femoral trochlear ridge obtained 3 months after the procedures. Cylindrical defects corresponding to graft plug harvest sites (*arrows*) can be seen within the subchondral aspect of the femoral trochlea perpendicularly oriented relative to the trochlear articular surface. Overlying defects in the articular cartilaginous surface of the trochlea corresponding to the articular surface of the graft plugs can be seen on the T2-weighted image, as can mild marrow edema surrounding the graft harvest sites. Corresponding follow-up sagittal, intermediate-weighted (TR/TE: 4000/20 ms) (**C**) and fat-suppressed, T2-weighted (TR/TE: 3500/70 ms) (**D**) fast spin-echo MR images 15 months postoperatively show resolution of the edematous changes and an apparent smooth articular contour at the harvest plug sites.

degree of subchondral edema-like signal has been observed at the transplantation site up to 2 to 3 years postoperatively in asymptomatic and stable grafts.[31,87] In contrast, prominent areas of persistent subchondral graft/perigraft edema–like signal changes or subchondral perigraft cysts are worrisome imaging findings suggestive of poor graft incorporation or graft necrosis (Fig. 4-11).[32,86,87]

Additional complications of AOT that may be observed on MRI include graft cartilage fissures, degeneration or delamination, as well as graft plug fracture (Fig. 4-12) and possible displacement.

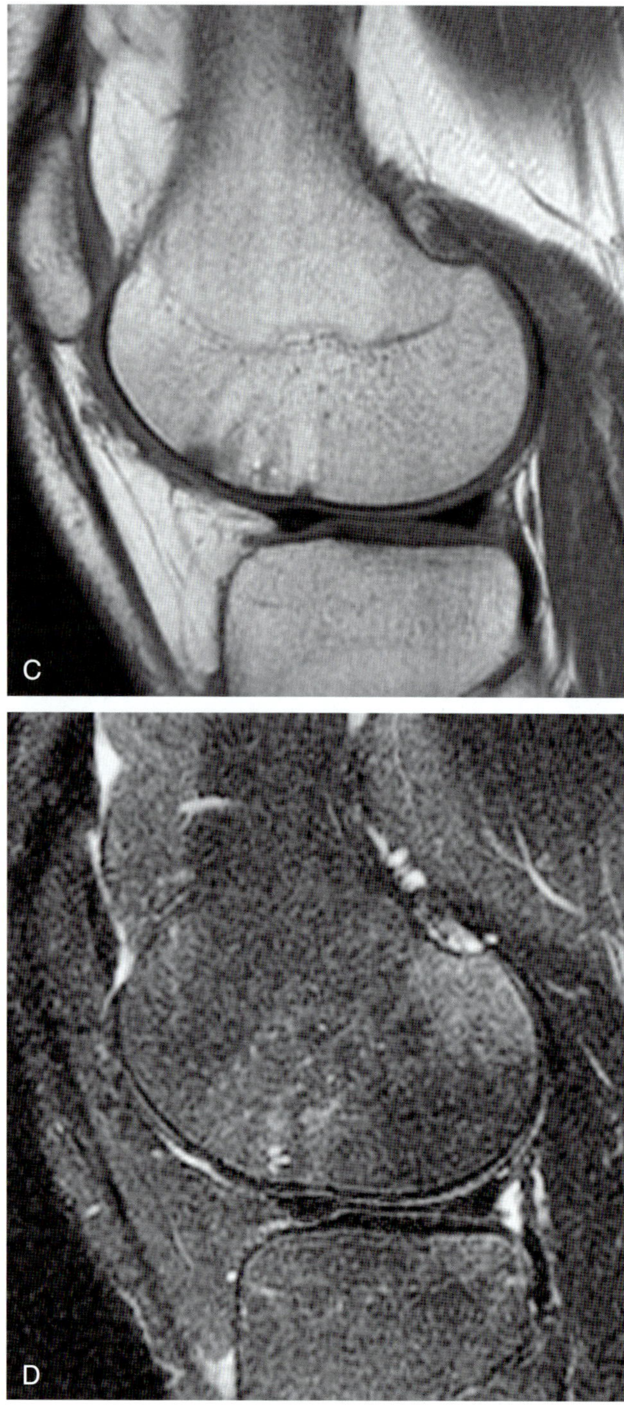

FIGURE 4-6, cont'd

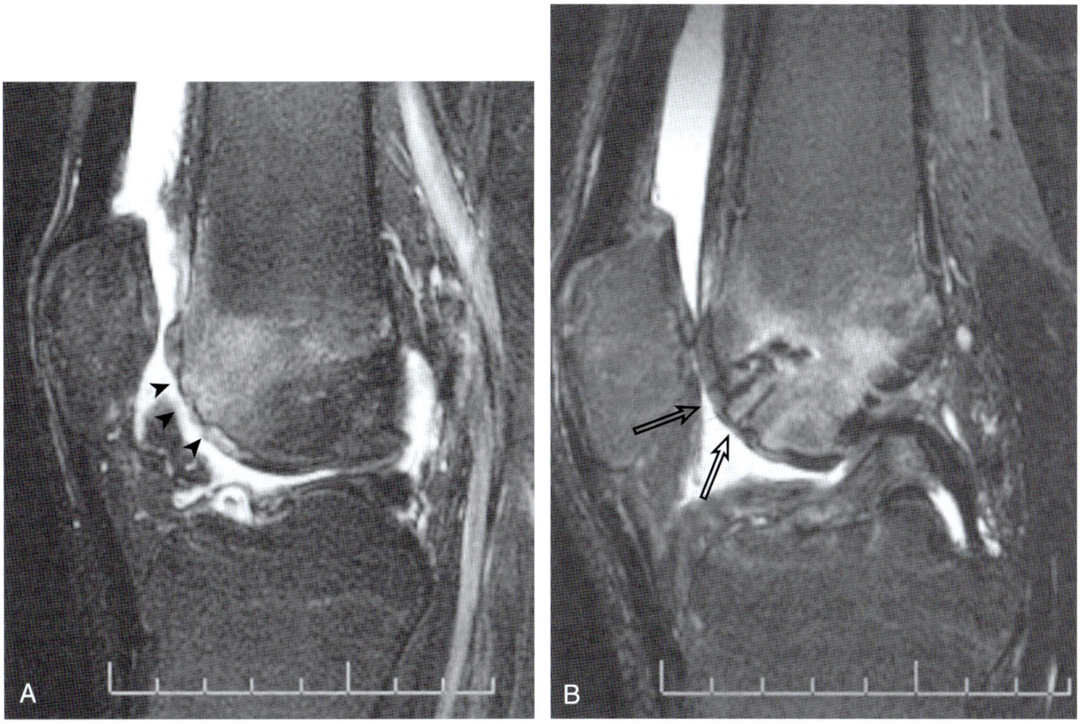

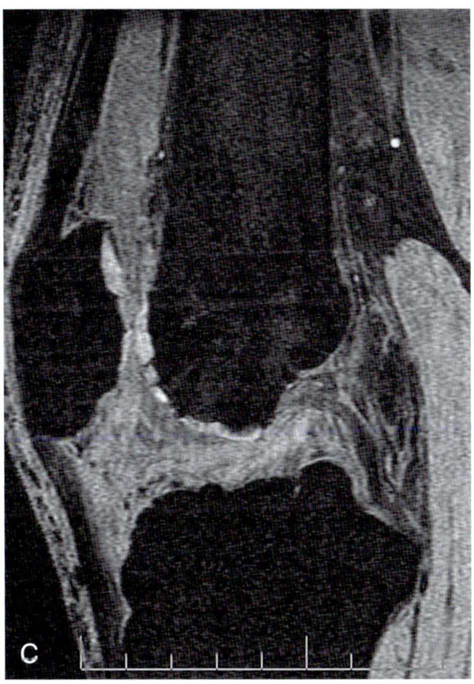

FIGURE 4-7. Mosaic autogenic osteochondral transplantation of the femoral trochlear articular surface in a 38-year-old male athlete. **A**, Preoperative sagittal, fat suppressed, T2-weighted (TR/TE: 3500/70 ms), fast spin-echo MR image illustrates an extensive full-thickness articular cartilage defect (*arrowheads*) along the central aspect of the femoral trochlea. Reactive edematous marrow signal changes are seen within the subchondral aspect of the trochlea. Postoperative sagittal, fat-suppressed, T2-weighted (TR/TE: 3500/70 ms), fast spin-echo (**B**) and 3D fat-suppressed, spoiled gradient-echo (SPGR) (TR/TE/FA: 47 ms/10 ms/45°) (**C**) MR images show a smooth neoarticular surface (**B**, *arrows*) 3 months after mosaicplasty repair and reconstruction of the trochlear articular surface with multiple transplantation osteochondral plugs.

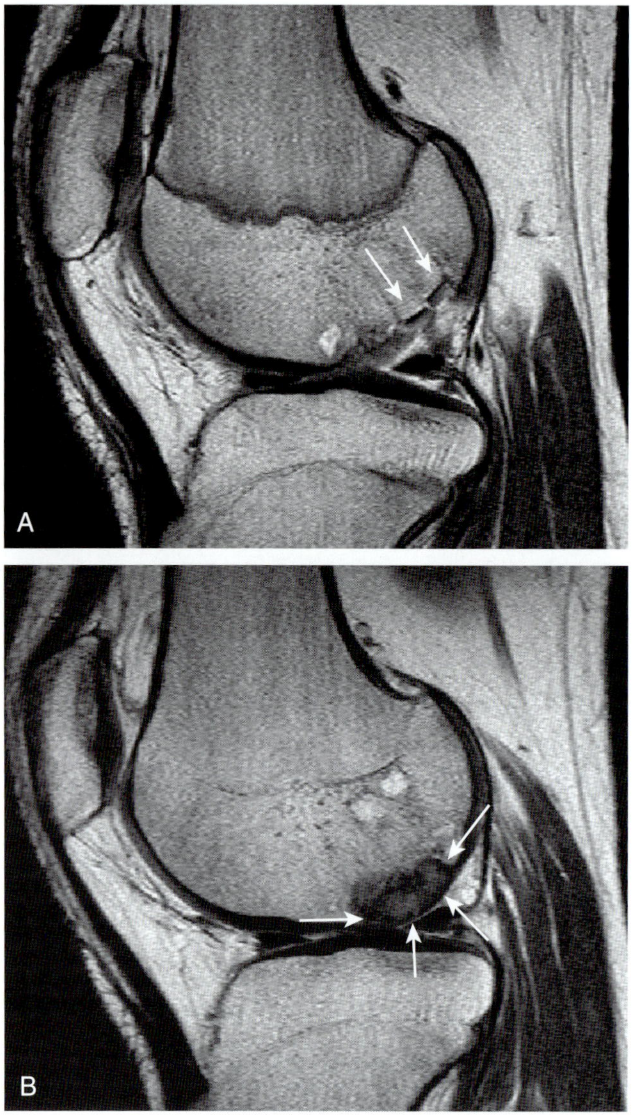

FIGURE 4-8. Autologous chondrocyte transplantation in a 20-year old. **A,** Sagittal, intermediate proton-density–weighted (TR/TE: 3000/44 ms), fast spin-echo image demonstrating incongruity of the cartilage/cartilage interface secondary to subsidence of the osteochondral plugs (*arrows*). **B,** At 3.5 years after surgery there is a decrease in the incongruity secondary to an increase in repair tissue (*arrows*) overlying the transplanted plugs.

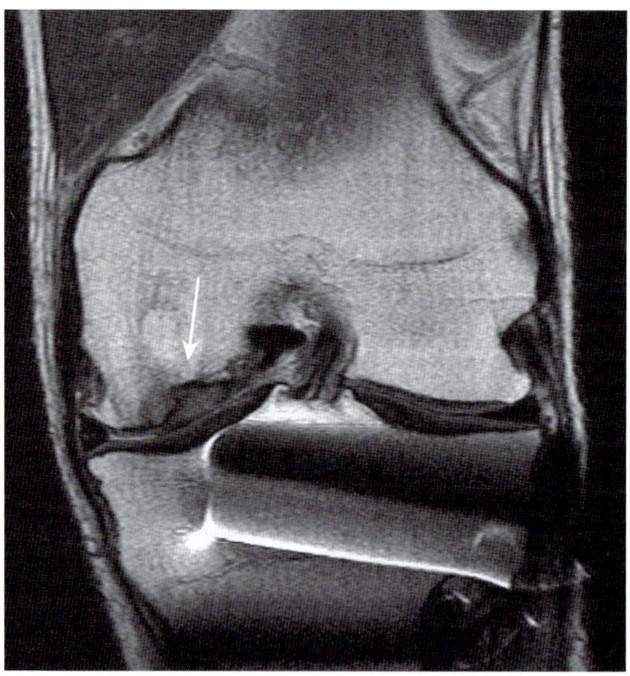

FIGURE 4-9. Coronal proton-density–weighted, fast spin-echo image (TR/TE: 3000/43 ms) in a 35-year-old man demonstrating stepoff of the bone/bone interface (*arrow*).

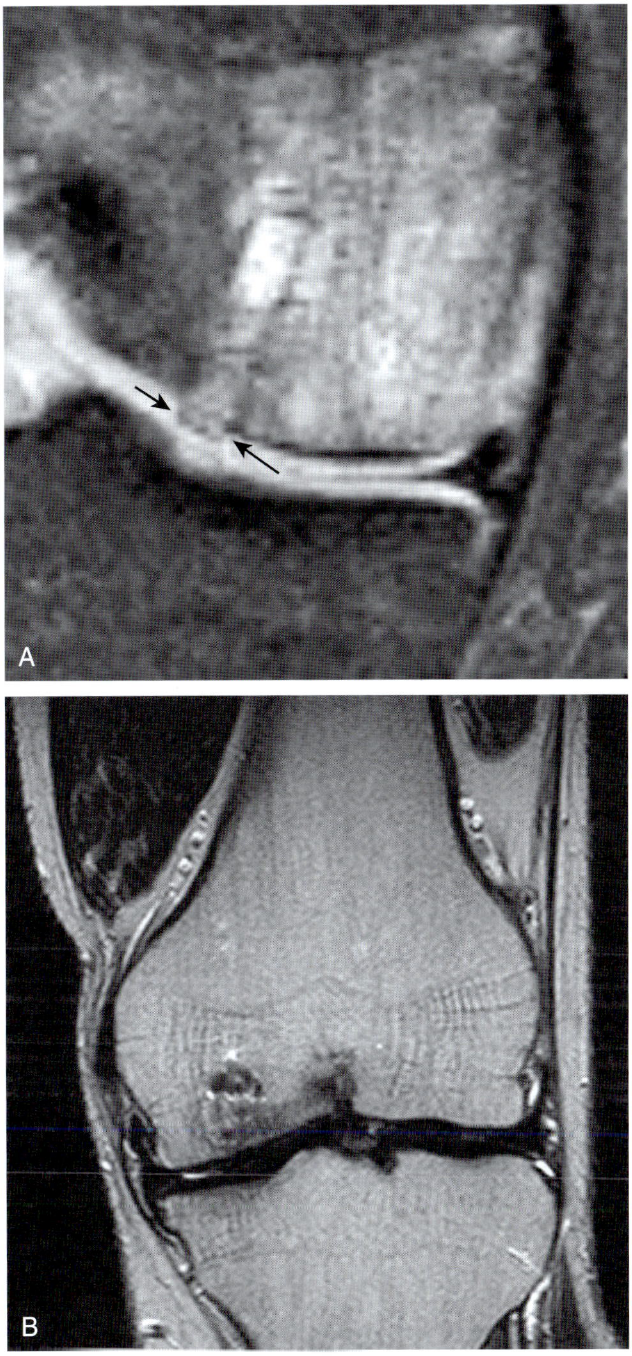

FIGURE 4-10. **A,** Fat-suppressed, coronal, T2-weighted, fast spin-echo image (TR/TE: 4200/70 ms) demonstrating bone marrow edema at the transplant site 4 months after autologous osteochondral transplant in a 35-year-old man. Also note the offset at the bone/bone interface (*arrows*). **B,** Coronal, fat-suppressed, T2-weighted (TR/TE: 6000/120 ms) image in a 34-year-old man demonstrating incorporation of bone plugs with minimal bone marrow edema 18 months after autologous osteochondral transplant. Note some susceptibility artifact in the region of the incorporated plugs.

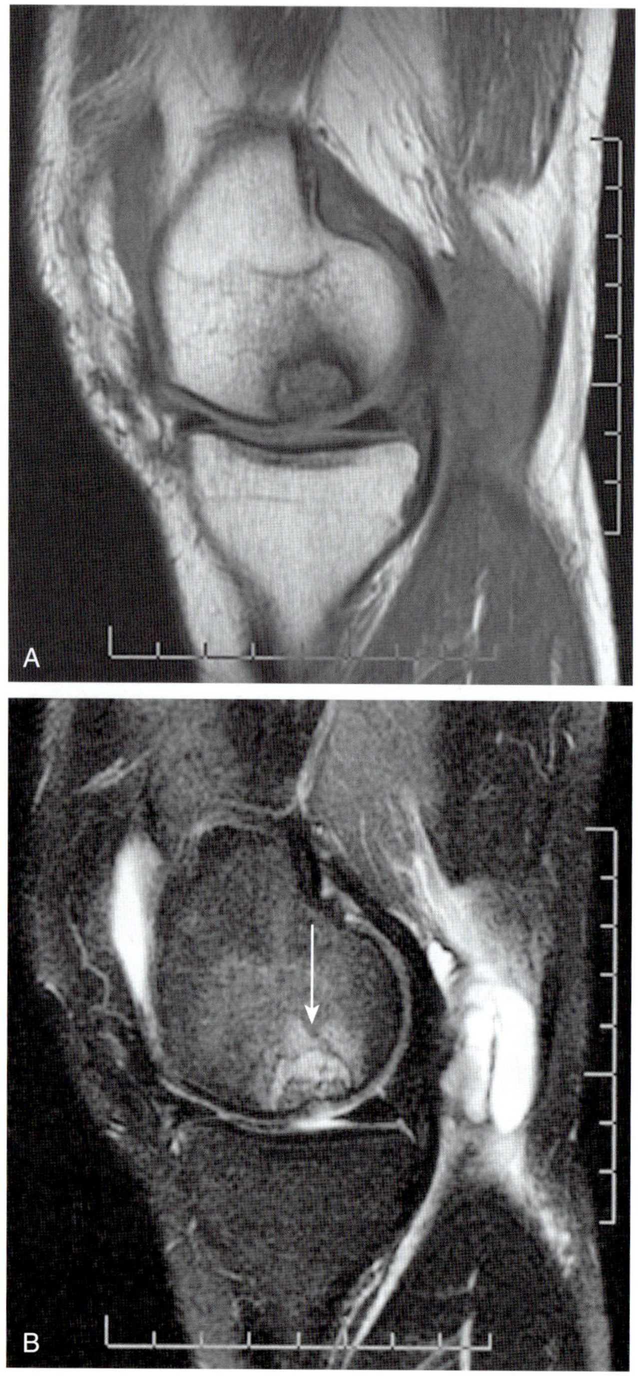

FIGURE 4-11. A 29-year-old man presented with recurrent pain after osteochondral autograft transplantation repair of a focal cartilage defect of the medial femoral condyle. Sagittal intermediate-weighted (TR/TE: 3700/20 ms) (**A**) and fat-suppressed T2-weighted (TR/TE: 3500/70 ms) (**B**) fast spin-echo MR images 23 months after the procedure show a well-demarcated area of subchondral heterogeneous signal, with persistent, irregular, increased T2-weighted signal at the transplantation/repair site (**B**, *arrow*). Flattening and irregularity of the repair site articular cartilage contour are seen in this patient with recurrent symptoms secondary to graft plug necrosis and collapse.

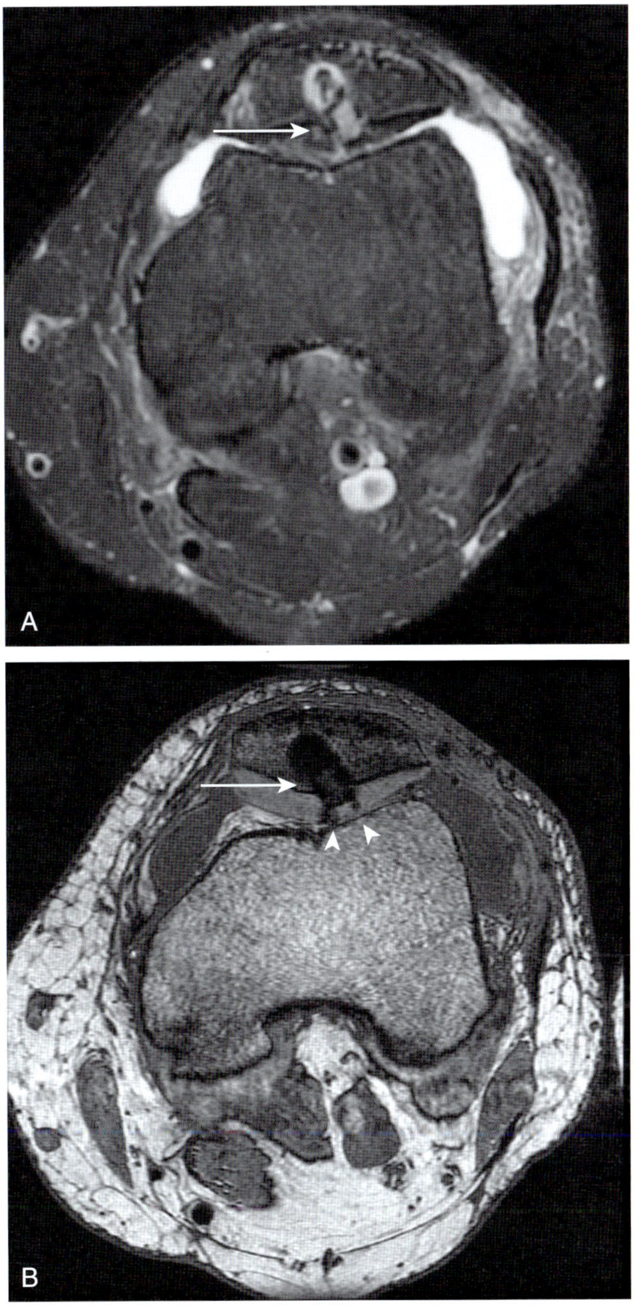

FIGURE 4-12. Early and follow-up MR images in a patient after osteochondral autograft transplantation repair of a focal cartilage defect of the patella. Axial, fat-suppressed, T2-weighted (TR/TE: 3500/70 ms) fast spin-echo (**A**) and 3D non–fat-suppressed spoiled gradient-echo (SPGR) (TR/TE/FA: 47 ms/10 ms/45°) (**B**) MR images 3 months postoperatively show a single osteochondral transplantation plug (*arrow*) after repair of a focal cartilage defect of the central aspect of the lateral patellar articular facet. Congruity is seen of the articular surface of the transplantation plug with the adjacent articular surface of the patella (*arrowheads*). **C,** Follow-up axial, 3D, fat-suppressed spoiled gradient-echo (SPGR) (TR/TE/FA: 47/10/450 ms) MR image illustrates interval fracture of the transplantation graft plug (*arrow*) with rotation of the graft articular surface (*arrowheads*) perpendicular to the articular surface of the patella.

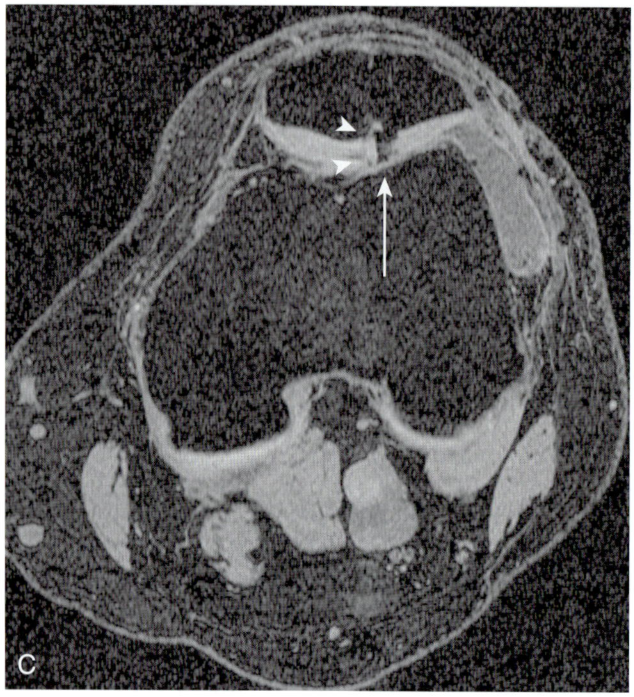

FIGURE 4-12, cont'd

Osteochondral Allograft Transplantation

Osteochondral allograft transplantation (OAT) involves the replacement of damaged segments of articular cartilage and underlying subchondral bone with anatomically matched segments of cadaveric graft composed of healthy viable articular cartilage and its attached nonliving subchondral bone. In contrast to autologous osteochondral transplants, allograft transplantation eliminates issues related to donor site morbidity and potential limitations related to reconstruction defect size. Potential drawbacks of osteochondral allograft transplants include limited graft availability, cost, immunogenic graft rejection, possibilities of disease transmission,[91,92] and demanding surgical techniques required for precise graft implantation. Given the unrestricted transplantable tissue volume osteochondral allografts offer, allogeneic osteochondral transplants are most commonly utilized for repair of large osteochondral defects, greater than 3 cm^2 in size and greater than 1 cm in depth, where autologous transplantation techniques and other repair procedures are impractical.

Osteochondral allograft material utilized for transplantation is typically "fresh," having been procured within 12 hours of a donor's death and transplanted within 1 week thereafter. To minimize potential immunogenic reaction, blood and marrow elements are washed from the donor tissue. Strict donor screening protocols, sterile graft procurement and processing, as well as storage of graft material in antibiotic solution are utilized to minimize risks of tissue disease transmission.

OAT is usually performed via an open surgical arthrotomy. Exposure and precise measurement of the morphology and size of the articular defect are matched to the allograft segment, and the surgically sized and trimmed graft is inserted with press-fit fixation (Fig. 4-13) and/or stabilization via bioabsorbable pins or fixation screws.

Postoperatively, biomechanical overload of the graft is avoided through an extended period of limited weight bearing. Continuous passive motion is often employed during this period to promote mechanical stimulation of chondrocytes, prevent joint adhesions, and regain joint range of motion.[37]

Clinical reviews of patients treated by OAT have shown excellent clinical results as long as 7 to 10 years postoperatively,[93-97] with viable hyaline cartilage confirmed on biopsy up to 17 years after transplantion.[98,99]

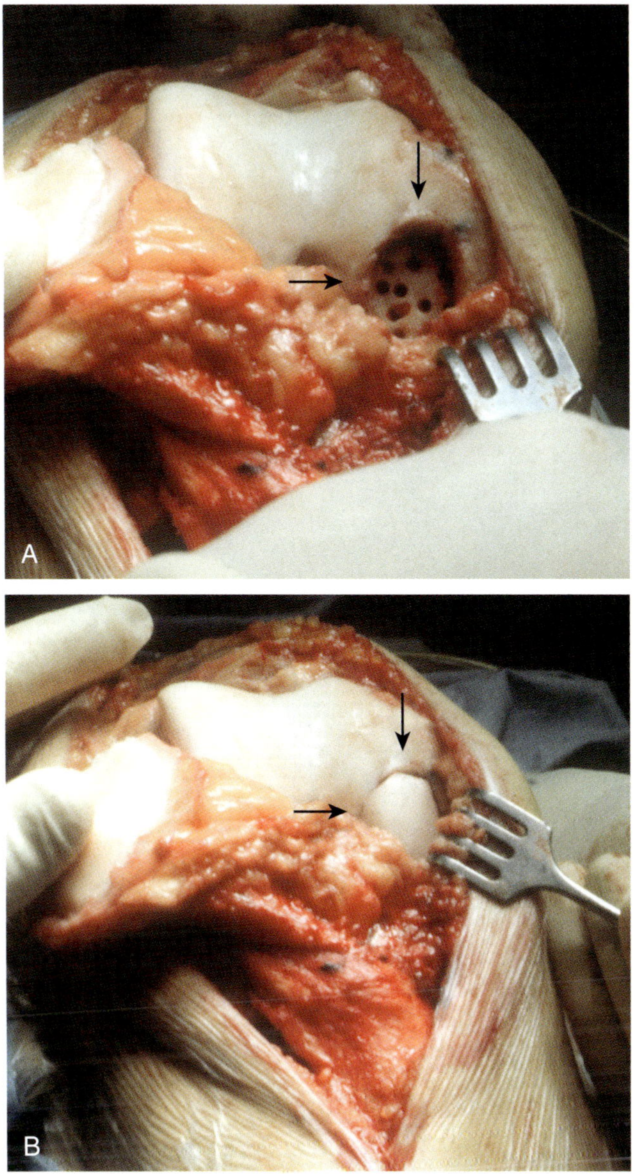

FIGURE 4-13. Intraoperative images during osteochondral allograft transplantation in a 29-year-old man who presented for treatment of a prior post-traumatic osteochondral defect of the medial femoral condyle. **A,** Intraoperative photograph illustrates the prepared transplantation site (*arrows*) along the weight-bearing aspect of the medial femoral condyle. **B,** Follow-up photograph shows the osteochondral allograft transplant in place resurfacing the prior defect site (*arrows*). (Courtesy of Allan Gross, MD.)

Factors identified that have been associated with a higher incidence of graft failure include advanced age (>50 years) at the time of transplantation, articular defects on opposing sides of the joint, and joint malalignment.[3,100,101]

MRI after Osteochondral Allograft Transplantation

MRI of osteochondral allografts may be complicated by metallic artifacts originating from graft fixation hardware or stabilization hardware associated with concomitantly performed realignment osteotomy. As such, MRI techniques to minimize metal-related imaging artifacts may be useful in the postoperative imaging assessment of patients after OAT.[102]

Postoperative MRI of osteochondral allografts can provide noninvasive assessment of graft position, status of the articular surface of the graft and adjacent native cartilage (Fig. 4-14), and status of graft incorporation. Early postoperative MRI clearly

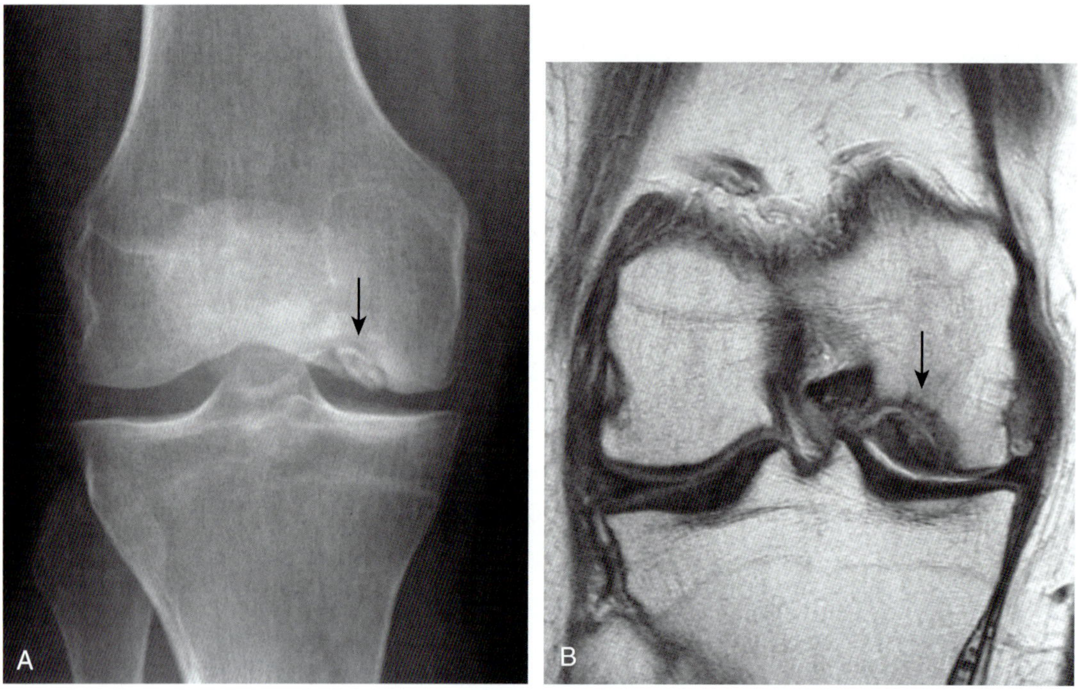

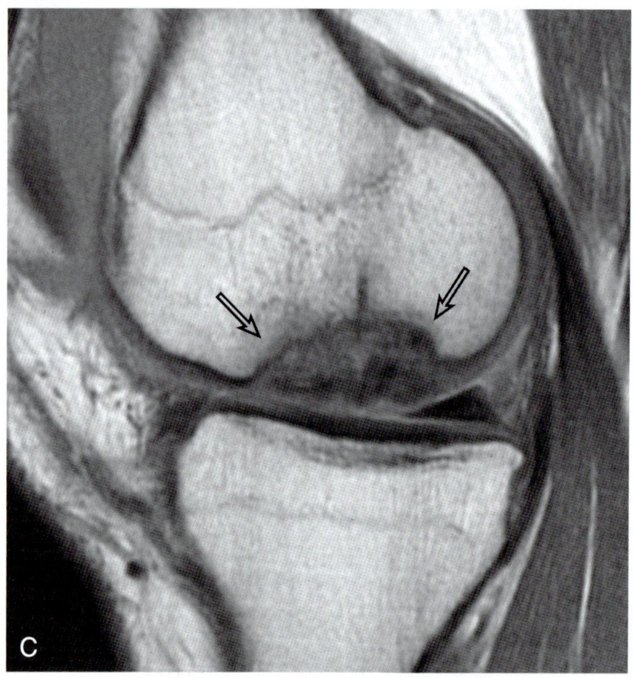

FIGURE 4-14. A 24-year-old man presented after allograft osteochondral transplantation of the medial femoral condyle. Anteroposterior radiograph (**A**) and coronal intermediate-weighted (TR/TE: 4000/34 ms), fast spin-echo (**B**) and sagittal intermediate-weighted (TR/TE: 3700/20 ms) (**C**) MR images show an osteochondral dissecans lesion along the central aspect of the medial femoral condyle (**A-C**, *arrows*). The lesion was unstable, with fluid signal traversing the articular surface, subchondral plate, and interface of the lesion and the underlying femoral condyle. Patient complaints included pain and mechanical symptoms of catching. Corresponding conventional radiograph (**D**), as well as coronal (**E**) and sagittal (**F**) intermediate-weighted (TR/TE: 4000/34), fast spin-echo MR images show repair of the prior osteochondral lesion with a press-fit osteochondral allograft (**D-F**, *arrows*). A smooth contour is seen of the reconstruction graft with a congruent interface with adjacent native articular cartilage of the medial femoral condyle. Stabilization hardware related to a concomitant high tibial valgus osteotomy is seen along the proximal tibial metaphysis.

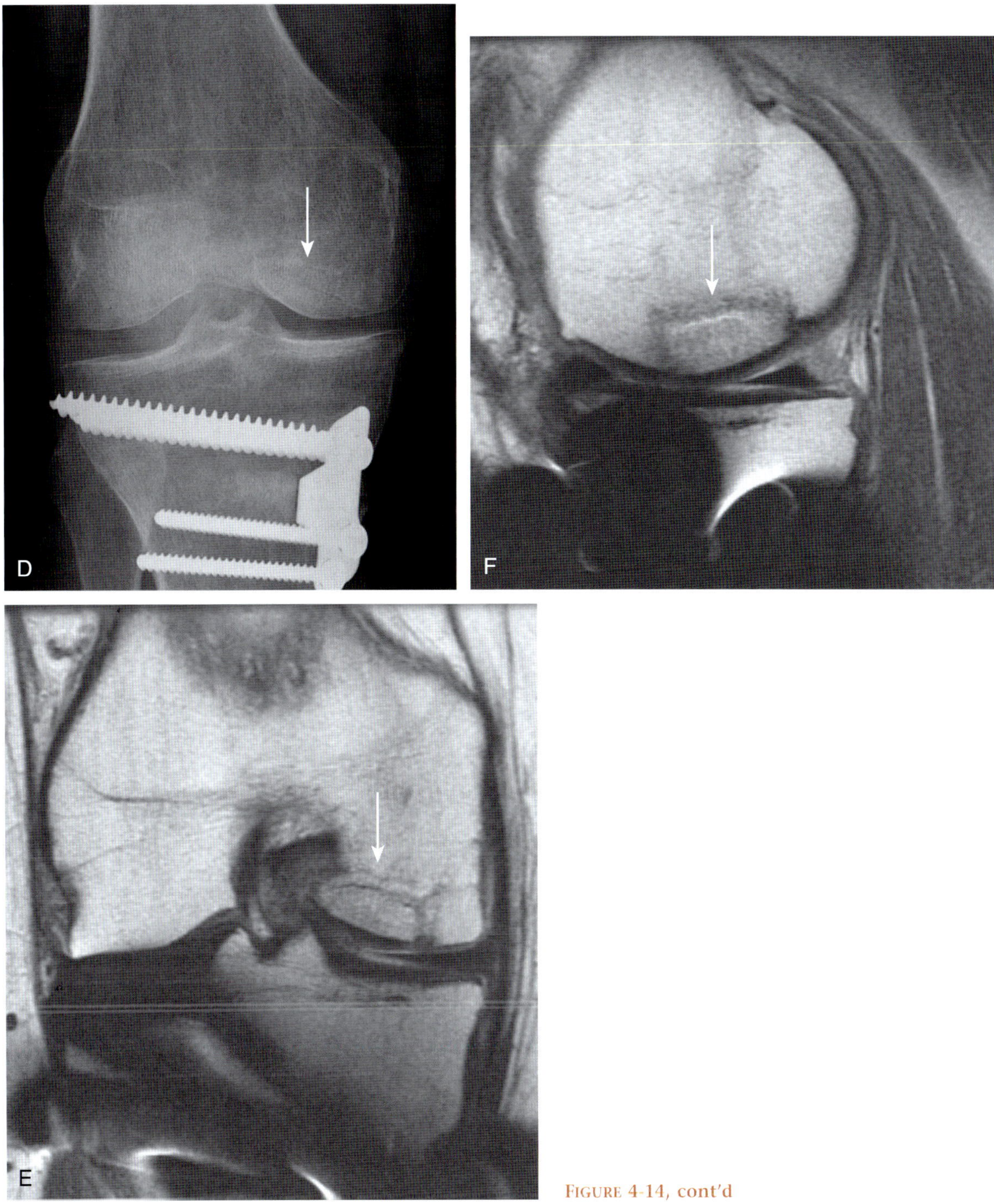

FIGURE 4-14, cont'd

depicts the graft/host interface with subjacent postoperative edematous changes with the host marrow. Progressive marrow edema signal changes are typically seen at the graft/host marrow interface and within the subjacent portions of the graft bone during the phase of graft incorporation. Histologic evidence of mature allograft remodeling and incorporation may take 3 to 4 years to fully complete.[95,103] Similar to the postoperative findings in osteochondral autograft transplants, the edema-like MR signal changes observed during this interval are presumed to be related to histologic changes of postoperative osseous remodeling, ingrowth of fibrovascular reparative tissue, and altered biomechanics. MRI findings reflective of mature allograft incorporation include resolution of subchondral graft marrow edema and progressive ill definition of the graft/host interface. In contrast, findings of persistent intense edematous signal changes within the graft and at the graft/host interface are seen in the setting of graft/host immune response,[26,104] graft rejection, or graft necrosis. Clinical graft failure in such cases may additionally be associated with MRI findings of graft collapse, fragmentation, or migration.[26,102,104]

Cartilage-sensitive MR acquisitions can allow for the assessment of integrity of graft articular cartilage and that of adjacent joint surfaces. MRI also allows for accurate assessment of congruity of the graft/host articular interface, which is crucial to ultimate successful graft incorporation and long-term clinical graft success.[105]

Autologous Chondrocyte Implantation

Autologous chondrocyte implantation (ACI) is a biologic technique of transplantation of autologous cells grown in culture into chondral and osteochondral defects. The classic ACI procedure was initially described in the mid 1990s[106,107] and is currently employed as a primary clinical repair technique for symptomatic medium-to-large (2 to 12 cm^2) defects with minimal involvement of subchondral bone or for treatment of lesions that have failed prior repair procedures, including débridement, marrow stimulation, or osteochondral autograft repair techniques.

ACI is a two-stage procedure. In the initial stage of the technique, arthroscopic assessment of the defect site is performed along with a harvesting biopsy of healthy articular hyaline cartilage. After harvesting, cells from articular cartilage are cultured and grown in vitro for 4 to 6 weeks. After this period of cell culturing, the second stage of the procedure involves an open surgical arthrotomy. At surgery, the articular surface of the defect site is débrided to stable margins and an autologous periosteal patch (usually harvested from the ipsilateral proximal tibia or distal femur) is sutured over the defect with its margins sealed to the edges of the defect with fibrin glue. After watertight sealing of the periosteal flap, the cultured cartilage cells are injected into the defect beneath the periosteal cover.

Variations of the classic ACI procedure have been subsequently developed and utilized in clinical practice.[108] "Second generation" ACI involves the use of a bioengineered bilayer collagen membrane instead of a periosteal patch for containment of the implanted cultured cartilage cells. Use of a collagen membrane in this manner reduces overall surgical morbidity and simplifies the second stage of the surgical procedure. Further technical developments have led to "third generation" ACI techniques, also referred to as matrix-induced autologous chondrocyte implantation (MACI).[109] In this variation of the ACI procedure, autologous chondrocytes are cultured within a 3D membrane scaffold. The cell-seeded membrane scaffold is subsequently trimmed to the size of the defect and implanted at the repair site with fibrin glue fixation (Fig. 4-15). Advantages of this variation of ACI include obviating the needs for a periosteal graft or fixation sutures and overall technical simplicity of the procedure.

Strict adherence to a postoperative rehabilitation protocol after ACI surgery is essential to the success of the procedure. Such rehabilitation protocols typically include initial use of continuous passive motion and protective weight bearing for 4 to 6 weeks, followed by slow advancement to full weight bearing.[37]

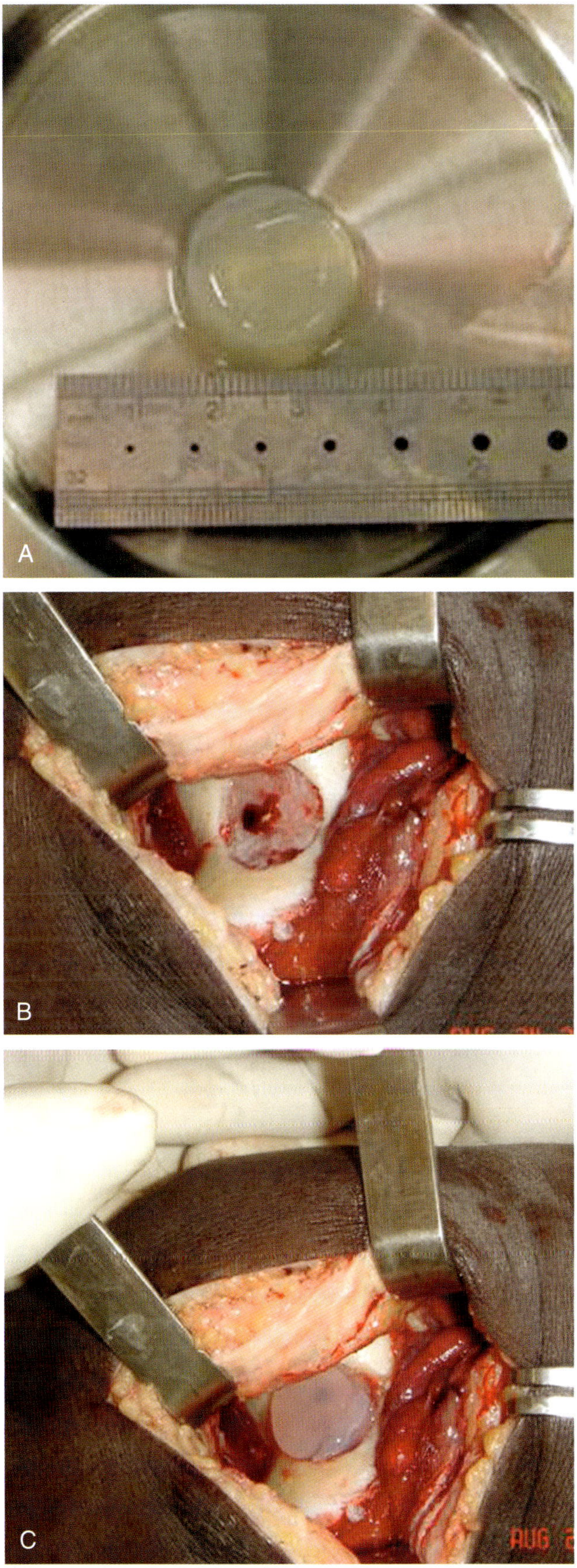

Figure 4-15. Autologous cell–seeded matrix chondrocyte implantation in a 39-year-old woman. **A,** The transplant ex vivo before the implantation. **B,** Intraoperative image demonstrating the débrided defect. **C,** Intraoperative image demonstrating the defect after implantation of the transplant.

Multiple studies have described the clinical outcomes of patients treated with ACI in the knee.[51,85,110-116] These studies have demonstrated good clinical outcomes in 74% to 92% of patients.[109-115] In general, younger and more active patients are more likely to have a better clinical outcome.[51] Lower success rates have been described for patients treated with multiple lesions and lesions treated with concomitant ligament repairs.[112] Although high overall clinical success rates have been reported after ACI, comparative studies to date have not shown a significant difference between clinical results obtained with ACI versus microfracture at 1 to 2 years postoperative follow-up.[51,117]

Histologic studies have illustrated variable results of ACI repair tissue analysis ranging from fibrocartilaginous to hyaline-like repair tissue, with all cases differing morphologically and/or histologically in some degree from normal hyaline cartilage. However, investigators have found that biopsy specimens obtained from repairs at a longer time interval postoperatively have shown a greater degree of hyaline-like morphology, suggesting that ACI transplants may become more hyaline-like in histologic appearance over time.[118] Despite these findings, comparative histologic studies have not shown an association between the quality of repair tissue at follow-up postoperative biopsy and overall clinical outcome.[51]

MRI after Autologous Chondrocyte Implantation

After ACI procedures, MRI can assess and define the degree of defect filling, appearance of the graft tissue surface morphology, integration of the graft to adjacent cartilage and subchondral bone, as well as potential complications of the procedure, including graft hypertrophy and delamination.[26,27,30-33,51,119-125]

The depth and volume of defect filling after ACI procedures can be readily assessed on MRI evaluation (Fig. 4-16).[26,31-33,119,124] In the initial postoperative period, the volume of repair tissue may decrease slightly within the defect site, with defect fill volume usually stabilizing by 3 months postoperatively.[118,123-125]

Graft tissue hypertrophy postoperatively is manifest by thickening of repair tissue protruding beyond the normal contour of the articular surface of adjacent hyaline cartilage and may be a reflection of hypertrophy of graft repair cartilage or the overlying periosteal flap. Graft hypertrophy is most commonly seen between 3 and 7 months postoperatively and has been reported to occur in up to 10% to 39% of cases.[112,126,127] Clinically, graft hypertrophy may be associated with symptoms and signs of joint catching, locking, and pain.[124] Graft hypertrophy has been described to be less common after MACI versus classic ACI repairs utilizing periosteal flaps.[109,128] Trattnig and coworkers reported a similar incidence of initial graft hypertrophy after MACI procedures as seen with classic ACI techniques; however, resolution of MACI graft hypertrophic changes was seen in the majority of cases by 1 year postoperatively, presumably as the result of progressive MACI graft remodeling.[125]

At postoperative MRI, uncomplicated ACI graft material typically shows fluid-like signal characteristics in the early postoperative period. Most studies have described a subsequent progressive change in graft signal characteristics to essentially equal those of native hyaline articular cartilage by 12 to 24 months postoperatively.[26,33,116] In contrast, other investigations have described persistent relative hyperintensity of graft material on intermediate-weighted fast spin-echo acquisitions more than 18 months postoperatively (Fig. 4-17).[27]

Graft surface morphology should normally appear smooth and contiguous with adjacent native articular cartilage. Surface fissures, clefts, and ulcerations may be seen as manifestations of graft complications. A smooth indiscernible interface of the ACI graft and native articular cartilage is also normally visualized in the setting of successful graft integration. Fissuring or fluid-like splits between graft and native cartilage (Fig. 4-18), particularly when fluid signal extends beneath the base of the ACI graft, have been described in the setting of incomplete incorporation and graft delamination. Delamination is described as a potential complication of 5% of all ACI

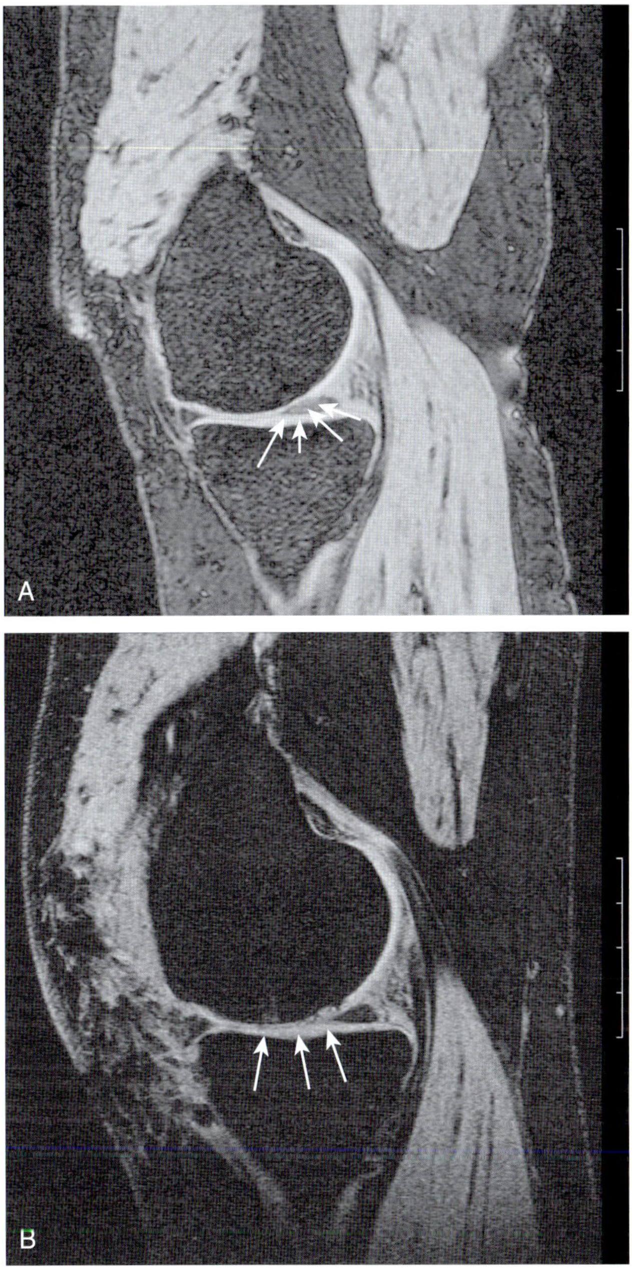

FIGURE 4-16. Autologous cell–seeded matrix chondrocyte implantation in a 39-year-old woman. Preoperative (**A**), 1 month postoperative (**B**), and 1 year postoperative (**C**) sagittal, fat-suppressed, T1-weighted gradient-echo (TR/TE/FA: 40 ms/10 ms/45°) images demonstrating the original full-thickness chondral lesion on the medial femoral condyle with progressive fill of repair tissue (*arrows*).

cases and is most commonly manifest within the first 6 months postoperatively.[112,119,126] Further complications of ACI graft delamination include the creation of unstable graft flap segments or graft tissue dislodgment and displacement into the joint space.

Varying degrees of subchondral edema-like signal changes at the site of an ACI repair is a normal finding in the early postoperative period.[26,27,32,116,119,123] Persistent subchondral marrow edema signal or subchondral cyst formation at the repair site beyond 1 year postoperatively has been suggested as a sign of failure of graft/bone incorporation and ultimately a poor prognostic indicator of graft outcome.[33,116,129] Additional complications that may be seen by MRI after ACI procedures include

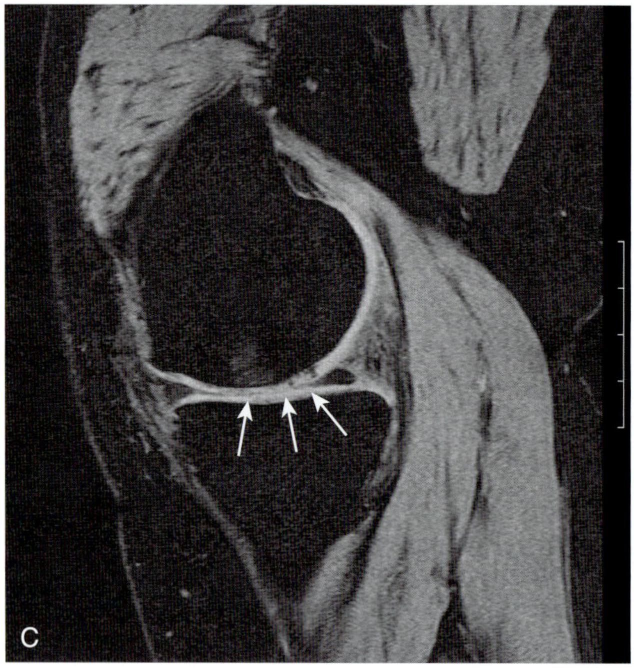

FIGURE 4-16, cont'd

synovitis, joint effusions, and joint adhesions, which occur in up to 10% of patients postoperatively.[26,33,112,130]

Surrogate MRI Measures of Cartilage Repair Tissue Composition

Conventional MRI techniques utilized in the routine clinical assessment of chondral lesions and cartilage repair allow for excellent depiction of preoperative and postoperative articular surface morphology as well as characterization of bulk temporal changes in signal characteristics of repair tissue, adjacent normal cartilage, and subjacent bone. Such imaging additionally allows for accurate assessment of other articular structures, the integrity of which may be critical in successful preoperative cartilage repair planning.

In addition to conventional imaging, a great deal of investigational interest has been focused on the evaluation and validation of adjuvant MRI strategies as potential surrogate markers of biomechanical and biochemical ultrastructural composition, both within normal healthy cartilage as well as within degenerative and traumatic cartilage disease. Among these MRI techniques are T2 mapping, delayed gadolinium-enhanced MRI of cartilage (dGEMRIC), diffusion imaging, T1 rho imaging, sodium imaging, and magnetization transfer imaging. Several of these investigational MRI strategies have been preliminarily evaluated in the setting of postoperative cartilage repair.

Quantitative T2 mapping and qualitative assessments of spatial variation of T2 within cartilage have been correlated to type II collagen matrix organization within normal hyaline articular cartilage. Investigators have utilized T2 mapping in the characterization of experimental and clinical models of cartilage repair.[22-25,131-134] Initial experimental studies have supported the potential of quantitative and qualitative analysis of T2 mapping of articular tissue to accurately differentiate histologically confirmed areas of postoperative fibrocartilage after microfracture from normal hyaline cartilage overlying plugs after AOT (Fig. 4-19).[49,135,136] T2 mapping has additionally been evaluated by other studies in the characterization of ACI grafts,

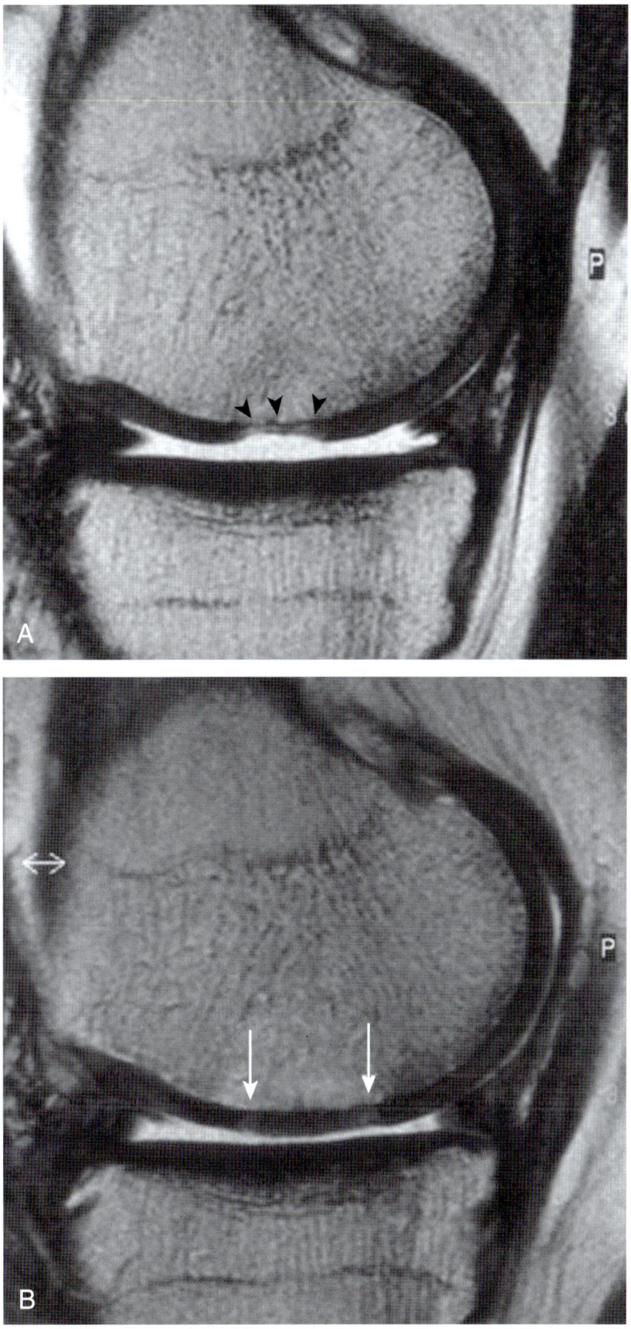

FIGURE 4-17. Matrix-induced autologous chondrocyte implantation (MACI). Preoperative (**A**) and 1 year postoperative (**B**), sagittal, intermediate-weighted (TR/TE: 4000/32 ms) fast spin-echo images. **A,** Preoperative imaging shows a near full-thickness articular cartilage defect along the weight-bearing aspect of the medial femoral condyle (*arrowheads*). **B,** Postoperative image demonstrates filling of the defect with repair tissue of slightly heterogeneous increased signal intensity relative to native articular cartilage. The repair site demonstrates a smooth congruent articular surface at 1 year postoperatively (*arrows*). (Courtesy of Siegfried Trattnig, MD.)

with temporal changes in T2 characteristics of cartilage repair tissue formed after classic ACI, as well as MACI procedures observed within the first 2 years postoperatively.[137,138]

Magnetization transfer imaging is an imaging technique that has been shown to be sensitive to macromolecular constituents, particularly the collagen network, within articular cartilage.[139,140] A preliminary investigation has studied the potential utility of magnetization transfer imaging in the analysis of cartilage repair tissue after microfracture and ACI surgery.[141] This preliminary study showed a trend toward

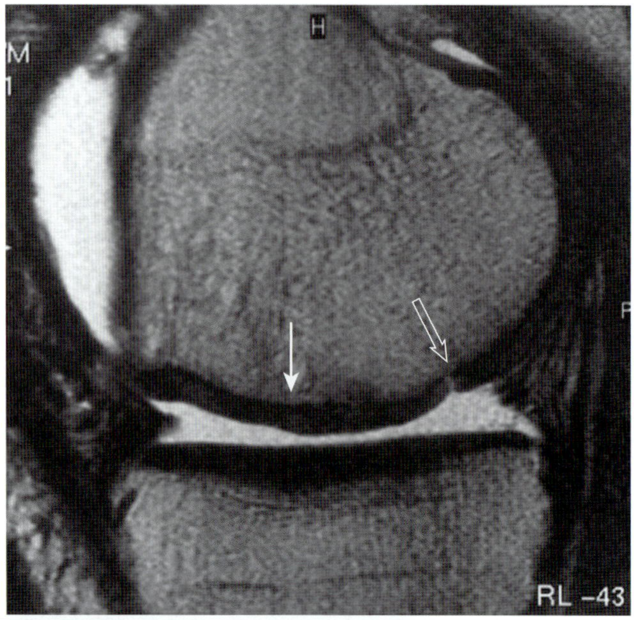

FIGURE 4-18. Matrix-induced autologous chondrocyte implantation (MACI). Sagittal, intermediate-weighted (TR/TE: 4000/32 ms), fast spin-echo image 1 year after MACI repair (*arrows*) of a prior full-thickness defect of articular cartilage. A fluid signal cleft is evident at the posterior margin of a MACI repair site (*open arrow*) indicative of poor integration of the repair tissue and adjacent native hyaline articular cartilage of the femoral condyle. (Courtesy of Siegfried Trattnig, MD.)

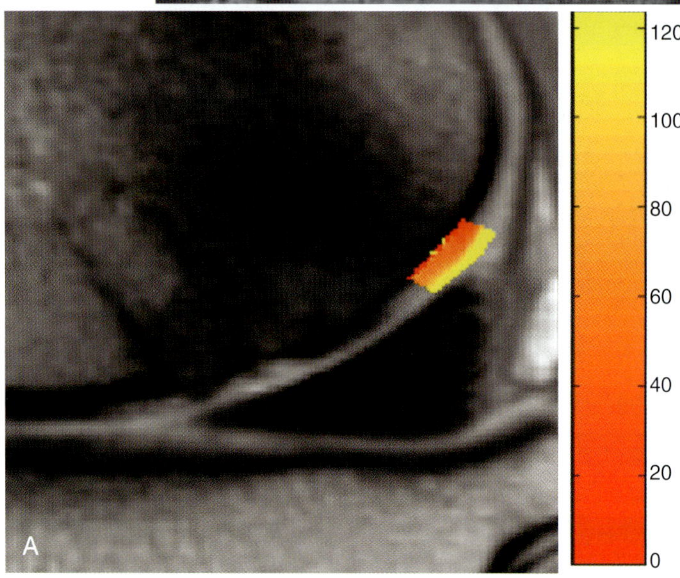

FIGURE 4-19. T2 mapping images of an equine knee articular surface at sites of normal articular cartilage, osteochondral autologous transplantation (OAT), osteochondral plug harvest, and microfracture repair. Sagittal intermediate-weighted (TR/TE: 2500/39.7 ms) MR images of the weight-bearing aspect of the medial femoral condyle with T2 maps of control normal articular cartilage (**A**) (1.5-cm posterior to a site of an osteochondral transplant graft [*arrow*]), articular cartilage overlying an OAT plug (**B**), articular tissue at an osteochondral graft harvest site (**C**), and articular cover at a site of microfracture (**D**) superimposed on the sagittal MR images. An organized cartilage T2 pattern is shown at the control site (**A**) and overlying an OAT plug (**B**), with a transition of low-to-high T2 values seen from deep to superficial aspects of the cartilage thickness corresponding to histologic findings of normal hyaline articular cartilage. In contrast, a disorganized T2 pattern of repair tissue is seen at the harvest site (**C**) and at the site of prior microfracture (**D**) with a lack of a normal transition of low-to-high T2 values from deep to superficial articular aspects of the region of interest corresponding to histologic findings of reparative fibrocartilage (**D**). (From White LM, Sussman MS, Hurtig M, et al. Cartilage T2 assessment: differentiation of normal hyaline cartilage and reparative tissue after arthroscopic cartilage repair in equine subjects. Radiology 2006; 241:407-414.)

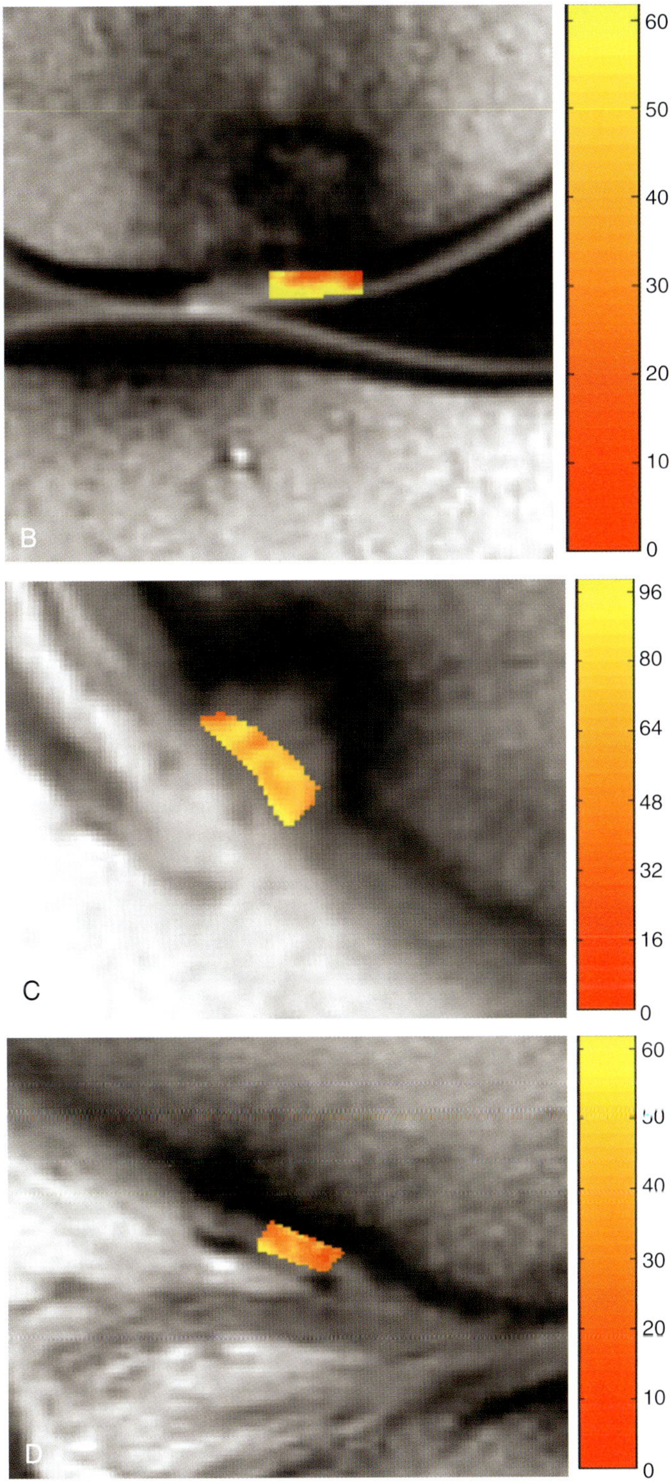

FIGURE 4-19, cont'd

normalization of magnetization transfer ratio values within cartilage repair tissue as compared with normal articular cartilage at 2 years postoperative follow-up. However, the overall magnitude of the magnetization transfer ratio differences observed in this study between histologically confirmed damaged hyaline articular cartilage and repair tissue was too small to enable confident evaluation of repair cartilage quality and collagen macromolecular content after repair of cartilage tissues.

Delayed gadolinium-enhanced MRI of cartilage (dGEMRIC) is an imaging technique in which the distribution of negatively charged gadolinium-based MR contrast material (gadopentetate dimeglumine) within cartilage has been validated as an accurate surrogate marker of cartilage tissue glycosaminoglycan (GAG) concentration.[142,143] dGEMRIC has been evaluated in the assessment of repair tissue after ACI and MACI procedures.[137,144,145] These studies have illustrated the clinical feasibility of dGEMRIC in the assessment of transplantation tissue after cartilage repair,[137,144-146] with some investigations showing a variable degree of apparent GAG replenishment within ACI transplant repair tissue over the course of the first year postoperatively,[137,144] correlating well to histologic analysis results of ACI repair tissue in the literature.[123]

References

1. Curl WW, Krome J, Gordon ES, et al. Cartilage injuries: a review of 31,516 knee arthroscopies. Arthroscopy 1997; 13:456-460.
2. Aroen A, Loken S, Hei S, et al. Articular cartilage lesions in 993 consecutive knee arthroscopies. Am J Sports Med 2004; 32:211-215.
3. Buckwalter JA. Articular cartilage injuries. Clin Orthop Relat Res 2002; (402):21-37.
4. Buckwalter JA, Hunziker EB, Rosenberg LC. Articular cartilage: composition and structure. In Woo SL, Buckwalter JA (eds). Injury and Repair of the Musculoskeletal Soft Tissues. Park Ridge, IL, American Academy of Orthopedic Surgeons, 1988, pp 405-425.
5. Buckwalter JA, Mankin HJ. Articular cartilage I: tissue design and chondrocyte-matrix interactions. J Bone Joint Surg Am 1997; 79:600-611.
6. Buckwalter JA, Mankin HJ. Articular cartilage II: degeneration and osteoarthrosis, repair, regeneration and transplantation. J Bone Joint Surg Am 1997; 79:612-632.
7. Buckwalter JA, Rosenberg LC, Coutts R. Articular cartilage: injury and repair. In Woo SL, Buckwalter JA (eds). Injury and Repair of the Musculoskeletal Soft Tissues. Park Ridge, IL, American Academy of Orthopedic Surgeons, 1988, pp 465-482.
8. Browne JE, Brance TP. Surgical alternatives for treatment of articular cartilage lesions. J Am Acad Orthop Surg 2000; 8:180-189.
9. Recht MP, Kramer J, Marcelis S, et al. Abnormalities of articular cartilage in the knee: analysis of available MR techniques. Radiology 1993; 187:473-478.
10. Disler DG, McCauley TR, Kelman CG, et al. Fat-suppressed three-dimensional spoiled gradient-echo MR imaging of hyaline cartilage defects in the knee: comparison with standard MR imaging and arthroscopy. AJR Am J Roentgenol 1996; 167:127-132.
11. Yao L, Gentili A, Thomas J. Incidental magnetization transfer contrast in fast spin-echo imaging of cartilage. J Magn Reson Imaging 1996; 1:180-184.
12. Potter HG, Linklater JM, Allen AA, et al. MR imaging of articular cartilage in the knee: a prospective evaluation utilizing fast spin-echo imaging. J Bone Joint Surg Am 1998; 80:1276-1284.
13. Sonin AH, Roychowdhury S, Fonner BT, Fitzgerald SW. Grading the articular cartilage of the patellofemoral joint with a double-echo spin-echo sequence pair [Abstract]. Presented before the 5th scientific meeting of the International Society of Magnetic Resonance Medicine, 1997, p 341.
14. Broderick LS, Turner DA, Renfrew DL, et al. Severity of articular cartilage abnormality in patients with osteoarthritis: evaluation with fast spin-echo MR vs. arthroscopy. AJR Am J Roentgenol 1994; 162:99-103.
15. Bredella MA, Tirman PFJ, Peterfy CG, et al. Accuracy of T2-weighted fast spin-echo MR imaging with fat saturation in detecting cartilage defects in the knee: comparison with arthroscopy in 130 patients. AJR Am J Roentgenol 1999; 172:1073-1080.
16. Recht MP, Piraino DW, Paletta GA, et al. Accuracy of fat-suppressed three-dimensional spoiled gradient-echo FLASH MR imaging in the detection of patellofemoral articular cartilage abnormalities. Radiology 1996; 198:209-212.
17. Disler DG, McCauley TR, Wirth CR, Fuchs MD. Detection of knee hyaline articular cartilage defects using fat suppressed three dimensional spoiled gradient-echo MR imaging: comparison with standard MR imaging and correlation with arthroscopy. AJR Am J Roentgenol 1995; 165:377-382.

18. Konig H, Sauter R, Deimling M, Vogt M. Cartilage disorders: comparison of spin-echo, CHESS, and FLASH sequence MR images. Radiology 1987; 164:753-758.
19. Chandnani VP, Ho C, Chu P, et al. Knee hyaline cartilage evaluated with MR imaging: a cadaveric study involving multiple imaging sequences and intraarticular injection of gadolinium and saline solution. Radiology 1991; 178:557-561.
20. Burstein D, Velyvis J, Scott KT, et al. Protocol issues for delayed Gd (DTPA)2– enhanced MR imaging (dGEMRIC) for clinical evaluation of cartilage. Magn Reson Med 2001; 45:36-41.
21. Bashir A, Gray M, Boutin RD, Burstein D. Glycosaminoglycan in articular cartilage: in vivo assessment with delayed Gd(DTPA)2– enhanced MR imaging. Radiology 1997; 205:551-558.
22. Rubenstein JD, Kim JK, Morava-Protzner I, et al. Effects of collagen orientation on MR imaging characteristics of bovine articular cartilage. Radiology 1993; 188:219-226.
23. Mosher TJ, Dardzinski BJ, Smith MB. Human articular cartilage: influence of aging and early symptomatic degeneration on the spatial variation of T2: preliminary findings at 3T. Radiology 2000; 214:259-266.
24. Nieminen MT, Rieppo J, Toyras J, et al. T2 relaxation reveals spatial collagen architecture in articular cartilage: a comparative quantitative MRI and polarized light microscopy study. Magn Reson Med 2001; 46:487-493.
25. Xia Y, Moody JB, Burton-Wurster N, Lust G. Quantitative in situ correlation between microscopic MRI and polarized light microscopy studies of articular cartilage. Osteoarthritis Cartilage 2001; 9:393-406.
26. Alparslan L, Winalski CS, Boutin RD, Minas T. Postoperative magnetic resonance imaging of articular cartilage. Semin Musculoskel Radiol 2001; 5:345-363.
27. Brown WE, Potter HG, Marx RG, et al. Magnetic resonance imaging appearance of cartilage repair in the knee. Clin Orthop Relat Res 2004; 422:214-223.
28. Link TM, Stahl R, Woertler K. Cartilage imaging: motivation, techniques, current and future significance. Eur Radiol 2007; 17:1135-1146.
29. Marlovits S, Striessnig G, Resinger CT, et al. Definition of pertinent parameters for the evaluation of articular cartilage repair tissue with high-resolution magnetic resonance imaging. Eur J Radiol 2004; 52:310-319.
30. Polster J, Recht M. Postoperative MR evaluation of chondral repair in the knee. Eur J Radiol 2005; 54:206-213.
31. Recht MP, White LM, Winalski CS, et al. MR imaging of cartilage repair procedures. Skeletal Radiol 2003; 32:185-200.
32. Recht MP, Goodwin DW, Winalski CS, White LM. MRI of articular cartilage: revisiting current status and future directions. AJR Am J Roentgenol 2005; 185:899-914.
33. Alparslan L, Minas T, Winalski CS. Magnetic resonance imaging of autologous chondrocyte implantation. Semin Ultrasound CT MR 2001; 22:341-351.
34. Woertler K, Strothmann M, Tombach B, Reimer P. Detection of articular cartilage lesions: experimental evaluation of low- and high-field-strength MR imaging at 0.18 and 1.0T. J Magn Reson Imaging 2000; 11:678-685.
35. Kladny B, Bluckert K, Swoboda B, et al. Comparison of low-field (0.2 Tesla) and high-field (1.5 Tesla) magnetic resonance imaging of the knee joint. Arch Orthop Trauma Surg 1995; 114:281-286.
36. Vahlensieck M, Schneiber O. (Performance of an open low-field MR unit in routine examination of knee lesions and comparison with high field systems). Orthopade 2003; 32:175-178.
37. Lewis PB, McCarty LP, Kang RW, Cole BJ. Basic science and treatment options for articular cartilage injuries. J Orthop Sports Phys Ther 2006; 36:717-727.
38. Simon TM, Jackson DW. Articular cartilage: injury pathways and treatment options. Sports Med Arthrosc Rev 2006; 14:146-154.
39. Gill TJ, Asnis PD, Berkson EM. The treatment of articular cartilage defects using the microfracture technique. J Orthop Sports Phy Ther 2006: 36:728-738.
40. Mithoefer BK, Williams RJ, Warren RF, et al. Chondral resurfacing of articular cartilage defects in the knee with the microfracture technique: surgical technique. J Bone Joint Surg Am 2006; 88:S294-304.
41. Steadman JR, Rodkey WG, Singleton SB, Briggs KK. Microfracture technique for full thickness chondral defects: technique and clinical results. Oper Tech Orthop 1997; 7:300-304.
42. Steadman JR, Rodkey WG, Rodrigo JJ. Microfracture: surgical technique and rehabilitation to treat chondral defects. Clin Orthop Relat Res 2001: (391 Suppl):362-369.
43. Mithoefer BK, Williams RJ, Warren RF, et al. The microfracture technique for the treatment of articular cartilage lesions in the knee: a prospective cohort study. J Bone Joint Surg Am 2005; 87:1911-1920.
44. Kreuz PC, Steinwachs MR, Erggelet C, et al. Results after microfracture of full-thickness chondral defects in different compartments in the knee. Osteoarthritis Cartilage 2006; 14:1119-1125.
45. Steadman JR, Briggs KK, Rodrigo JJ, et al. Outcomes of microfracture for traumatic chondral defects of the knee: average 11 year follow-up. Arthroscopy 2003; 19:477-484.
46. Nehrer S, Spector M, Minas T. Histologic analysis of tissue after failed cartilage repair procedures. Clin Orthop Relat Res 1999; 365:149-162.

47. Frisbie DD, Trotter GW, Powers BE, et al. Arthroscopic subchondral bone plate microfracture technique augments healing of large chondral defects in the radial carpal bone and medial femoral condyle of horses. Vet Surg 1999; 28:242-255.
48. Frisbie DD, Oxford JT, Southwood L, et al. Early events in cartilage repair after subchondral bone microfracture. Clin Orthop Relat Res 2003; 407:215-227.
49. White LM, Sussman MS, Hurtig M, et al. Cartilage T2 assessment: differentiation of normal hyaline cartilage and reparative tissue after arthroscopic cartilage repair in equine subjects. Radiology 2006; 241:407-414.
50. Gobbi A, Nunag P, Malinowski K. Treatment of full thickness chondral lesions of the knee with microfracture in a group of athletes. Knee Surg Sports Traumatol Arthrosc 2005; 13:213-221.
51. Knutsen G, Engebretsen L, Ludvigsen TC, et al. Autologous chondrocyte implantation compared with microfracture in the knee. J Bone Joint Surg Am 2004; 86:455-464.
52. Shapiro F, Koide S, Glimcher MJ. Cell origin and differentiation in the repair of full-thickness defects of articular cartilage. J Bone Joint Surg Am 1993; 75:532-553.
53. Neher S, Dorotka R, Bindreiter U, et al. Microfracture in the treatment of chondral defects in a sheep model [Abstract]. Presented before the 5th Symposium of the International Cartilage Repair Society, Ghent, Belgium, 2004, p 42.
54. Simon W. Scale effects in animal joints: articular cartilage thickness and compressive stress. Arthritis Rheum 1970; 13:244-256.
55. Schinagl RM, Gurskis D, Chen AC, Sah RL. Depth-dependent confined compression modulus of full thickness bovine articular cartilage. J Orthop Res 1997; 15:499-506.
56. Rasanen T, Messner K. Regional variations of indentation stiffness and thickness of normal rabbit knee articular cartilage. J Biomed Mater Res 1996; 31:519-524.
57. Hangody L, Kish G, Karpati Z, Eberhart R. Osteochondral plugs: autogenous osteochondral mosaicplasty for the treatment of focal chondral and osteochondral articular defects. Oper Tech Orthop 1997; 7:312-322.
58. Hangody L, Kish G, Karpati Z, et al. Mosaicplasty of the treatment of articular cartilage defects: application in clinical practice. Orthopedics 1998; 21:751-756.
59. Bartha L, Vajda A, Duska Z, et al. Autologous osteochondral mosaicplasty grafting. J Orthop Sports Phys Ther 2006; 36:739-750.
60. Barber FA, Chow JC. Arthroscopic chondral osseous autograft transplantation (COR procedure) for femoral defects. Arthroscopy 2006; 22:10-16.
61. Hangody L. The mosaicplasty technique for osteochondral lesions of the talus. Foot Ankle Clin 2003; 8:259-273.
62. Hangody L, Kish G, Modis L, et al. Mosaicplasty for the treatment of osteochondritis dissecans of the talus: two to seven year results in 36 patients. Foot Ankle Int 2001; 22:552-558.
63. Karataglis D, Green MA, Learmonth DJA. Autologous osteochondral transplantation for the treatment of chondral defects of the knee. Knee 2006; 13:32-35.
64. Duchow J, Hess T, Kohn D. Primary stability of press-fit-implanted osteochondral grafts: influence of graft size, repeated insertion, and harvesting technique. Am J Sports Med 2000; 28:24-27.
65. Nakagawa Y, Suzuki T, Kuroki H, et al. The effect of surface congruity of grafted plugs in osteochondral grafting: a report of five cases. Knee Surg Traumatol Arthrosc 2007; 15:591-596.
66. Barber FA, Chow JC. Arthroscopic osteochondral transplantation: histologic results. Arthroscopy 2001; 17:832-835.
67. Leo BM, Turner MA, Diduch DR. Split-line pattern and histologic analysis of a human osteochondral plug graft. Arthroscopy 2004; 20S:39-45.
68. Bobic V, Morgan CD, Carter T. Osteochondral autologous graft transfer. Op Tech Sports Med 2000; 8:168-178.
69. Hangody L, Kish G, Karpati Z, et al. Treatment of osteochondritis dissecans of the talus: use of the mosaicplasty technique—a preliminary report. Foot Ankle Int 1997; 18:628-634.
70. Jacob R, Franz T, Gautier E, Mainil-Varlet P. Autologous osteochondral grafting in the knee: indication, results and reflections. Clin Orthop 2002; 401:170-184.
71. Hangody L, Feczko P, Bartha L, et al. Mosaicplasty for the treatment of articular defects of the knee and ankle. Clin Orthop Relat Res 2001; (391 Suppl):328-336.
72. Hangody L, Fules P. Autologous osteochondral mosaicplasty for the treatment of full-thickness defects of weight-bearing joints: ten years of experimental and clinical experience. J Bone Joint Surg Am 2003; 85 SII: 25-32.
73. Hangody L, Kish G, Karpati Z, et al. Arthroscopic autogenous osteochondral mosaicplasty for the treatment of femoral condylar articular defects: a preliminary study. Knee Surg Sports Traumatol Arthrosc 1997; 5:262-267.
74. Hangody L, Rathonyi GK, Duska A, et al. Autologous osteochondral mosaicplasty: surgical technique. J Bone Joint Surg Am 2004; 86S:65-72.
75. Marcacci M, Kon E, Zaffagnini S, Visani A. Use of autologous grafts for reconstruction of osteochondral defects of the knee. Orthopedics 1999; 22:595-600.
76. Morelli M, Nagomori J, Miniaci A. Management of chondral injuries of the knee by osteochondral autogenous transfer (mosaicplasty). J Knee Surg 2002; 15:185-190.
77. Meneche DS, Vangsness CT Jr, Pitman M, et al. The treatment of isolated articular cartilage lesions in the young individual. Instr Course Lect 1998; 47:505-515.

78. Marcacci M, Kon E, Delcogliano M, et al. Arthroscopic autologous osteochondral grafting for cartilage defects of the knee: prospective study results at a minimum 7-year follow-up. Am J Sports Med 2007; 35:2014-2021.
79. Chow JC, Hantes ME, Houle JB, Zalavras CG. Arthroscopic autogenous osteochondral transplantation for treating knee cartilage defects: a 2- to 5-year follow-up study. Arthroscopy 2004; 20:681-690.
80. Ozturk A, Ozdemir MR, Ozkan Y. Osteochondral autografting (mosaicplasty) in grade IV cartilage defects in the knee joint: 2- to 7-year results. Int Orthop 2006; 30:200-204.
81. Agneskirchner JD, Brucker P, Burkart A, Imhoff AB. Large osteochondral defects of the femoral condyle (MEGA-OATS). Knee Surg Sports Traumatol Arthrosc 2002; 10:160-168.
82. Laprell H, Petersen W. Autologous osteochondral transplantation using diamond bone-cutting system (DBCS): 612 years follow-up of 35 patients with osteochondral defects at the knee joint. Arch Orthop Trauma Durg 2001; 121:248-253.
83. Gudas R, Kalesinskas RJ, Kimtys V, et al. A prospective randomized clinical study of mosaic osteochondral autologous transplantation versus microfracture for the treatment of osteochondral defects in the knee joint in young athletes. Arthroscopy 2005; 21:1066-1075.
84. Dozin B, Malpeli M, Cancedda R. Comparative evaluation of autologous chondrocyte implantation and mosaicplasty: a multicentered randomized clinical trial. Clin J Sport Med 2005; 15:220-226.
85. Horas U, Pelinkovic D, Herr G, et al. Autologous chondrocyte implantation and osteochondral cylinder transplantation in cartilage repair of the knee joint: a prospective, comparative trial. J Bone Joint Surg Am 2003; 85:185-192.
86. Pearce SG, Hurtig MB, Clarnette R, et al. An investigation of 2 techniques for optimizing joint surface congruency using multiple cylindrical osteochondral autografts. Arthroscopy 2001; 17:50-55.
87. Link TM, Mischung J, Wortler K, et al. Normal and pathological MR findings in osteochondral autografts with longitudinal follow-up. Eur Radiol 2006; 16:88-96.
88. Sanders TG, Mentzer KD, Miller M, et al. Autogenous osteochondral "plug" transfer for the treatment of focal chondral defects: postoperative MR appearance with clinical correlation. Skeletal Radiol 2001; 30:570-578.
89. Dew TI, Martin RA. Functional, radiographic, and histologic assessment of healing of autogenous osteochondral grafts and full thickness cartilage defects in the talus of dogs. Am J Vet Res 1992; 53:2141-2152.
90. Lane JM, Brighton CT, Ottens HR, Lipton M. Joint resurfacing in the rabbit using autologous osteochondral graft. J Bone Joint Surg Am 1977; 59:218-222.
91. Buck BE, Malinin TI, Brown MD. Bone transplantation and human immunodeficiency virus: an estimate of risk of acquired immunodeficiency syndrome (AIDS). Clin Orthop Relat Res 1989; 240:129-136.
92. Schreiber GB, Busch MP, Kleinman SH, Korelitz JJ. The risk of transfusion-transmitted viral infections: the retrovirus epidemiology donor study. N Engl J Med 1996; 334:1685-1690.
93. Ghazavi MT, Pritzker KP, Davis AM, Gross AE. Fresh osteochondral allografts for post-traumatic osteochondral defects of the knee. J Bone Joint Surg Br 1997; 79:1008-1013.
94. Chu CR, Convery FR, Akeson WH, et al. Articular cartilage transplantation: clinical results in the knee. Clin Orthop Relat Res 1999; 360:159-168.
95. Oakeshott RD, Farine I, Pritzker KP, et al. A clinical and histological analysis of failed fresh osteochondral allografts. Clin Orthop Relat Res 1988; (233):283-294.
96. Aubin PP, Cheah HK, Davis AM, Gross AE. Long-term follow up of fresh femoral osteochondral allografts for posttraumatic knee defects: long term follow up of femoral osteochondral allografts. Clin Orthop Relat Res 2001; (391 Suppl):318-327.
97. Czitrom AA, Keating S, Gross AE. The viability of articular cartilage in fresh osteochondral allografts after clinical transplantation. J Bone Joint Surg Am 1990; 72:574-581.
98. Convery FR, Akeson WH, Amiel D, et al. Long-term survival of chondrocytes in an osteochondral articular cartilage allograft. J Bone Joint Surg Am 1996; 78:1082-1088.
99. McGoveran BM, Pritzker KP, Shasha N, et al. Long-term chondrocyte viability in a fresh osteochondral allograft. J Knee Surg 2002; 15:97-100.
100. Gross AE. Cartilage resurfacing: filling defects. J Arthroplasty 2003; 18:14 17.
101. Hennig A, Abate J. Osteochondral allografts in the treatment of articular cartilage injuries in the knee. Sports Med Arthrosc Rev 2007; 15:126-132.
102. Pressman A, White LM, Gross AE. MR imaging evaluation of fresh osteochondral allografts: a pilot study. Presented before the International Cartilage Repair Society Symposium, June 2002.
103. Cain EL, Clancy WG. Osteochondral injuries of the knee: treatment algorithm for osteochondral injuries of the knee. Clin Sports Med 2001; 20:321-342.
104. Sirlin CB, Brossmann J, Boutin RD, et al. Shell osteochondral allografts of the knee: comparison of MR imaging findings and immunologic responses. Radiology 2001; 219:35-43.
105. Kusnick C, Hayward I, Sartoris DJ, et al. Radiographic evaluation of joints resurfaced with osteochondral shell allografts. AJR Am J Roentgenol 1987; 149:743-748.
106. Peterson L, Minas T, Brittberg M, Lindahl A. Treatment of osteochondritis dissecans of the knee with autologous chondrocyte transplantation: results in two to ten years. J Bone Joint Surg Am 2003; 85(Suppl 2):17-24.

107. Brittberg M, Lindahl A, Nilsson A, et al. Treatment of deep cartilage defects in the knee with autologous chondrocyte transplantation. N Engl J Med 1994; 331:889-895.
108. Marlovits S, Zeller P, Singer P, et al. Cartilage repair: generations of autologous chondrocyte transplantation. Eur J Radiol 2006; 57:24-31.
109. Bartlett W, Skinner JA, Gooding CR, et al. Autologous chondrocyte implantation for osteochondral defects of the knee: a prospective, randomized study. J Bone Joint Surg Br 2005; 87:640-645.
110. Gillogly SD. Treatment of large full thickness chondral defects of the knee with autologous chondrocyte implantation. Arthroscopy 2003; 19(Suppl):147-153.
111. Minas T, Chiu R. Autologous chondrocyte transplantation. Am J Knee Surg 2000; 13:41-50.
112. Peterson L, Minas T, Brittberg M, et al. Two to nine year outcomes after autologous chondrocyte transplantation of the knee. Clin Orthop Relat Res 2000; (374):212-234.
113. Bahuaud J, Maitrot RC, Bouvet R, et al. [Implantation of autologous chondrocytes for cartilaginous lesions in young patients: a study of 24 cases.] Chirurgie 1998; 123:568-571.
114. Richardson JB, Caterson B, Evans EH, et al. Repair of human articular cartilage after implantation of autologous chondrocytes. J Bone Joint Surg Br 1999; 81:1064-1068.
115. Bentley G, Biant LC, Carrington RW, et al. A prospective, randomized comparison of autologous chondrocyte implantation versus mosaicplasty for osteochondral defects of the knee. J Bone Joint Surg Br 2003; 85:223-230.
116. Henderson IJP, Tuy B, Connell D, et al. Prospective clinical study of autologous chondrocyte implantation and correlation with MRI at three and 12 months. J Bone Joint Surg Br 2003; 85:1060-1066.
117. Jakobsen RB, Engebretsen L, Slauterbeck JR. An analysis of the quality of cartilage repair studies. J Bone Joint Surg Am 2005; 87:2232-2239.
118. Roberts S, McCall IW, Darby AJ, et al. Autologous chondrocyte implantation for cartilage repair: monitoring its success by magnetic resonance imaging and histology. Arthritis Res Ther 2003; 5:60-73.
119. Ho YY, Stanley AJ, Hui JHP, Wang SC. Postoperative evaluation of the knee after autologous chondrocyte implantation: what radiologists need to know. RadioGraphics 2007; 27:207-222.
120. James SLJ, Connell DA, Saifuddin A, et al. MR imaging of autologous chondrocyte implantation of the knee. Eur Radiol 2006; 16:1022-1030.
121. Marlovits S, Singer P, Mandl I, et al. Magnetic resonance observation of cartilage repair tissue (MOCART) for the evaluation of autologous chondrocyte transplantation: determination of interobserver variability and correlation to clinical outcome after 2 years. Eur J Radiol 2006: 57:16-23.
122. Takahashi T, Tins B, McCall IW, et al. MR appearance of autologous chondrocyte implantation in the knee: correlation with the knee features and clinical outcome. Skeletal Radiol 2006; 35:16-26.
123. Tins BJ, McCall IW, Takahashi T, et al. Autologous chondrocyte implantation in knee joint: MR imaging and histologic features at 1-year follow-up. Radiology 2005: 234:501-508.
124. Trattnig S, Millington SA, Szomolanyi P, Marlovits S. MR imaging of osteochondral grafts and autologous chondrocyte implantation. Eur Radiol 2007; 17:103-118.
125. Trattnig S, Pinker K, Krestan C, et al. Matrix-based autologous chondrocyte implantation for cartilage repair with Hyalograft C: two-year follow-up by magnetic resonance imaging. Eur J Radiol 2006; 57:9-15.
126. Minas T, Peterson L. Advanced techniques in autologous chondrocyte transplantation. Clin Sports Med 1999; 18:13-44.
127. Azer NM, Winalski CS, Minas T. MR imaging for surgical planning and postoperative assessment in early osteoarthritis. Radiol Clin North Am 2004; 42:43-60.
128. Haddo O, Mahroof S, Higgs D, et al. The use of chondrogide membrane in autologous chondrocyte implantation. Knee 2004; 11:51-55.
129. Brittberg M, Winalski CS. Evaluation of cartilage injuries and repair. J Bone Joint Surg Am 2003; 85(Suppl 2):58-69.
130. Minas T, Peterson L. Autologous chondrocyte transplantation. Oper Techniques Sport Med 2000; 8:144-157.
131. Xia Y, Farquhar T, Burton-Wurster N, Lust G. Origin of cartilage laminae in MRI. J Magn Reson Imaging 1997; 7:887-894.
132. Dardzinski BJ, Mosher TJ, Li S, et al. Spatial variation of T2 in human articular cartilage. Radiology 1997; 205:546-550.
133. Smith HE, Mosher TJ, Dardzinski BJ, et al. Spatial variation in cartilage T2 of the knee. J Magn Reson Imaging 2001; 14:50-55.
134. Mosher TJ, Dardzinski BJ. Cartilage MRI T2 relaxation time mapping: overview and applications. Semin Musculoskelet Radiol 2004; 8:355-368.
135. Watrin-Pinzano A, Ruaud JP, Cheli Y, et al. Evaluation of cartilage repair tissue after biomaterial implantation in rat patella by using T2 mapping. MAGMA 2004; 17:219-228.
136. Watrin-Pinzano A, Ruaud JP, Cheli Y, et al. T2 mapping: an efficient MR quantitative technique to evaluate spontaneous cartilage repair in rat patella. Osteoarthritis Cartilage 2004; 12:191-200.
137. Kurkijarvi JE, Mattila L, Ojala RO, et al. Evaluation of cartilage repair in the distal femur after autologous chondrocyte transplantation using T2 relaxation time and dGEMRIC. Osteoarthritis Cartilage 2007; 15:372-378.

138. Trattnig S, Mamisch TC, Welsch GH, et al. Quantitative T2 mapping of matrix-associated autologous chondrocyte transplantation at 3 tesla. Invest Radiol 2007; 42:442-448.
139. Kim DK, Ceckler TL, Hascall VC, et al. Analysis of water-macromolecular proton magnetization transfer in articular cartilage. Magn Reson Med 1993; 29:211-215.
140. Gray ML, Burstein D, Lesperance LM, Gehrke L. Magnetization transfer in cartilage and its constituent macromolecules. Magn Reson Med 1995; 34:319-325.
141. Palmieri R, De Keyzer F, Maes F, Van Breuseghem I. Magnetization transfer analysis of cartilage repair tissue: a preliminary study. Skeletal Radiol 2006; 35:903-908.
142. Trattnig S, Mlynárik V, Breitenseher M, et al. MRI visualization of proteoglycan depletion in articular cartilage via intravenous administration of Gd-DTPA. Magn Reson Imaging 1999; 17:577-583.
143. Bashir A, Gray ML, Hartke J, Burstein D. Nondestructive imaging of human cartilage glycosaminoglycan concentration by MRI. Magn Reson Med 1999; 41:857-865.
144. Gillis A, Bashir A, McKeon B, et al. Magnetic resonance imaging of relative glycosaminoglycan distribution in patients with autologous chondrocyte transplants. Invest Radiol 2001; 36:743-748.
145. Watanabe A, Wada Y, Obata T, et al. Delayed gadolinium-enhanced MR to determine glycosaminoglycan concentration in reparative cartilage after autologous chondrocyte implantation: preliminary results. Radiology 2006; 239:201-208.
146. Trattnig S, Marlovits S, Gebetsroither S, et al. Three-dimensional delayed gadolinium-enhanced MRI of cartilage (dGEMRIC) for in vivo evaluation of reparative cartilage after matrix-associated autologous chondrocyte transplantation at 3.0T: preliminary results. J Magn Reson Imaging 2007; 26:974-982.

Chapter 5

Ultrasound Evaluation of Rheumatoid Arthritis

Michael A. Bruno and Richard J. Wakefield

In this chapter we focus on the application of ultrasound imaging for the assessment of rheumatoid arthritis (RA), both as a means of identifying structural joint changes (e.g., joint erosions, subluxations, loss of cartilage, osteophytes) and of evaluating the degree of inflammatory activity (e.g., synovial proliferation, joint fluid, and hyperemia) within a joint. In this way, ultrasonography can serve as both a structural and functional imaging tool. Ultrasound evaluation has a number of specific attributes that make it an especially desirable imaging tool for patients with RA. First, it is able to scan multiple joints in a relatively short period of time. This is of value because RA is a polyarticular disease. Second, it is relatively inexpensive and very widely available (as compared with MRI). Third, it is able to simultaneously image bone and soft tissue. Finally, ultrasound imaging uniquely allows dynamic, real-time examination.

The aims of this chapter are to (1) review key pathologic and clinical features of RA and especially those that lend themselves to imaging assessment and therapeutic intervention and (2) discuss the role of ultrasonography in relation to other imaging modalities in the management of RA.

RHEUMATOID ARTHRITIS

Rheumatoid arthritis is a severe, progressive, and debilitating multisystem autoimmune disease with an overall prevalence of approximately 1% worldwide. Thus, it affects tens of millions of people, with approximately a 3:1 female-to-male incidence ratio. Manifestations of the disease, which may begin at any age (peak 30-50 years), are highly variable between affected persons and tend to follow a relapsing and remitting course; if untreated, the disease will progress to irreversible joint damage and, potentially, premature death. The primary site of pathology in RA is the synovium. In normal joints, the synovium is a thin membrane that lines the joint capsule and does not encroach on the articular cartilage. At arthroscopy it appears almost translucent with a few blood vessels barely visible. In RA, however, there is expansion of the synovial tissue as the superficial layers become hyperplastic, while the deeper layers are infiltrated by abundant inflammatory cells and new blood vessels. This thickened synovium, known as *pannus* (L., "cloth" or "covering"), begins to migrate in a tumor-like fashion toward the center of the joint, resulting in initial cartilage loss and then subsequent bone loss (erosions). The first bony erosions occur in the periarticular region of a joint where the cartilage is at its thinnest—the so-called bare area. Subsequent invasion by the pannus leads to central erosions and, ultimately, to joint failure. Persistent inflammation within the joint also results in permanent capsule and collateral ligament damage that contributes to the many deformities seen in RA.

Clinical Presentation and Diagnosis

RA usually manifests as a polyarthritis (of six or more involved joints) with pain, stiffness, and swelling in the wrists and small joints of the hands (the metacarpophalangeal [MCP] and proximal interphalangeal [PIP] joints) and the feet (metatarsophalangeal [MTP] joints) in over 90% of patients. It subsequently progresses to involve most of the other synovial joints, including the knees, shoulders, hindfeet, and neck. It is relatively rare for RA to manifest as a monoarthritis (single joint) or oligoarthritis (five or fewer joints). Systemic symptoms such as fatigue, night sweats, and/or weight loss are common at disease presentation or during a flare. The clinical diagnosis of RA is based on criteria devised by the American College of Rheumatology.[1] These criteria, which were most recently revised in 1987, require a minimum of four specific indices to be fulfilled out of a possible seven to permit the diagnosis of RA. These include early morning stiffness lasting more than an hour, hand involvement, swelling of more than three joints, joint symmetry of three or more joint groups, presence of rheumatoid nodules, positive rheumatoid factor, and presence of radiographic bone erosions on radiographs of the hands and feet. The symptoms and signs need to be present for at least 6 weeks to exclude self-limited diseases, such as postinfectious arthritis (viral or streptococcal), which generally resolve within this period. The early physical signs of RA may be difficult to identify because the joints may only appear puffy; however, if left untreated or if inadequately treated, irreversible deformities may occur (Fig. 5-1). This progression may take only 2 to 5 years.

Although RA is a multisystem disease and potentially affects many organs, these manifestations are now fortunately rare, because in current practice patients are much more aggressively treated with immunosuppressive agents. However, situations do arise when a knowledge of these extra-articular manifestations is important, especially in the minority of patients who appear resistant to drug treatments. The most frequent extra-articular manifestation is that of soft tissue nodules, which classically occur at the elbows but also are evident on the hands; occasionally, they involve the sclera and lungs, where they may cavitate, resembling lung cancer. The kidneys are relatively spared in RA, although renal impairment may result from the use of drugs such as nonsteroidal anti-inflammatory agents. Renal amyloidosis is now fortunately very rare owing to earlier and more effective medical control of inflammation. In children, an RA pattern of disease may be seen with juvenile inflammatory arthritis that appears to have a different cluster of systemic and characteristic joint manifestations from that of adults and may be treated less aggressively.

Erythrocyte sedimentation rate (ESR) and C-reactive protein (CRP) are useful markers of inflammation. They increase, however, in the presence of any inflammation in the body and are therefore nonspecific. Rheumatoid factor (RF) is an antibody found in the blood of approximately 75% of patients with RA. Not all people with the condition, therefore, will have the antibody in their serum. Approximately 1 in 20 normal volunteers (5%) will have RF in their serum, and other inflammatory conditions may also cause a positive result. For this reason, results of the blood test must be interpreted with the clinical findings. Anti–cyclic citrullinated peptide antibody (anti-CCP Ab) is a newer laboratory test for RA. It is as sensitive as RF but much more specific and therefore can distinguish RA from other conditions. Furthermore, the anti-CCP antibody may predict who will develop the condition and identify who will be affected more severely.

Pathogenesis

RA appears to be a uniquely human disease, although limited animal models exist and have been used in research. RA synovitis has characteristic patterns of joint involvement but can potentially affect all of the synovial joints. It is triggered by unknown factors in an individual who is probably genetically susceptible and results

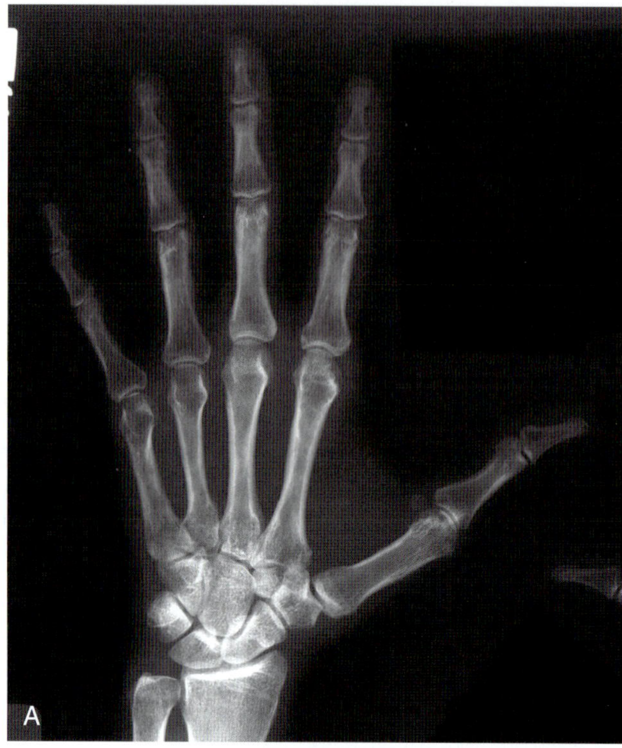

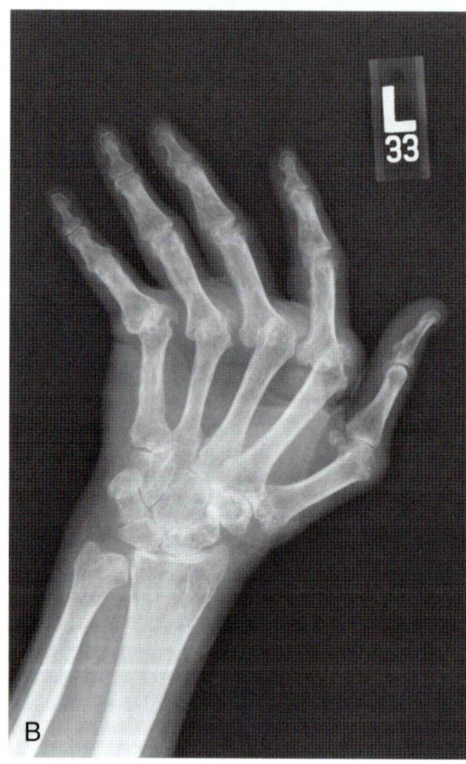

FIGURE 5-1. **A** and **B,** Radiographs of an untreated patient with RA, separated by a period of 8 years. The progression of radiographic findings illustrated would be reflected in a rising Sharp or Larsen score (see text).

in a complex interplay of inflammatory cells and chemical mediators. A significant body of research has demonstrated key roles for both cellular and humoral factors, most notably macrophages, fibroblasts, lymphocytes, tumor necrosis factor-alpha (TNF-α), interleukins 1 and 2 (IL-1 and IL-2), prostaglandins (PG), amines, vascular endothelial growth factor (VEGF), neuropeptides, various chemoattractant molecules, and nitric oxide, although other inflammatory cell lines and cytokines are also known to play perhaps significant roles in the pathophysiologic process. Many of these cellular and humoral disease mediators provide avenues both for imaging and laboratory evaluation of patients with RA, as well as for the pharmacologic intervention. The role of autoantibodies such as RF and anti-CCP Ab is still unknown; they may have a pathogenic role or merely represent an epiphenomenon due to the prolonged inflammation in RA.

Angioneogenesis, a feature more commonly associated with the growth and proliferation of malignancy, is seen within affected joints at the earliest stages of the disease. This includes pathologic small vessel proliferation within the synovium, a process that significantly increases overall blood flow in proportion to the severity and "activity" of the disease process. Small vessel permeability is also increased. There is, in fact, a close coupling between the disease state or "clinical disease activity" and the degree of abnormally increased synovial vascularity, with more severe symptoms and joint damage associated with higher degrees of abnormally increased vascularization, essentially one occurring in proportion to the other.[2] Furthermore, it has been demonstrated that, with effective treatment, the angioneogenesis ceases and resultant synovial vascularization rapidly diminishes. For example, treatment with corticosteroids and anti–TNF-α agents (e.g., etanercept [Enbrel]) are known to antagonize factors that promote angioneogenesis, and thus the benefit of steroids and biologic response modifying agents may be largely due to inhibition of the neovascularization.[3]

Therapeutic Options

Over the past decade it has been unequivocally proven that if inflammation in RA is identified and suppressed as soon as possible,[4,5] then joint damage can be minimized and function maintained. The place of modern imaging, therefore, has been to optimize inflammation assessment over what is already currently available (e.g., clinical examination, blood tests, and radiography). The general aim of RA management is to treat patients with immunosuppressive agents from the outset. Conventionally, this will include treatments such as corticosteroids, methotrexate, or sulfasalazine. Recently, as noted earlier, more targeted antibody therapies (the so-called biologics, or biologic response modifiers) that inhibit different parts of the inflammatory pathway have been developed as a direct result of our improved basic understanding of the pathophysiology of the disease. The most noticeable success has been with the anti–TNF-α agents, such as etanercept, but more recently agents that inhibit the B-cell production of autoantibodies, such as rituximab,[6] or the co-stimulation of B and T cells (anti-CLTA4Ig)[7] have been used successfully. The timing of initiation of biologic response modifiers is controversial because they are very expensive and pose other risks to patients, such as a heightened risk of infection. However, there is a compelling and growing body of evidence that in early disease their effect may be sustained after withdrawal after only 1 year of treatment. This raises the possibility that the drugs may not be required over the long term for all patients.[8]

ULTRASOUND IMAGING FOR RHEUMATOID ARTHRITIS

Ultrasonography is an imaging technique that evolved from World War II submarine SONAR technology and was first introduced to the radiologic community for the purpose of medical diagnostic imaging in the 1960s. Images are generated by analyzing the echo reflections of high-frequency sound waves that are both generated and received by an electronic probe, or transducer, that is applied directly to the skin, usually along with a small amount of acoustic coupling gel. Since its introduction, ultrasonography has benefited from continuous technological improvements occurring over the past decade, most especially improvements in transducer (probe) design and computerized image processing. Currently, ultrasonography is the second most commonly utilized imaging method overall, after plain film radiography, and has also become the predominant imaging modality in obstetrics. As a direct result of these relatively recent technological advances, musculoskeletal ultrasonography in general and the sonographic imaging of small joints in particular have become viable clinical tools. Evaluation with ultrasound was perhaps first applied to patients with RA in 1988,[9] and now a significant body of literature supports the use of ultrasound for a variety of musculoskeletal applications, including evaluating injuries and internal derangements of joints, guiding interventional procedures, and so on. These topics are the subjects of their own comprehensive textbooks.[10-13] As regards the care of patients with RA, ultrasound imaging technology is also a powerful and versatile asset for rheumatologists and radiologists; it is valuable indeed for the evaluation of all types of inflammatory arthritis but relatively few clinicians currently avail themselves of its benefits in clinical practice.

Since the first report by De Flaviis and associates,[9] ultrasound imaging has been evaluated as applied to all human arthritides and enthesopathies, including both degenerative and erosive joint diseases; however, its use has been best studied in RA. Like MRI, ultrasonography is a cross-sectional imaging modality and one that utilizes no ionizing radiation. It has shown greater utility in the detection of erosions than plain radiography, but it is less sensitive in this regard than MRI.[14] Because ultrasound imaging requires physical placement and manipulation of a transducer, or probe, that is placed directly onto or close to the region of anatomic interest, stearic hindrance can interfere. As such, several authors have noted the presence of relative "blind spots" for the sonographic detection of joint erosions in RA, most notably including significant portions of the third and fourth MCP joints of the hand, which are situated such that the probe cannot be placed in close enough proximity. MRI, which is a tomographic tool, does not have this disadvantage.

Ultrasound Technique

There is incomplete consensus regarding standard examination techniques or technical parameters, but guidelines for ultrasound techniques for the evaluation of RA have been offered.[14,15] Patients are scanned by direct application of a transducer optimized for musculoskeletal imaging, typically a high-frequency broadband (usually ranging from 18-5 MHz) electronically steered, linear small-footprint transducer with good near-field focus, such as the "hockey stick" or Entos probe transducer type illustrated in Figure 5-2. A standoff pad is thus obviated, but a small amount of acoustic coupling gel is used. It is important, particularly when using Doppler imaging, to examine joints in a relaxed position without too much joint flexion or overlying transducer pressure, because the findings of abnormally increased blood flow to the joint may be obliterated.

Ultrasonography vs. Radiography in Rheumatoid Arthritis: Diagnosis vs. Evaluation

The plain radiograph in RA remains the primary radiologic means for the establishment of the initial diagnosis of RA. It is the cornerstone of the diagnostic classification of all of the arthritides and is still a superb tool for the detection and characterization of erosive disease. Although ultrasonography is a more sensitive

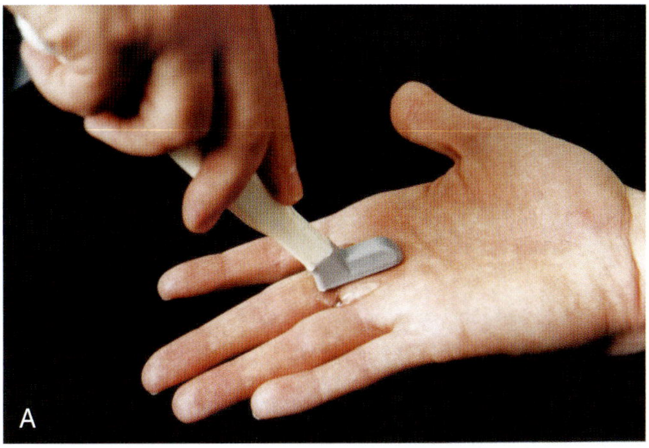

A

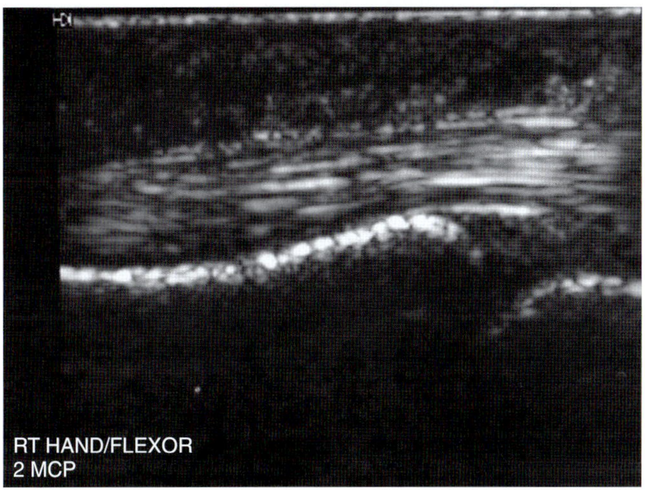

B

FIGURE 5-2. **A,** Generally, direct application of a dedicated high-frequency, small-footprint linear musculoskeletal probe to the affected joint is easily tolerated by patients and nearly every joint can be rapidly and comfortably imaged. Evaluation of the entire hand and wrist can usually be completed in less than 10 minutes. **B,** Normal ultrasonographic appearance of a finger tendon, as scanned in **A**. (**A** from Tsou I, Peh W, Bruno MA: Rheumatoid arthritis: Hand. In: eMedicine Radiology Online Peer-Reviewed Radiology Journal, April 6, 2004; updated December 15, 2006. Available at http://www.emedicine.com/radio/topic877.htm. Reprinted with permission from eMedicine.com.)

diagnostic tool, it lacks the specificity of plain radiographs for recognition of the specific manifestations and disease patterns that allow the radiologist and rheumatologist to readily discriminate RA from other prevalent inflammatory arthropathies. Many studies, however, have demonstrated that plain films are relatively insensitive in the earliest stages of the disease and have only very limited utility in evaluating response to treatment. For example, Backhaus and associates[14] showed that both MRI and ultrasonography can detect evidence of RA in patients with completely normal radiographs.

Dr. Robert Lopez-Ben and colleagues at the University of Alabama at Birmingham[16] studied 168 joints in 21 patients with RA and found that ultrasonography detected 15-fold more erosions than plain films at baseline and more than 6-fold more erosions on follow-up than did radiography. In their series, the use of power Doppler imaging also allowed the detection of synovitis in 100% of affected patients at baseline and in most patients on follow-up. Interobserver reliability for erosions was excellent, with Cohen's κ value for inter-reader agreement equal to 0.98 and that for the severity of synovitis on power Doppler imaging of 0.96. Surprisingly, in their series, the interobserver agreement for the detection of erosions on radiographs, which is something the readers had much more experience doing, was not as good ($\kappa = 0.86$)! Wakefield and associates[17] compared radiography and ultrasonography for the detection of erosions in the MCP joints of 100 patients with RA (Figs. 5-3, 5-4, and 5-5). They found that ultrasonography was able to detect smaller erosions

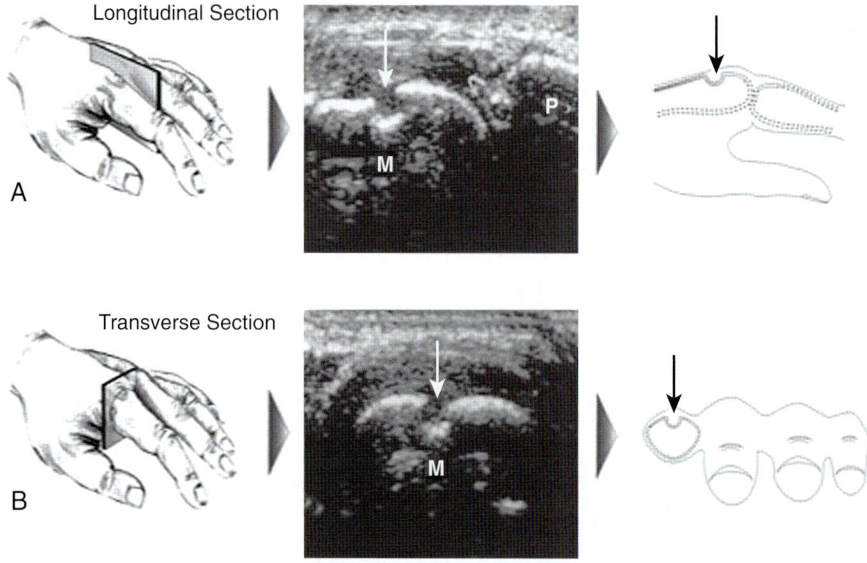

FIGURE 5-3. Illustration of the appearance of the joint erosions of rheumatoid arthritis, as seen on ultrasonography. **A,** Longitudinal section through the second MCP joint; note cortical defect (*straight arrow*) in metacarpal head (M). *Curved arrow* indicates joint space. P, proximal phalanx of the second digit. **B,** Transverse image confirming the defect as a definite erosion. (From Wakefield FJ, Givvon WW, Conaghan PG, et al. The value of sonography in the detection of bone erosions in patients with rheumatoid arthritis. Arthritis Rheum 2000; 43:2762-2770. Used with permission from John Wiley & Sons.)

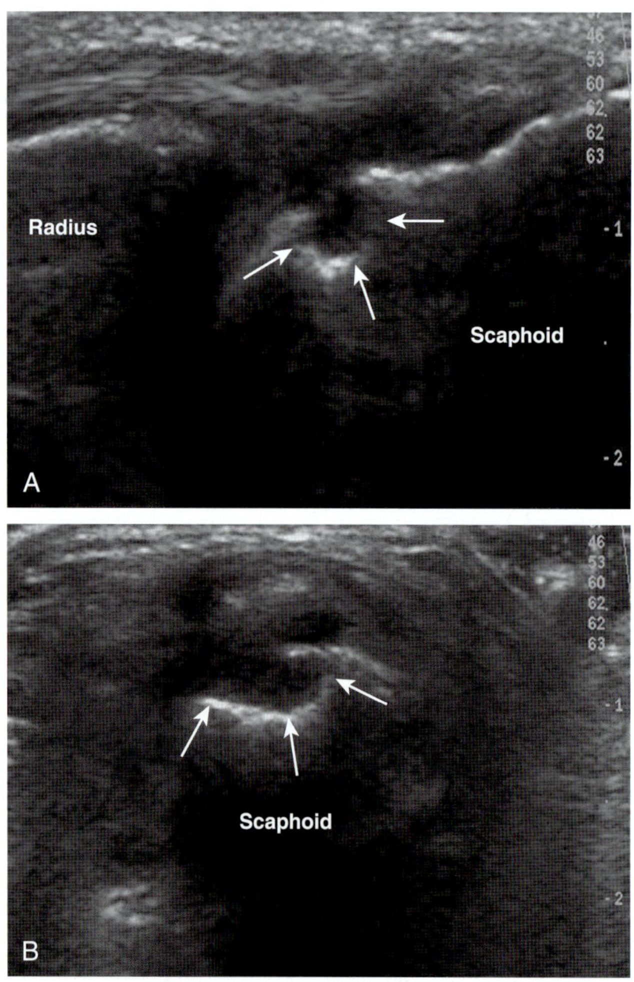

FIGURE 5-4. **A,** Longitudinal section through the radiocarpal joint showing an erosion in the scaphoid (*arrows*). **B,** The same erosion was confirmed in transverse section (*arrows*). Note the "undercutting" profile of the erosion in this case.

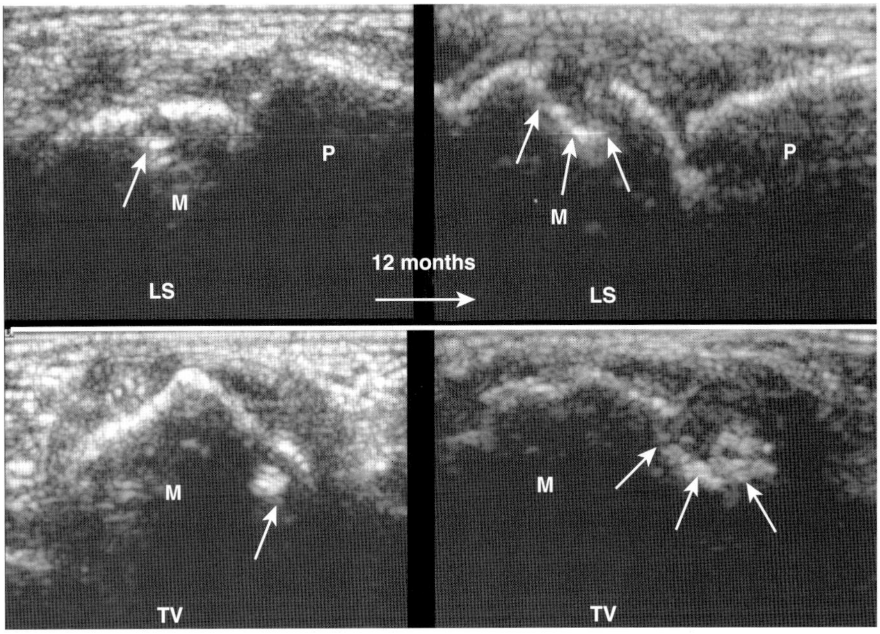

FIGURE 5-5. Progression of bone erosion over a 12-month period in a patient with RA. A small cortical break or erosion (*arrows*) is seen in longitudinal and transverse views on the left; this erosion enlarges in the 12-month interval, a relatively short period of time. M, metacarpal; P, phalanx; LS, longitudinal section; TV, transverse section.

than radiography, particularly if the erosions were en face, that is, lost in a 2D radiographic image. It was also noted that "blind spots" existed where the probe did not have acoustic access, which meant the ultrasonography failed to detect some abnormalities, most notably between the third and fourth MCP joints. In clinical practice, serial radiographs are used somewhat sparingly in the long-term management of RA patients. In the short term, radiographic changes can be quite subtle, although over longer time periods very significant differences are readily apparent on radiographs.

For the radiologist, characteristic bone erosions on the plain films of the hands and feet have been the sine qua non of diagnosis in RA, and for many research studies the identification of characteristic erosions is essential to allow the classification of a joint process in a particular patient as being erosive. Indeed, studies examining RA by MRI and ultrasound have often used the radiographic erosion as their gold standard.

For research purposes, plain film–based rating scales of varying degrees of complexity have been developed to assess the progression of RA findings and to infer the response to treatment. In recent years, simplified or modified versions of the Sharp and/or Larsen scoring systems have been most commonly used,[18-23] although their true predictive value has been questioned.[24] Each of the several published methods relies on the recognition and scoring of a large number of the radiographic manifestations of RA, including counting the erosions in target joints. A relatively large number of discrete radiographic observations contribute to the final score, which provides an index for comparison and grading the progress of the disease over time. The natural history of RA is for the manifestations to worsen, and thus for the score to inexorably rise. A favorable response to treatment is inferred when the scores stabilize over time or if the scores progress more slowly than expected. The problem with radiography is simply as it relates to the assessment of the effects of ongoing therapy, in that the plain film response is significantly delayed and is relatively sluggish as an indicator of treatment response. Indeed, the radiograph itself can be thought of as a relatively static record of the cumulative effects of joint damage; there is only limited depiction of the salutary effects of treatment, or lack thereof. In essence, changes that are visible on plain radiographs evolve too slowly to be of good clinical use in the management of RA patients.

There are indeed reliable radiographic manifestations of treatment success, such as partial healing of RA erosions, as shown in Figure 5-6. The regrowth of cortical bone margins within erosions, and increased mineralization of the periarticular bone, however, are examples of changes seen only late in the treatment process; and at least initially their absence does not indicate treatment failure. In the early stages of treatment these findings will not yet be present to reassure the clinician and patient that the current treatment plan is an adequate one. Often these radiographic changes are both very subtle and significantly delayed with respect to the onset of effective therapies.

Tenosynovitis in Rheumatoid Arthritis

Tenosynovitis in RA is a complex pathophysiologic processes involving various cytokines (IL-1, TNF-α, VEGF, and other chemical and cellular mediators, with a significant role played by macrophages. Ultrasound and MRI studies have both independently confirmed that tenosynovitis has an extremely high prevalence in RA but relatively little data exist in early disease.[25] Tendon pathology is readily demonstrated by ultrasound, and its contribution to the morbidity of RA has previously been underestimated. Fuchs and Pincus and their colleagues at the Vanderbilt University Medical Center[26] have shown that joint destruction in RA follows a first-order kinetics model, and several studies[2,27] have shown that, in early RA, synovitis is the primary abnormality and bone damage is subsequent and occurs in proportion to the level of synovitis and never in its absence.

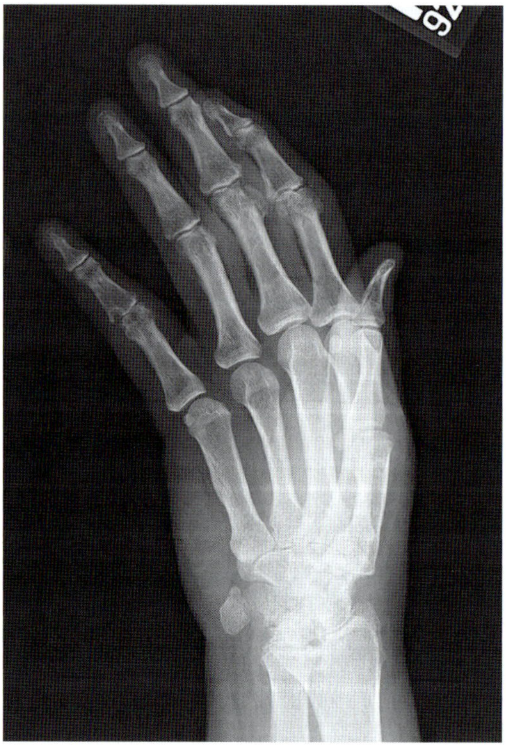

FIGURE 5-6. Healing erosion in RA. Note the sclerotic margin surrounding the erosion at the PIP joint of the small finger in this patient with RA.

Normal tendons have a characteristic "fibrillary" appearance on ultrasound evaluation, as shown in Figures 5-2 and 5-7, owing to their composition of highly organized linear collagen bundles; as a result of this high level of linear orientation, tendons demonstrate isotropic echogenicity with respect to the angle of insonation by the ultrasound beam.

In early inflammatory change, one of the first manifestations is edema within the tendon, which alters the echogenicity (usually reducing it). This is because interstitial fluid intercalates between the collagen bundles, effectively reducing the density of their sonographic interfaces, and their degree of regularity, dampening their overall echogenicity and the isotropic effect. Widening or thickening of the tendon is also a frequent early finding, and fluid or debris in the tendon sheath is commonly seen (Fig. 5-8). In early ultrasound publications describing the ultrasound characteristics of RA, this fluid layer was erroneously offered as a pathognomonic finding in RA. It is not, however, the frequency of its observation in patients with RA that underscores the extremely high prevalence of tenosynovitis as a manifestation of the disease in its early phases.[25]

Either MRI, as is illustrated in Chapter 6, or ultrasonography can be used to measure imaging findings of tenosynovitis in RA. As with joint pannus, both synovial volume and vascularity can be assessed. Wakefield and colleagues[25] compared gray-scale ultrasonography with gadolinium-enhanced MRI for the detection of finger

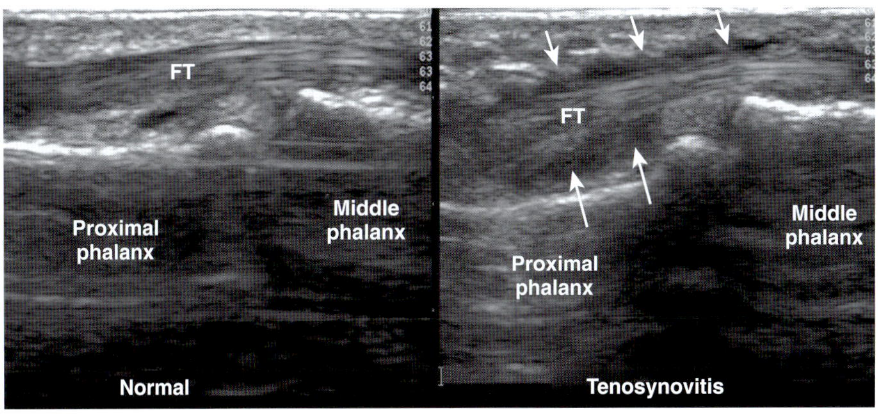

FIGURE 5-7. Longitudinal ultrasound images demonstrating a normal tendon (left) and a case of tenosynovitis (right). Synovial fluid accumulation within the tendon sheath is illustrated in the image on the right. The small fluid gap fills the potential space between the flexor tendon (FT) and its sheath (*arrows*). This is not a pathognomonic feature of RA, as was suggested in some early articles, but rather is a finding commonly associated with all causes of tenosynovitis.

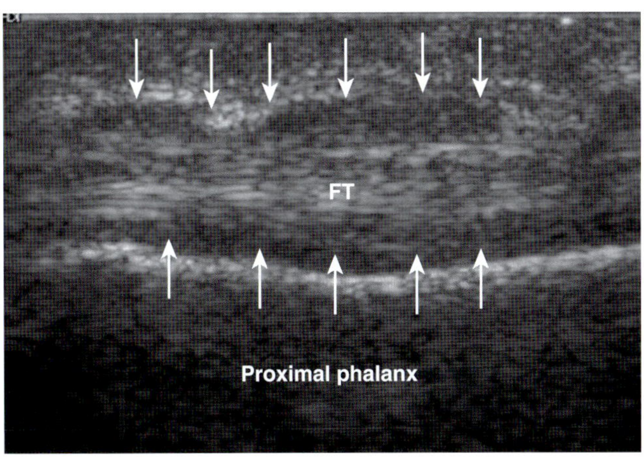

FIGURE 5-8. Boggy, echogenic synovial debris surrounds the flexor tendon (FT) of the fourth digit, within the tendon sheath (*arrows*). There is significant expansion of the potential space.

tenosynovitis in 50 patients with early RA and 20 normal controls. Flexor tenosynovitis was found in 57 (28.5%) of 200 joints in 24 (48%) of 50 patients on ultrasonography compared with 128 (64%) of 200 joints in 41 (82%) of 50 patients on MRI. Peri-extensor tenosynovitis was found in 14 (7%) joints in 9 (18%) patients on ultrasonography compared with 80 (40%) joints in 36 (72%) patients on MRI. No controls had imaging tenosynovitis. By using MRI as the gold standard, the sensitivity, specificity, and negative and positive predictive values for ultrasonography were 0.44, 0.99, 0.49, and 0.98, respectively, for flexor tenosynovitis and 0.15, 0.98, 0.63, and 0.86 for extensor tenosynovitis, respectively. The inter-reader reliability κ values were good: 0.85 and 0.8 for ultrasonography and MRI, respectively. The most frequently involved joints on ultrasonography and MRI were the second and third MCP joints. The authors concluded that a negative gray-scale ultrasound scan does not exclude inflammation and that, if clinically suspected, an MRI study should be considered. Further work is recommended to standardize definitions and image acquisition for both ultrasound and MR images. It was considered that Doppler imaging would have increased the specificity of the sonographic findings but decreased the sensitivity further, because abnormal Doppler signal rarely occurred in joint areas with gray-scale abnormalities.

Ultrasonography vs. MRI in Rheumatoid Arthritis: Structure vs. Function

In comparison of the modalities of ultrasonography and MRI, it has become clear that MRI allows earlier detection of joint erosions than is possible by either ultrasonography or plain radiographs. Ultrasonography does detect *most* joint erosions in RA, although not as many as can be visualized by MRI on a site-by-site basis. As noted earlier, in the hands of patients with RA, erosions are well visualized sonographically in some locations but not as well in others owing to limitations in probe positioning and placement, whereas all joint erosions are equally well depicted by MRI. Conversely, where ultrasonography has good visualization, it corresponds very accurately with MRI.[17] For this reason, ultrasonography performs less well for detecting erosions in deeper joints (e.g., the hip, where only the anterior part can be seen) and complex joints (e.g., the intercarpal region of the wrist). In addition, in some joints where there many be concomitant degenerative changes, distinguishing an erosion from a depression between two adjacent osteophytes may be difficult. This problem is commonly encountered in the wrist, proximal interphalangeal joints, and mid foot.

As functional imaging methods, both ultrasonography and MRI have the ability to depict active synovitis; however, with MRI, detection of synovitis is accomplished indirectly, by injecting an intravenous contrast agent and inferring the degree of inflammatory activity on the basis of T1 contrast enhancement of the joint tissues on fat-saturation images (see Chapter 6). In the case of Doppler ultrasonography, the relationship between measurable abnormal blood flow and synovitis is more direct and the effect is quite robust (Figs. 5-9 and 5-10). In our own work, we have observed as much as a 10-fold difference between a normal degree of synovial blood

---

FIGURE 5-9. **A,** Comparison of radiography (CR), scintigraphy, ultrasonography, MRI, and clinical examination for detection of erosions. Note that MRI is superior for detection of erosions but ultrasonography outperforms MRI, conventional radiography, and clinical examination for detection of synovitis. **B,** Patients were divided into two groups: group 1 (n = 32) included those without any radiographic evidence of arthritis, and group 2 included patients with radiographically apparent erosions (n = 28). For each imaging modality, the *bar* indicates the percentage of visualized joints where evidence of pathology was detected between each group and method. TS, tenosynovitis. (From Backhaus T, Kamradt D, Sandrock D, et al. Arthritis of the finger joints. Arthritis Rheum 1999; 42:1232-1245. Used with permission from John Wiley & Sons.)

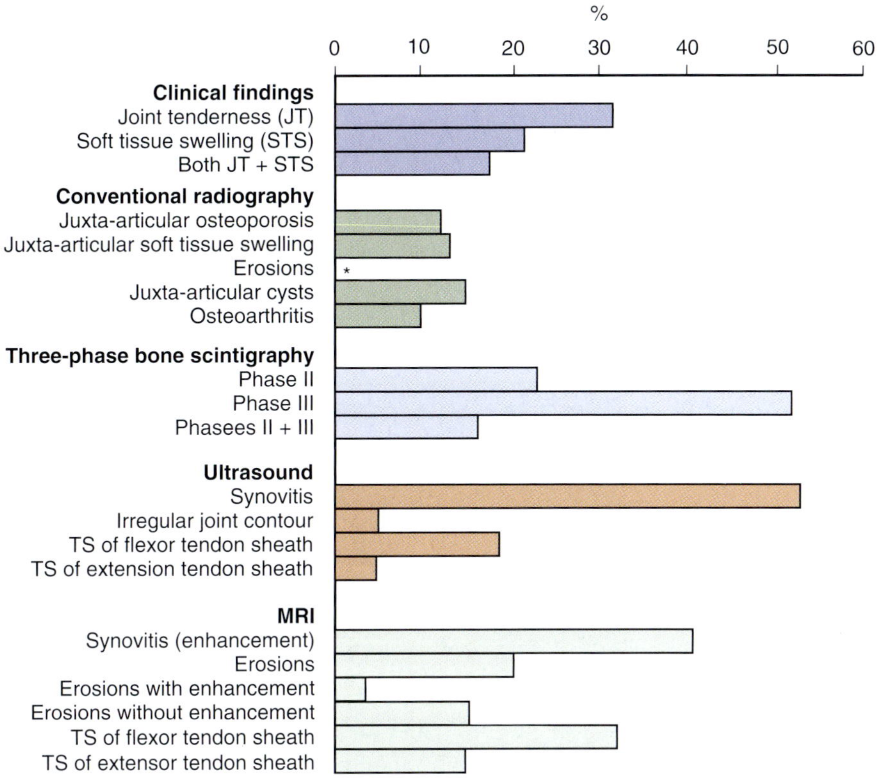

*Larsen grade I, no erosions

A

Finger joints (n = 448)

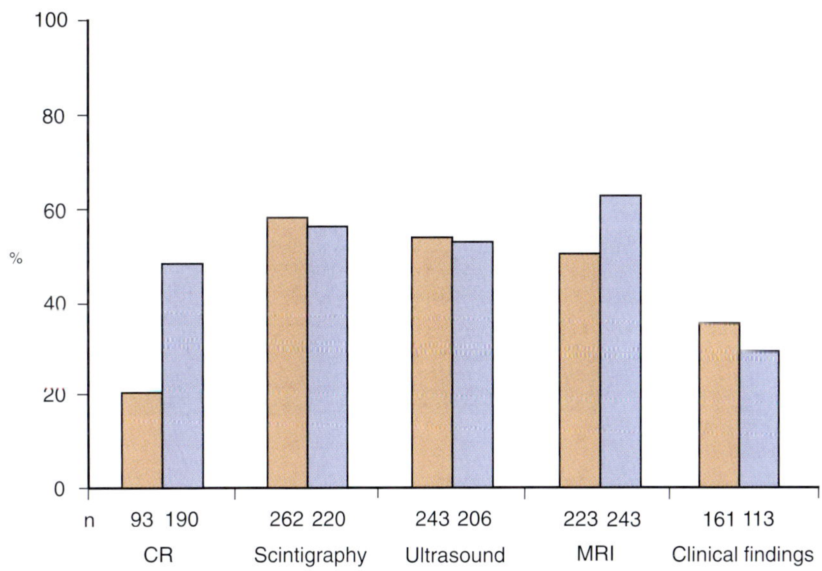

	$P < .001$ highly significant	$P < .01$ very significant	$P < .05$ significant
Group 1	Scintigraphy 1) Ultrasound 1) MRI 1)	Scintigraphy 2) Ultrasound 2)	Clinical findings 1) MRI 2)
Group 2	Scintigraphy 2) Ultrasound 2) MRI 2)	CR 2)	MRI 1) MRI 3)

Wilcoxon's signed rank test:
1) compared with CR (conventional radiography)
2) compared with clinical findings
3) compared with ultrasound

B

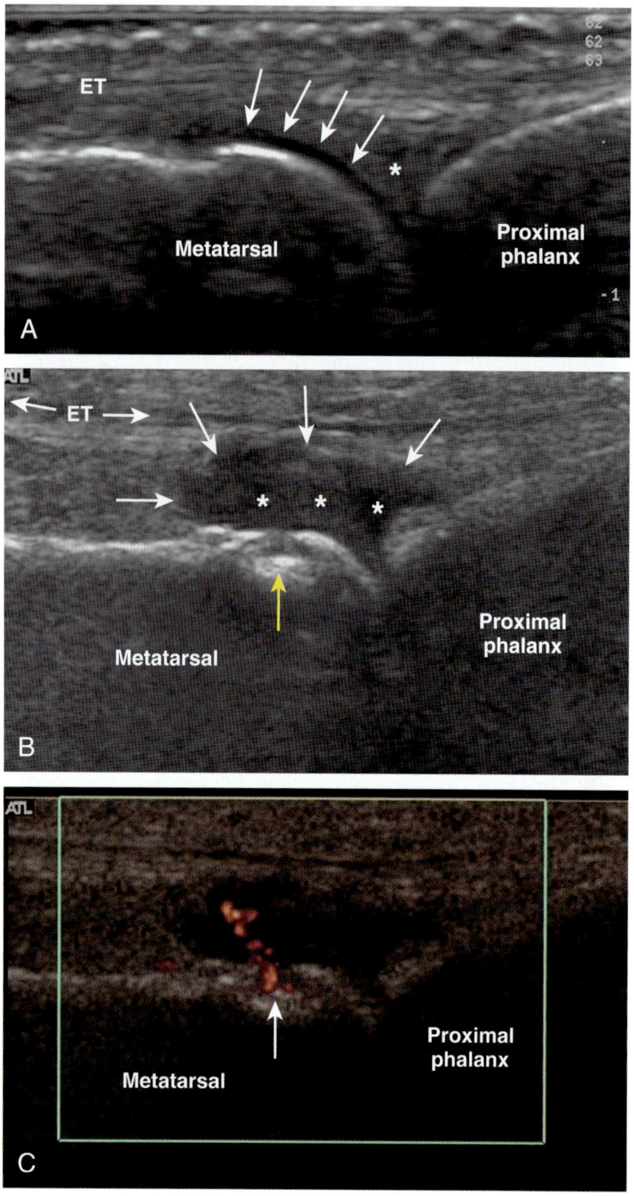

FIGURE 5-10. **A,** Longitudinal ultrasound image through an MCP joint of a patient with RA. Note the cartilage overlying the metacarpal head (*arrows*). The inverted triangular area (*asterisk*) represents loose connective tissue. ET, extensor tendon. **B,** Longitudinal gray-scale image through an MTP joint of a patient with RA. There is marked distention of the joint capsule (*white arrows*). Ultrasonographic evidence of synovitis, with joint fluid and synovial hypertrophy, is shown (*asterisks*). The *yellow arrow* indicates an erosion. ET, extensor tendon. Note the cartilage that is not clearly seen as fluid within the joint has a similar acoustic impedance as cartilage, such that there is no reflection at the interface. **C,** Corresponding image to **B**, with power Doppler superimposition. Note the Doppler signal extending down into the erosion.

flow and pathologic synovial hyperemia in RA,[28] a finding that has subsequently been confirmed by several others using varying techniques for quantification, including Hau and associates,[29] who demonstrated a very high degree of statistical significance in their series ($P < .001$) and Teh and colleagues,[30] who had similar results from different methods. Studies comparing ultrasonography and MRI in RA of the hands have shown a high level of agreement for synovitis; a study by Backhaus and coworkers[14] in 60 patients showed that ultrasonography was more sensitive than MRI in detecting synovitis, whereas MRI was more sensitive for detection of erosions (see Fig. 5-9). Szkudlarek and associates[31] published similar results, in which they found that power Doppler imaging has a sensitivity of 89% and a specificity of 98% for RA in the MCP joints, significantly outperforming the clinical examination.

A considerable literature exists on the evaluation of erosions on plain film and MRI, a topic that is addressed in detail in Chapter 6 and elsewhere.[32,33] However, it is worth emphasizing here that the unique ability to detect erosions *and* pre-erosive changes early in the course of disease is a significant advantage of MRI over ultrasonography. By extension, this line of reasoning would suggest that the role of MRI in RA may be best focused on the initial workup and rare/occasional periodic reevaluation of the joints, whereas a more frequent use of ultrasonography aimed at ongoing treatment assessment is appropriate. Ultrasonography may thus have greater clinical utility for frequent applications (e.g., as with every clinical office visit) in that patients spend less time and experience lower cost, and more joints can be evaluated in a single encounter when compared with MRI. It is noteworthy in this regard that the sonographically detected erosive changes are not always in accord with the findings on MRI,[34] which supports a role for both modalities because neither can completely replace the other.

Musculoskeletal sonographic images are, for most practitioners, significantly more difficult to interpret than MR images, and this is true for several reasons: (1) sonographic images are not limited to the standard three anatomic planes, which are respected in MRI by convention; (2) the "perspective" of ultrasonography is an unusual one, in which the image "fans out" from the point of probe contact to terminate at a variable depth within the tissue being studied, as opposed to MRI or radiographs that depict tissues in a way in which anatomic landmarks are more easily recognized; and (3) although they contain information with very high spatial resolution, sonographic images appear more "fuzzy," with a relatively poor signal-to-noise ratio when compared with radiographs, CT, or MRI and are thus visually less pleasing.

Because of these features it is not only more difficult for the clinician to appreciate the significance of the findings on sonographic images, it is also considerably more difficult for the clinician to share the images and discuss the findings directly with patients, in contrast to MRI and radiographs, which are much more familiar and visually accessible, even to laypersons, if viewed with appropriate physician guidance. Furthermore, as an imaging modality, ultrasonography has generally not been embraced by the community of musculoskeletal radiologists in the United States, who as a group are much more comfortable with MRI, CT, and conventional radiographs. There is a widespread impression that ultrasonography is somehow less reliable and trustworthy than MRI, owing to its "operator dependence," inconsistencies between machines, and other technical factors. Although these concerns are not completely without validity,[35] the resultant negative impression regarding ultrasonography is in fact not justified by the actual data, which support the use of ultrasound in the evaluation of a wide variety of musculoskeletal indications.[12,13] Musculoskeletal ultrasound evaluation is more widely accepted and much more heavily used outside the United States, where in many locations, especially in the United Kingdom and Australia, it has become an integral and routine part of the rheumatologist's clinical examination, in some centers being used at each and every patient encounter.

Ultrasound Functional Imaging in Rheumatoid Arthritis

The basis of ultrasound functional imaging in RA is (1) the fact that the severity of inflammation is physiologically correlated with the volume of regional blood flow in the effected synovial tissues; (2) that the pathologically increased blood flow states, caused by synovial angiogenesis and capillary leakage,[36] are reversible with effective treatment; and (3) that the Doppler method is sufficiently sensitive and reliable in reflecting these changes. The synovial hyperemia seen in RA is a fundamental pathophysiologic feature of the disease; it is most likely the principal factor underlying the "hallmark" radiographic observation of periarticular demineralization on radiographs of patients with RA and is generally accepted to occur in proportion to joint-destructive disease activity. By extension, the Doppler flow signal is thus an excellent surrogate marker for joint-destroying disease activity in RA. Doppler imaging can directly assess the hyperemic blood flow state within the inflamed joint, and a quantitative or semi-quantitative measure of the degree of severity can be derived, as we will illustrate.

This type of functional or physiologic assessment is primarily performed with the use of the amplitude, or "power," Doppler mode, which should be distinguished from other ultrasound techniques, especially conventional color Doppler sonography, which is a method in which the direction and velocity information from the Doppler interrogation is "encoded" and integrated into the gray-scale image as a color signal. In this mode the color hue is assigned based on the velocity of the moving reflectors (higher speeds are usually brighter hues). In general, by convention, red signals of all hues indicate flow that is directed *toward* the ultrasound probe, while blue signals indicate flow that is directed *away* from the probe. For quantification purposes, an angle correction is needed, because the strength of the signal is related to the cosine of the angle of the reflected sound wave. A corollary to this fact is that, as the Doppler angle of the reflected sound waves approaches 90 degrees, the cosine approaches zero, so the signal rapidly diminishes (the signal vanishes at 90 degrees). In duplex ultrasonography, a method commonly used for vascular assessment, the velocity of flow is estimated from the Doppler shift, usually in combination with a cross-sectional image and a Doppler angle correction.

Power Doppler imaging is generally believed to be more sensitive to small blood flows and has the significant advantage in that it is not direction dependent, although some experts insist that conventional (directional) pulsed Doppler techniques with current equipment have a similar level of sensitivity to low-level flows. Although some disagreement on this issue remains in the literature, most experts concur that power Doppler imaging has heretofore been significantly more sensitive and reliable across multiple equipment platforms than has directional pulsed Doppler imaging for this application. Because the contribution of the reflectors' velocity to the power Doppler (color) signal is related to its square (thus negating its direction), all echo-generating flows contribute positively to the signal amplitude. Thus, the color intensity on the image reflects the overall strength, that is, the "milliwattage," or "power" generated by these moving reflectors. The color hue is encoded with the total "power" or amplitude of this signal, generally with dark orange or purple colors indicating a very low level of flow and bright orange-to-white hues indicating a very high amplitude of flow, such as in a major artery at peak systole. Power Doppler is, as a result of the underlying physics and engineering, an extremely sensitive method, one that is able to detect very low-level flow states in very small vessels and discriminate these small signals reliably from the background "noise." This already very high sensitivity is augmented further by the use of sonographic intravenous contrast agents (e.g., Levovist) that add many additional bloodborne reflector particles, in the form of harmless circulating partially stabilized microbubbles, to contribute substantially to the overall Doppler signal. With further technologic innovation in ultrasound instrumentation, it is possible that the large sensitivity advantages of power Doppler imaging over conventional spectral/pulsed (directional) Doppler methods, especially with regard to low flow states, may be diminished.

The use of power Doppler imaging for the purpose of evaluating the severity of inflammatory manifestations in RA was first described by Newman and coworkers,[37,38] and since that time over 100 related articles have been published. Currently the volume of evidence supporting the use of power Doppler imaging to assess synovitis is fairly overwhelming. These include very solid work by Hau and associates,[39] in which power Doppler quantification correlated with other measures of disease activity with a high degree of significance beyond chance ($P < .001$), a study by Rubin,[40] which showed power Doppler imaging had predictive value for therapeutic monitoring in RA and other types of inflammatory arthritis, and a report by Stone and associates,[41] which showed, in a small study involving 12 patients, that power Doppler imaging related quantitatively to other established measures of synovitis. Naredo and colleagues[42] showed that the power Doppler signal and synovial thickening correlates with clinically swollen joint counts and did so more effectively than laboratory measures such as CRP and ESR, probably because ultrasonography was capable of detecting subclinical levels of synovitis (Fig. 5-11).

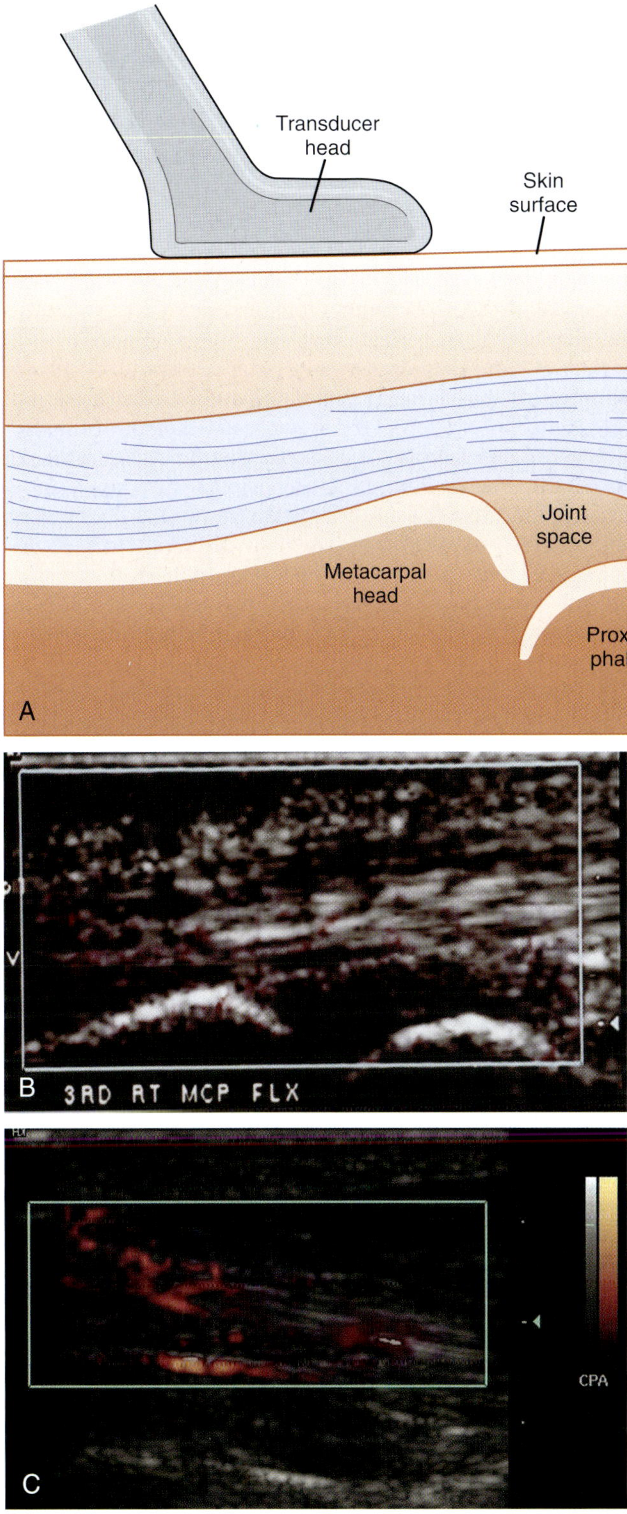

FIGURE 5-11. Artist's rendering (**A**) and a clinical image from an amplitude Doppler study (**B**) in a normal volunteer depicting normal blood flow within an MCP joint (flexor aspect). Note the normal fibrillary appearance of the flexor tendon and low degree of overlying color pixels indicating minimal capillary-type blood flow. **C,** Power Doppler ultrasound image of a typical patient with RA. Note the abnormally increased blood flow (synovial hyperemia) throughout, which is substantially greater than that seen in the image of the normal volunteer depicted in **B**.

Several experimental studies have provided histopathologic confirmation to the validity of the power Doppler signal as a surrogate marker for hypervascularization and synovitis, including those of Donnelly and Fleisher[43] and Walker and associates,[44] who found a highly significant correlation between the power Doppler results and histopathologic findings of synovial vascularization ($P < .01$). Strunk and coworkers,[45] also showed a highly significant correlation between microvascular power Doppler flow and both clinical and biochemical measures of synovitis ($P < .0001$) (Fig. 5-12).

Musculoskeletal Ultrasonography: Clinical Applications in Rheumatoid Arthritis

Despite its limitations and relative underutilization among musculoskeletal radiologists in the United States, ultrasound evaluation as an imaging modality may in fact have more to offer the patient with RA than radiography or even MRI. Numerous studies have unequivocally shown that, in patients with RA, ultrasonography is significantly more sensitive than is clinical examination for the detection of signs of inflammation and disease activity.[46] As discussed earlier, the unique contribution of ultrasonography in this setting is that it allows very accurate assessment of the day-to-day changes in the severity of rheumatoid synovitis by the indirect measure of small changes in synovial blood flow in multiple affected joints in a single, brief examination and in doing so it can provide semi-quantitative as well as quantitative measures of these small blood flow fluctuations in patients with RA that are readily compared with other quantifiable measures. The intrinsic sensitivity of the method to small changes in blood flow states may be even further augmented by the intravenous use of microbubble contrast agents, which have recently begun to be used in research studies.

Careful research over the past decade from numerous centers worldwide has supported the conclusion that the power Doppler signal is a very rapidly responsive indicator and predictor of therapeutic response in rheumatoid disease. As such, the

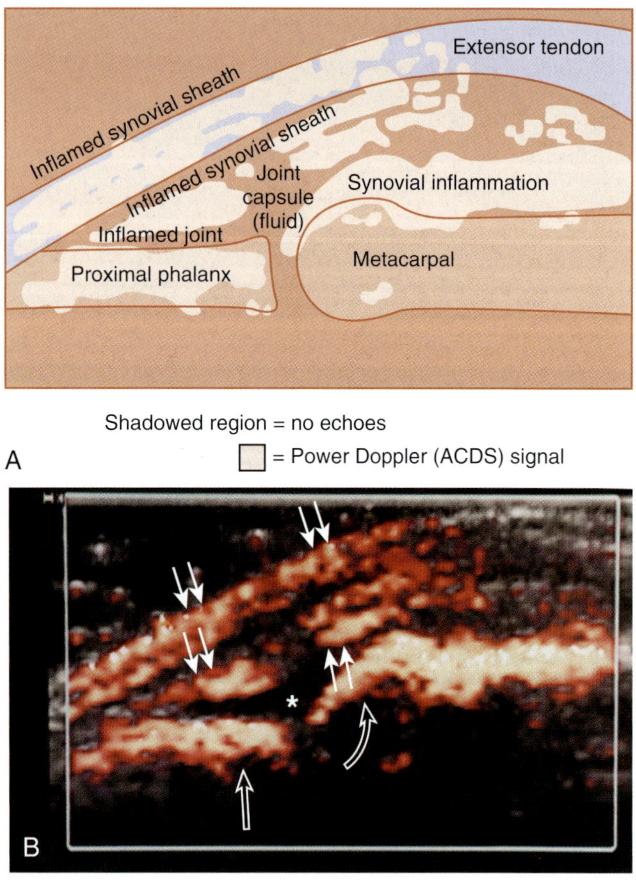

FIGURE 5-12. An example of severe hyperemia in a very severe case of RA, scanned from the dorsal aspect of the MCP joint. **A,** Artist's rendering. **B,** *Small arrows* demarcate the extensor tendon sheath; *large open arrow* indicates the bony surface. *Curved open arrow,* metacarpal head; *asterisk,* joint fluid/synovitis.

power Doppler signal can potentially be used clinically as a therapeutic "end point" for the titration of chemotherapeutic interventions, especially with regard to therapy with disease-modifying agents (DMARDs) such as methotrexate and the newer, extremely potent biologic response modifiers, the anti–TNF-α drugs such as etanercept (Enbrel), infliximab (Remicade), and adalimumab (Humira) discussed earlier. This point cannot be overemphasized. *It is the unique ability of power Doppler ultrasonography to reproducibly discriminate small changes in the severity of synovitis that allows its clinical use to monitor and modify the course of therapy long before a clinical or radiographic change might be detected.* The specific level of gray-scale synovitis that warrants treatment with biologic response modifiers is still in question, given that some pannus is likely to become fibrotic and effectively may leave "scar tissue" in the joint. Similarly, in patients with concomitant degenerative changes, some of the gray-scale changes (and sometimes Doppler signal) may be degenerative in origin and not inflammatory. In addition to being more sensitive than the clinical examination, the intraobserver reliability of ultrasonography has been shown to be much better than that of the rheumatologist's clinical examination.[42]

The primary criticism of ultrasonographic methods, which has become an extremely widely held misconception, is that there is too much "operator dependence" and, by extension, that reproducibility of the results and interobserver reliability must therefore be poor. This prejudice is held especially strongly regarding the use of quantitative or semi-quantitative methods. The existing data, however, overwhelmingly refute this supposition.[16] In evaluating the small joints of the hands of RA patients, Hau and coworkers[29] showed that pannus can be detected in 82% of joints with moderately active disease and that ultrasonography is even more sensitive than MRI in detection of synovitis in finger joints. In their series, ultrasonography detected more than 6.5 times more erosions than radiographs. Wakefield and Gibbon[17] found that ultrasonography is able to demonstrate finger erosions with a κ value of 0.75, which is significantly better than for two-reader double interpretations in screening mammography.[47] In fact, the data indicate that ultrasound in RA, in the hands of an experienced radiologist, is among the imaging studies with the *very highest degree of inter-reader reliability and reproducibility*. Interobserver reliability has also been shown to be excellent in the hands of relatively untrained examiners who were provided with a four-grade semi-quantitative scoring system.[48] We would also emphasize that MRI is not itself free of "operator dependence." Furthermore, it is not a trivial consideration that MRI systems are relatively limited in availability outside the United States, as compared with ultrasound systems, owing to their relatively higher acquisition, operational, and maintenance costs.

Semiquantitative vs. Quantitative Methods

With ultrasound, the use of semiquantitative methods (i.e., those in which the operator applies a rating scale for the Doppler flow signal [most commonly a 3-point or 4-point scale]) probably has the best clinical utility for routine practice; these methods have been used in several published studies since 1994. Typically, a score of 0 is given when no measurable power Doppler signal is present and a score of 3 or 4 is given for a large abnormal flow signal covering most or all of the synovium, with proportionate intermediate grades. For most research purposes, however, more intensive quantitative methods are needed, and several good computer-assisted methods have been developed, approaching this problem in various ways using widely available commercial or shareware image-processing software. The added step of image quantification extracts yet a deeper layer of information from the images as to the immediate severity of disease activity at the time of each assessment. In so doing, anatomic data (i.e., the presence of a disease manifestation in a specific anatomic location) is combined with functional/physiologic data in the form of a numerical index for synovial blood flow. This is typically a unitless numerical measure tied to the volume or density of overall blood flow within a selected region of interest. This measure can be used to quantifiably track major and minor fluctuations of disease activity over time and in response to treatment. Such a numerical index can be readily compared with other quantifiable indices of disease activity and treatment response, and thus the ultrasound assessment lends itself to statistical analysis and a higher degree of analytical rigor than would otherwise be possible. Quantification (more so than the more commonly used semi-quantitative approach) allows power Doppler ultrasonography to be more effectively used in research and clinical trials.

Quantification has been accomplished using a variety of methods, all arriving at very similar results. These methods have included (1) automated pixel counting methods, (2) the generation of time-intensity curves from real-time scanning and then subsequently calculating the area under the curve of these time-intensity plots, and (3) estimation of the Doppler resistive index,[49] and others. The "resistive index" is calculated by measuring the peak systolic and diastolic velocities using pulsed Doppler; a ratio of the two that is greater than 0.8 is indicative of the presence of inflammation.[50] Most methods require a manual selection of regions of interest for analysis, such as the "power weighted pixel density" of Meyerowitz and Fleisher[51] used in our own work.[28] The PWPD flow index provides a reproducible measure, one that can be compared both between patients and over time within the same patient to assess the patient response to a particular treatment. The relative degree of operator dependency and error introduced by the hand selection of the region of interest is overwhelmed by the large quantitative differences in disease states (in essence, the "signal" overwhelms the "noise") inherent in the measurement (Fig. 5-13A).

Each quantification method has advantages and disadvantages; however, results from any of these methods appear to be equivalent, reflecting an average 10-fold difference between patients with active RA and normal controls, with no overlap between the groups (see Fig. 5-13B).

This 10-fold difference between normal volunteers and patients with active RA has since been confirmed by several researchers using a number of different methods for quantification, which lends further credibility to the quantification process. It remains to be demonstrated that the more labor-intensive quantification methods will add value to the clinical care of patients. Nonetheless, it is widely believed that image quantification is useful in both basic research and in clinical trials of new therapeutic agents in comparison with existing agents. Ribbens and coworkers[52] developed a composite index that combined clinical and ultrasound data into a "Disease Activity Score," which is a unique innovation. The DAS is determined from measures of the synovial thickness, Doppler signal, clinical tenderness, and swelling. In their intriguing study there was less than a 3% interobserver variation in determining the DAS, which proved to be a good predictor of treatment response. Although reliable and reproducible, ultrasound quantification methods are widely believed to be too labor intensive for routine clinical practice. If automated quantification methods can be developed in the future, that is, those not requiring operator selection of regions of interest for analysis, the acceptance of a quantification standard for routine clinical use would likely be expedited.

For individual patients with RA, this added degree of reliability and ability to discern subtle fluctuations in their individual disease activity may lead directly to more effective treatment. With a rapid means of assessment available, treating physicians and their patients are able to learn quickly whether their disease process is sensitive or refractory to particular medications or treatments, for example, as determined by use of "target" levels of quantitative Doppler signal response. These patients then may benefit from more timely adjustment of their chemotherapeutic regimens, rather than suffering ongoing, progressive joint destruction from "smoldering" disease that lies beneath the level of (relatively insensitive) clinical and radiographic detection.

Because joint damage in RA is cumulative and clinical examination has been shown to be relatively insensitive, and because delays of months or years may be needed to evaluate treatment by conventional radiographic means, the beneficial impact on the individual patient in such a scenario could be quite substantial. Indeed, it can be argued that any means to accelerate the implementation of optimal

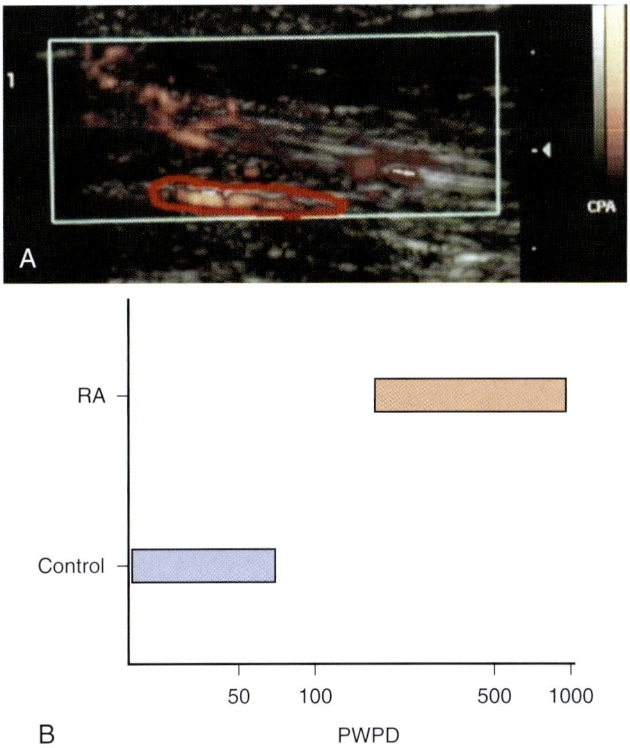

FIGURE 5-13. **A,** Selection of a region of interest (ROI) for quantification. In our own studies, quantification was performed after the method of Meyerowitz and colleagues,[51] by manual selection of an ROI, and color pixel values within the ROI are counted and averaged utilizing a specialized software package (Insight, version 5.9, GT Software, Bothell, WA). The quotient of the average pixel value within the ROI and the area of the ROI itself provide a reproducible flow index value, known as the "Power Weighted Pixel Density (PWPD)," which has been shown to be proportional to total regional blood flow and correlates extremely well with histologic findings of tissue neovascularity in animal models.[43] **B,** Bar chart comparing patients with RA and normal volunteer controls[28] using the computed flow index. PWPD is displayed in a log scale. Note a relatively larger range of values for patients with RA but no overlap between the two groups. There was an approximately 10-fold difference between the means of the two groups using this method. (**A** from Tsou I, Peh W, Bruno MA: Rheumatoid arthritis: hand. In: eMedicine Radiology Online Peer-Reviewed Radiology Journal, April 6, 2004; updated December 15, 2006. Available at http://www.emedicine.com/radio/topic877.htm. Reprinted, with permission from eMedicine.com.)

treatment, whether it be on the basis of directing an adjustment of dosages of medications already prescribed, supporting the addition of medications or combination therapies, or even merely allowing the patient and rheumatologist to weigh any undesirable side effects against tangible data demonstrating the benefit of a particular treatment regimen, may well be expected to have a favorable effect toward reducing the long-term morbidity in RA.

Quantification of Power Doppler Signal in Rheumatoid Arthritis using Contrast Agents

Not unexpectedly, the addition of ultrasound contrast agents appears to increase both the accuracy and sensitivity of ultrasonography in the evaluation of synovitis. These contrast agents are administered by intravenous injection and have a limited circulation time during which imaging must be performed. A full discussion of the history, physical and chemical properties, pharmacology, and imaging characteristics of ultrasonographic contrast agents is beyond our scope here but most consist of relatively stable gas microbubbles that serve as very efficient reflectors of the ultrasound beam, thus generating very intense Doppler signals when present in tissues and small vessels. The oldest and perhaps best studied of these agents is the so-called "first generation" ultrasound contrast agent Levovist, a microbubble stabilizing compound composed of galactose and palmitic acid, and most of the work published on this topic has utilized this agent. A newer, "second-generation" ultrasound contrast agent, SonoVue, which consists of stabilized microbubbles of sulfur hexafluoride gas, has also been studied for this purpose.

Time/intensity curves and calculation of the area under the curve and other dynamic quantitative indices of the contrast-enhanced power Doppler signal have been shown to significantly increase both the sensitivity and accuracy of the assessment of rheumatoid synovitis.[53]

One of the first uses of ultrasound microbubble contrast in RA was reported by Klauser and colleagues[54] using Levovist and showed markedly improved detection of intra-articular vascularization. Interestingly, this group's data showed that ultrasonographic contrast agents significantly improved detection of vascularization in the joints of patients with RA but seemed to have no effect at all on the Doppler signal measured from healthy joints. In a particularly elegant study, Teh and associates[30] utilized an intravenous contrast injection of Levovist and a computer-assisted pixel-counting method that correlated therapeutic response quantitatively to the Health Assessment Questionnaire and other clinical measures. Their technique takes into account the phasic blood flow that is usually observed in synovitis (see Figs. 5-15 and 5-16). In this study, the response to treatment was calculated from the difference in the area under each individual patient's curve, that is, their pretreatment and their post-treatment curves, a difference that was significant beyond chance at the $P < .001$ level. Future investigations should help establish whether there is any role for these agents in clinical practice (Figs. 5-14 and 5-15).

Schueller-Weidekamm and colleagues[55] studied a series of 14 patients using a different ultrasound microbubble contrast agent known as SonoVue and was able to quantitatively estimate the interarticular vascularization by deriving time-intensity curves following bolus contrast injection and determining the area under the curve before and after corticosteroid therapy. The gray area represents the change in vascularity that occurred as a response to treatment. In this regard it should be noted

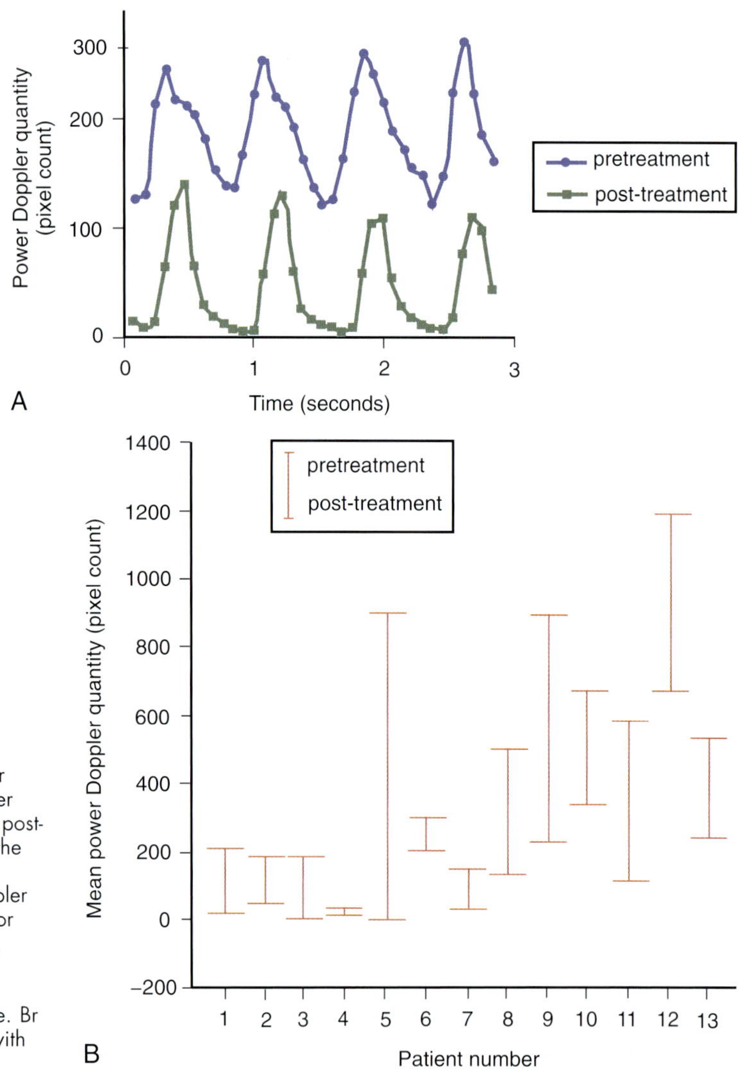

FIGURE 5-14. **A,** The power Doppler spectrum, representing power Doppler quantity over time. Pretreatment and post-treatment spectra are compared for the same patient. **B,** High-low graph demonstrating the mean power Doppler quantity before and after treatment for each patient. (From Teh J, Stevens K, Williamson L, et al. Power Doppler ultrasound of rheumatoid synovitis: quantification of therapeutic response. Br J Radiol 2003; 76:875-879. Used with permission.)

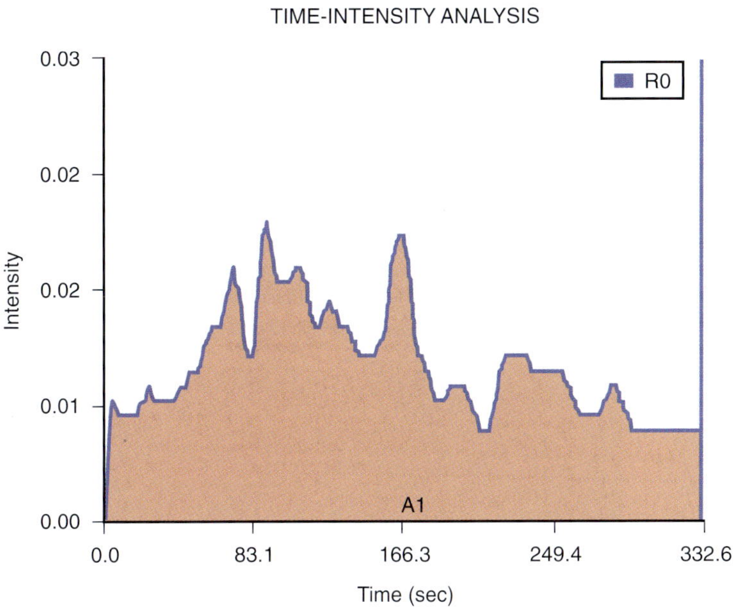

FIGURE 5-15. Quantification of the power Doppler signal after intravenous administration of Levovist. The area under the time-intensity curve is used to derive a numerical index from which pretreatment and post-treatment synovial vascularity is compared. (From Salaffi F, Carotti M, Manganelli P, et al. Contrast-enhanced power Doppler sonography of knee synovitis in rheumatoid arthritis: assessment of therapeutic response. Clin Rheumatol 2004; 23:285-290. With permission from Springer Science and Business Media.)

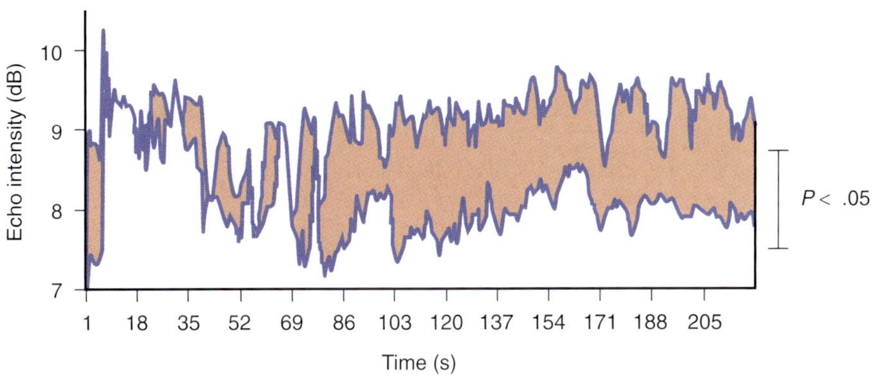

FIGURE 5-16. Change in the time-intensity curve after intravenous infusion of SonoVue as a quantified measure of response to treatment (see text for discussion).

that SonoVue does not diffuse into the extravascular space and is rapidly removed from the blood via the lungs and without any tissue perfusion. Thus, the results seen are believed to truly reflect changes in blood vessel volume and flow. The unique method, which the authors' called contrast-enhanced pulse-inversion harmonic imaging (PIHI) is believed to be a good quantitative estimate of synovial vascularization and was shown to be responsive to treatment. It is similar to the method used previously by Salaffi and associates[56] using Levovist (Fig. 5-16) that illustrates that for this particular purpose the various sonographic contrast agents may well be utilized interchangeably.

CASE EXAMPLE

A 42-year-old woman with severe RA underwent therapy with the biologic response modifier etanercept (Enbrel). This patient had been refractory to DMARD therapy with methotrexate. The pre-etanercept sonogram (Fig. 5-17A) demonstrated thickened tendons and subcutaneous tissues with substantial abnormal power Doppler signal indicative of severe tenosynovitis. The power Doppler signal reverted to the normal range soon after initiation of treatment with etanercept (see Fig. 5-17B).

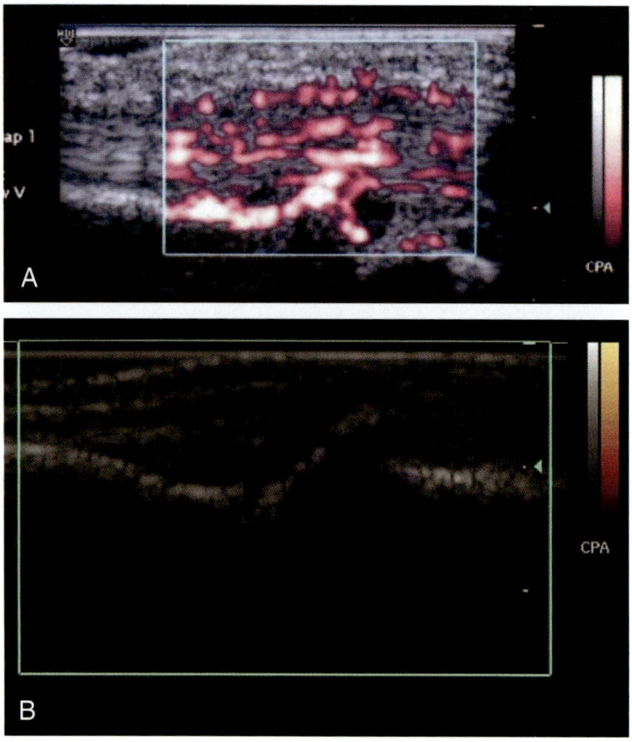

FIGURE 5-17. Power Doppler ultrasound of the third MCP joint of the dominant hand of an RA patient before (**A**) and after (**B**) initiation of etanercept. Both images of the same patient show complete resolution of the abnormal power Doppler signal. Shortly after this result was obtained, the patient developed a profound clinical remission, that is, Doppler signal changes preceded clinical remission. Quantitative indices of synovial blood flow on power Doppler derived from these images differed by more than 10-fold. This typical result illustrates the large relative size of the treatment effect, which is substantially greater than the relatively small degree of interoperator variability. (**A** from Schueller-Weidekamm C, Krestan C, Schueller G, et al. Power Doppler sonography and pulse-inversion harmonic imaging in evaluation of rheumatoid arthritis synovitis. AJR Am J Roentgenol 2007; 188:504-508. Used with permission.)

THE NEED FOR STANDARDIZATION AND THE OMERACT GROUP

In 1992, an informal international research group known as OMERACT (Outcome MEasurement in Rheumatoid Arthritis Clinical TRials) was formed with the goal of developing standardized outcome measures for RA. Initially this focused on clinical and imaging parameters but later went into standardizing techniques, definitions, and scoring systems in arthritis imaging, with the goal of achieving an international, data-driven consensus. The membership spans three continents, and the focus has been primarily on the development of an international consensus for the standardization of all forms of patient assessment in RA, including development of standardized scoring systems for all modalities of imaging, as well as to development of consensus standards for laboratory values and clinical questionnaires and examination techniques. Within the larger organization there are several focus groups composed of experts in each of the subtopics of overall interest. One of us (RJW) is the co-chair for the ultrasound working/study group of OMERACT, which was first established in 2004. Meetings are held every 2 years.

From the earliest days of its inception, the organization developed the concept of a measure having validity only when it passes the OMERACT Filter in its intended setting. The OMERACT Filter is summarized broadly as follows: Truth, Discrimination, and Feasibility. For this purpose, the words "truth," "discrimination," and "feasibility" have very specific connotations:

Truth: Does the index or measurement truly reflect what it intends to measure? Is the result unbiased and relevant?

Discrimination: Does the proposed measure discriminate between situations that are of actual clinical interest?

Feasibility: Can the measure be applied easily, given constraints of time, money, and interpretability?

Normal synovium is not visible as a discrete element on conventional ultrasound imaging. As such, almost any joint findings that depict synovial tissue in RA can be interpreted as abnormal. The OMERACT criteria for ultrasound[57] direct the observer to evaluate the synovial tissues in terms of their thickness, vascularity as shown by

Doppler imaging, and two other gray-scale features that are unique to synovitis: *incompressibility* of synovial tissues and their *nondisplaceability* both with regard to the application of pressure by the operator onto the joint via the ultrasound transducer itself. The aim of this maneuver is to distinguish between synovitis and the presence of synovial debris floating within the joint fluid. For the purpose of standardization, the OMERACT definition of rheumatoid synovitis evident on ultrasonography is *the presence of thickened intra-articular tissue that is nondisplaceable and poorly compressible and that may exhibit a Doppler signal.* This definition, although rigorous, is extremely circumspect considering the large volume of data supporting the use of power Doppler imaging for evaluation of synovitis in RA. It is extremely valuable, however, if for no other reason than to serve to illustrate the inherent difficulties in establishing a multinational consensus of experts!

Standardized Definitions for Ultrasound in Rheumatoid Arthritis

The OMERACT Ultrasound Special Interest Group was formed at the 7th OMERACT International Meeting in Asimolar, California, in 2004. This *ad hoc* committee established the following definitions for ultrasonographic pathology in inflammatory arthritis, constituting the first international standardized definitions for the use of ultrasound in RA. These were published in a report coauthored by the entire working group (lead author RJW), which appeared in the *Journal of Rheumatology*.[57] The proposed definitions are as follows:

RA erosion—An intra-articular discontinuity of the bone surface that is visible in two perpendicular planes

Synovial fluid—Abnormal hypechoic or anechoic intra-articular material that is displaceable and compressible and does not exhibit a Doppler signal

Synovial hypertrophy—Abnormal hypoechoic intra-articular tissue that is nondisplaceable and poorly compressible and that may exhibit a Doppler signal

Tenosynovitis—Hypoechoic or anechoic thickened tissue with or without fluid within the tendon sheath, which is seen in two perpendicular planes and which may exhibit a Doppler signal

The OMERACT group has also conducted systematic reviews on the role of ultrasound for the detection of synovitis. It has highlighted a paucity of robust data regarding issues such as reliability. This has led to a number of international exercises in an attempt to standardize and test the grading, acquisition, and interpretation of ultrasound images with respect to gray-scale and Doppler synovitis.

Ultrasound Technical Pitfalls

Several technical pitfalls in the use of power Doppler for assessment of RA have been demonstrated.[58,59] Foremost, there is indeed considerable variability in equipment that can confound serial measurements of individual patients/subjects if they are scanned on different types of ultrasound machines (especially different manufacturers' machines). This has been documented by several groups and is now a widely accepted pitfall in the method.[60] Patient and evaluator movement can also be a problem with power Doppler imaging, especially at the high gain settings needed to detect very low flows. The slightest unintended motion of the transducer in such a situation may result in a bright "flash" artifact. Breath holding, both on the part of the patient and the scanning sonographer, can become a necessity when using power Doppler imaging at the very high gain settings needed for detection of low-flow states. A common artifact is an "edge" effect that occurs at strong specular (mirror-like) reflectors, such as bone/soft tissue interfaces. It can be recognized as a steady color line along the rim of cortical bone. Most experts recommend setting the gain so that there is no observable signal in bone.[40,61] The color gain should generally be set as high as possible without producing artifacts.

Many observers have noted that manual application of pressure to the transducer can compress small vessels and reduce or even obliterate the visualized signal. Motion artifacts can be a significant problem as well. Standardizing probe/patient positioning remains a critical factor when comparing scans, especially when comparing serial examinations of the same patient. Increased flow can be seen with exercise and with skin heating, and it is helpful to perform these examinations within a reasonably narrow range of room temperatures. This has not been a significant problem in our own experience.

Although inter-scan, inter-machine, and interobserver variabilities have all been carefully documented—and as a result of these factors the reliability of comparisons between sonographic studies has been rightly questioned—we believe that this is a misplaced concern in the use of serial examinations to assess the efficacy of treatment, because the treatment effect is so much greater, by as much as 10-fold, than the interobserver or inter-platform variability.[28] Nonetheless, the sonographer, radiologist and rheumatologist are all well advised to control as many operator-dependent variables as is reasonably possible in the application of power Doppler imaging in the assessment of patients undergoing treatment for RA.[59]

SUMMARY

In the clinical evaluation of patients with RA ultrasonography can:

- Predict future response to therapy before any clinically evident response
- Reflect clinical changes and predict outcomes in longitudinal series, especially with regard to TNF-α antagonists, and thus can serve as an end point for determining treatment efficacy or directing changes in chemotherapy
- Surpass the accuracy and predictive value of the clinical examination, which is particularly important in early disease
- Correlate with outcomes better than biochemical markers and thus has potential prognostic significance
- Lend itself more readily to frequent utilization and to the evaluation of multiple joints than MRI or other imaging methods
- Detect more erosions than plain films, although fewer than can be seen on MRI
- Can be used to expedite clinical trials of novel therapeutic agents in RA

Future research directions for ultrasonography in RA should include:

- Further clarification of the role and scope of ultrasound contrast agents in RA
- Greater consensus on standardization of measures and techniques and quantification methods in Doppler ultrasound as applied to the ongoing assessment of patients undergoing treatment for RA using biologic response modifiers and disease-altering agents
- Development of easily applied standardized automated methods for image data quantification with greater cross-platform reproducibility

Acknowledgments

Some of the research described in this chapter was supported by a 1998 RSNA seed grant to Dr. Bruno. The authors also wish to acknowledge the invaluable manuscript assistance of Mrs. Debbie Pavone.

References

1. Arnett FC, Edworthy SM, Bloch DA, et al. The American Rheumatism Association 1987 revised criteria for the classification of rheumatoid arthritis. Arthritis Rheum 1988; 31:315-324.
2. Conaghan P, O'Connor P, McGonagle D, et al. Elucidation of the relationship between synovitis and bone damage: a randomized MRI study of individual joints in patients with early rheumatoid arthritis. Arthritis Rheum 2003; 48:64-71.
3. Nauch M, Karakiulakis G, Perruchoud AP, et al. Corticosteroids inhibit the expression of the vascular endothelial growth factor gene in human vascular smooth muscle cells. Eur J Pharmacol 1998; 341:309-315.

4. Quinn MA, Emery P. Window of opportunity in early rheumatoid arthritis: possibility of altering the disease process with early intervention. Clin Exp Rheumatol 2003; 21(Suppl 31):S154-S157.
5. Emery P. Treatment of rheumatoid arthritis. BMJ 2006; 332:152-155.
6. Edwards JCW, Szczepariski L, Szechinski J, et al. Efficacy of B-cell–targeted therapy with rituximab in patients with rheumatoid arthritis. N Engl J Med 2004; 350:2572-2581.
7. Kremer JM, Westhovens R, Leon M, et al. Treatment of rheumatoid arthritis by selective inhibition of T-cell activation with fusion protein CTLA4Ig. N Engl J Med 2003; 349:1907-1915.
8. Quinn MA, Conaghan PG, O'Connor PJ, et al. Very early treatment with infliximab in addition to methotrexate in early, poor-prognosis rheumatoid arthritis reduces magnetic resonance imaging evidence of synovitis and damage, with sustained benefit after infliximab withdrawal. Arthritis Rheum 2005; 52:27-35.
9. De Flaviis L, Scaglione P, Nessi R, et al. Ultrasonography of the hand in rheumatoid arthritis. Acta Radiol 1988; 29:457-460.
10. Fornage B, Bruno D (eds). Musculoskeletal Ultrasound. New York, Churchill Livingstone 1995.
11. Chhem RK, Cardinal E. Guidelines and Gamuts in Musculoskeletal Ultrasound. New York, Wiley-Liss, 1999.
12. Van Holsbeeck MT, Intracaso JH. Musculoskeletal Ultrasound, 2nd ed. Philadelphia, Mosby, 2001.
13. Bianchi S, Martinoli C. Ultrasound of the Musculoskeletal System. Heidelberg, Springer, 2007.
14. Backhaus T, Kamradt D, Sandrock D, et al. Arthritis of the finger joints: a comprehensive approach comparing conventional radiography, scintigraphy, ultrasound, and contrast-enhanced magnetic resonance imaging. Arthritis Rheum 1999; 42:1232-1245.
15. Tsao I, Peh W, Bruno MA. Rheumatoid arthritis: hand. In: e-medicine Radiology Online Peer-Reviewed Radiology Journal, April 6, 2004; updated December 15, 2006. Available at http://www.emedicine.com/radio/topic877.htm. Reprinted, with permission from eMedicine.com.
16. Lopez-Ben R, Bajaj S, Alarcon G. Utilizing ultrasound in early RA to establish progression of erosive disease [Abstract]. Presented at the RSNA annual meeting, Chicago, November 27, 2005.
17. Wakefield RJ, Gibbon WW, Conaghan PG, et al. The value of sonography in the detection of bone erosions in patients with rheumatoid arthritis: a comparison with conventional radiography. Arthritis Rheum 2000; 43:2762-2770.
18. Sharp JT, Young DY, Bluhm GB, et al. How many joints in the hands and wrists should be included in a score of radiologic abnormalities used to assess rheumatoid arthritis? Arthritis Rheum 1985; 28:1326-1335.
19. Sharp JT, Wolfe F, Mitchell DM, et al. The progression of erosion and joint space narrowing scores in rheumatoid arthritis during the first twenty-five years of disease. Arthritis Rheum 1991; 34:660-668.
20. Kaye JJ, Nance EP Jr, Callahan LF, et al. Observer variation in quantitative assessment of rheumatoid arthritis: II. A simplified scoring system. Invest Radiol 1987; 22:41-46.
21. Fuchs HA, Kaye JJ, Callahan LF, et al. Evidence of significant radiographic damage in rheumatoid arthritis within the first two years of disease. J Rheumatol 1989; 16:585-591.
22. Fuchs HA, Pincus T. Reduced joint counts in controlled clinical trials in rheumatoid arthritis. Arthritis Rheum 1994; 37:470-475.
23. Pincus T, Larsen A, Brooks RH, et al. Comparison of 3 quantitative measures of hand radiographs in patients with rheumatoid arthritis: Steinbrocker stage, Kaye Modified Sharp score, and Larsen score. J Rheumatol 1997; 24:2106-2112.
24. Brower AC. Use of the radiograph to measure the course of rheumatoid arthritis: the gold standard versus fool's gold. Arthritis Rheum 1990; 33:316-324.
25. Wakefield RJ, O'Connor PJ, Conaghan PG, et al. Finger tendon disease in untreated early rheumatoid arthritis: a comparison of ultrasound and magnetic resonance imaging. Arthritis Rheum 2007; 57:1158-1164.
26. Fuchs HA, Pincus T. Radiographic damage in rheumatoid arthritis: description by nonlinear models [Editorial]. J Rheumatol 1992; 19:1655-1658.
27. Kirwan JR. The relationship between synovitis and erosions in rheumatoid arthritis. Br J Rheumatol 1997; 36:225-228.
28. Bruno MA, Fuchs HA. Quantification of amplitude color Doppler (ACD) ultrasound for assessment of rheumatoid arthritis: preliminary findings and description of a new technique [Abstract]. Invited presentation at the Special Scientific Session of the 27th annual meeting of the International Skeletal Society, Barcelona, Spain, September 10, 2000.
29. Hau M, Shultz H, Hans-Peter T, et al. Evaluation of pannus and vascularization of the metacarpophalangeal and proximal interphalangeal joints in rheumatoid arthritis by high-resolution ultrasound (multidimensional linear array). Arthritis Rheum 1999; 42:2303-2308.
30. Teh J, Stevens K, Williamson L, et al. Power Doppler ultrasound of rheumatoid synovitis: quantification of therapeutic response. Br J Radiol 2003; 76:875-879.
31. Szkudlarek M, Narvestad E, Klarlund M, et al. Ultrasonography of the metatarsophalangeal joints in rheumatoid arthritis. Arthritis Rheum 2004; 50:2103-2112.
32. Hazy MD, Slavotinek J, Smith MD. Role of ultrasound in assessment of early rheumatoid arthritis. Australas Radiol 2007; 51:120-126.
33. ØstergaardM, Døhn UM, Ejbjerg BJ, McQueen FM. Ultrasonography and magnetic resonance imaging in early rheumatoid arthritis: recent advances. Curr Rheumatol Rep 2006; 8:378-385.

34. Hoving JL, Buchbinder R, Hall S, et al. A Comparison of magnetic resonance imaging, sonography and radiography of the hand in patients with early rheumatoid arthritis. J Rheumatol 2004; 31:663-675.
35. Farrant JM, O'Connor PJ, Grainger AJ. Advanced imaging in rheumatoid arthritis: II. Erosions. Skeletal Radiol 2007; 36:381-389.
36. Hirohata S, Sakakibara J. Angioneogenesis as a possible elusive triggering factor in rheumatoid arthritis. Lancet 1999; 353:1331.
37. Newman JS, Adler RS, Bude RO, et al. Detection of soft-tissue hyperemia: value of power Doppler sonography. AJR Am J Roentgenol 1994; 163:385-389.
38. Newman JS, Laing TJ, et al. Power Doppler sonography of synovitis: assessment of therapeutic response—preliminary observations. Radiology 1996; 198:582-584.
39. Hau M, Kneitz C, Tony HP, et al. High resolution ultrasound detects a decrease in pannus vascularization of small finger joints in patients with rheumatoid arthritis receiving treatment with soluble tumor necrosis factor alpha receptor (etanercept). Ann Rheum Dis 2002; 61:55-58.
40. Rubin JM. Musculoskeletal power Doppler. Eur Radiol 1999; 9(Suppl 3):S403-S406.
41. Stone M, Bergin D, Whelan B, et al. Power Doppler ultrasound assessment of rheumatoid hand synovitis. J Rheumatol 2001; 28:1979-1982.
42. Naredo E, Bonilla G, Gamero F, et al. Assessment of inflammatory activity in rheumatoid arthritis: a comparative study of clinical evaluation with grey-scale and power Doppler ultrasonography. Ann Rheum Dis 2005; 64:375-381.
43. Donnelly EF, Geng L, Wojcicki WE, et al. Quantified power Doppler US of tumor blood flow correlates with microscopic quantification of tumor blood vessels. Radiology 2001; 219:166-169.
44. Walther M, Harms H, Krenn V, et al. Correlation of power Doppler sonography with vascularity of the synovial tissue of the knee joint in patients with osteoarthritis and rheumatoid arthritis. Arthritis Rheum 2001; 44:331-338.
45. Strunk J, Heinemann E, Neeck G, et al. A new approach to studying angiogenesis in rheumatoid arthritis by means of power Doppler ultrasonography and measurement of serum vascular endothelial growth factor. Rheumatology 2004; 43:1480-1483.
46. Joshua F, Lassere M, Bruyn GA, et al. Summary findings of a systemic review of the ultrasound assessment of synovitis. Proceedings of OMERACT 8. J Rheumatol 2007; 34:839-847.
47. Taplin SH, Rutter CM, Elmore JG, et al. Accuracy of screening mammography using single vs. independent double interpretation. AJR Am J Roentgenol 2000; 174:1257-1262.
48. Szkudlarek M, Court-Payen M, Jacobsen S, et al. Interobserver agreement in ultrasonography of the finger and toe joints in rheumatoid arthritis. Arthritis Rheum 2003; 48:955-962.
49. Terslev L, Torp-Pedersen S, Qvistgaard E, et al. Spectral Doppler and resistive index: a promising tool in ultrasonographic evaluation of inflammation in rheumatoid arthritis. Acta Radiol 2004; 44:645-652.
50. Terslev L, Torp-Pedersen S, Savnick P, et al. Doppler ultrasound and MRI of synovial inflammation of the hand in rheumatoid arthritis: a comparative study. Arthritis Rheum 2003; 48:2434-2441.
51. Meyerowitz C, Fleisher AC, Pickens DR, et al. Quantification of tumor vascularity and flow with amplitude color Doppler sonography in an experimental model. J Ultrasound Med 1996; 15:827-833.
52. Ribbens C, Andrew B, Marcelis S, et al. Rheumatoid hand joint synovitis: gray-scale and power Doppler US quantifications following anti-tumor necrosis factor-α treatment: pilot study. Radiology 2003; 229:562-569.
53. Carotti M, Salaffi F, Manganelli P, et al. Power Doppler sonography in the assessment of synovial tissue of the knee joint in rheumatoid arthritis: a preliminary experience. Ann Rheum Dis 2002; 61:877-882.
54. Klauser A, Frauscher F, Schirmer M, et al. The value of contrast-enhanced color Doppler ultrasound in the detection of vascularization of finger joints in patients with rheumatoid arthritis. Arthritis Rheum 2002; 46:647-653.
55. Schueller-Weidekamm C, Krestan C, Schueller G, et al. Power Doppler sonography and pulse-inversion harmonic imaging in evaluation of rheumatoid arthritis synovitis. AJR Am J Roentgenol 2007; 188:504-508.
56. Salaffi F, Carotti M, Manganelli P, et al. Contrast-enhanced power Doppler sonography of knee synovitis in rheumatoid arthritis: assessment of therapeutic response. Clin Rheumatol 2004; 23:285-290.
57. Wakefield RJ, Balint PV, Szkudlarek M, et al. Musculoskeletal ultrasound including definitions for ultrasonographic pathology. OMERACT 7 Special Interest Group Whitepaper, J Rheumatol 2005; 32:2485-2487.
58. Teh J. Applications of Doppler imaging in the musculoskeletal system. Curr Probl Diagn Radiol 2006; 35:22-34.
59. Torp-Pedersen ST, Terslev L. Settings and artefacts relevant in colour/power Doppler ultrasound in rheumatology. Ann Rheum Dis 2008; 67:143-149.
60. Farrant JM, O'Connor PJ, Grainger AJ. Advanced imaging in rheumatoid arthritis: I. Synovitis. Skeletal Radiol 2007; 36:269-279.
61. Schmidt W. Technology insight: the role of color and power Doppler ultrasonography in rheumatology. Nature Clin Pract Rheumatol 2007; 3:35-42.

Chapter 6

MRI IN RHEUMATOID ARTHRITIS

Michael A. Bruno

Magnetic resonance imaging has been applied to the study of rheumatoid arthritis (RA) for more than 15 years, and a large body of clinical and research experience on its use has contributed to a growing understanding of the important role of this modality, both in helping to develop our basic understanding of the disease and in the ongoing clinical management of patients with RA and juvenile RA (JRA).

There are two principal areas in which MRI has been shown to have particular utility and for which there is considerable clinical experience: (1) in the detection and measurement (quantification) of erosions and pre-erosive changes, especially in early disease, and (2) in the evaluation (quantitative and semi-quantitative) of synovitis, primarily by using intravenous gadolinium-based contrast agents. As with Doppler ultrasonography, MRI can evaluate an individual patient's response to treatment and help to guide day-to-day therapeutic decision making. Current research also suggests a developing role for MRI in depicting the basic cellular and molecular processes in RA, which may improve our basic understanding of the disease itself, as well as provide the highest degree of accuracy in evaluating the destructive activity of the disease and response to treatment that is possible with currently available methods. For each of these roles MRI overlaps with other modalities, including ultrasonography and molecular imaging.

EROSIONS IN RHEUMATOID ARTHRITIS: COMPARISON OF MRI VS. ULTRASONOGRAPHY VS. RADIOGRAPHY

Perhaps the most significant role for MRI in rheumatoid disease is in the early detection, measurement, and characterization of joint erosions and pre-erosive changes. The characteristic erosions of rheumatoid arthritis occur at the margins of joints, at synovial reflections, and at sites of insertion of interosseous ligaments. On MRI, these are best seen on coronal spin-echo images. As with ultrasonography, MRI is a cross-sectional imaging modality, and one with very high intrinsic tissue contrast. Despite having lower spatial resolution than plain radiographs, MRI has shown much greater sensitivity in the detection of joint destruction at an early stage and, in repeated studies, has been proven to detect and identify erosions, even very small ones, with greater sensitivity and efficiency than plain film radiography or, for that matter, any other available imaging modality. In terms of comparative sensitivity, evaluation with ultrasound has been shown to detect more erosions than are visible on plain radiographs,[1] and MRI detects still more than ultrasound in the same patient populations.[2] As such, MRI may be valuable even in patients who have normal findings on radiography. In a study involving 46 patients with early RA, Hoving and coworkers[3] showed that MRI is significantly more sensitive for the detection of erosions than either ultrasonography or radiography and has high inter-reader reliability. More than twice the number of erosions were detected on MRI than by either ultrasonography or radiography in their series. In early RA, MRI represents an especially significant advance in the detection of erosive changes as compared with the previous gold standard, plain film radiography, even when optimized radiographic methods are employed.[4,5]

In common clinical practice, most rheumatologists and radiologists over the past approximately 40 years have relied on conventional film-screen radiography using standard equipment and film for the detection and scoring of erosions. However, in many research studies and in some clinical practices, specialized high-resolution x-ray methods were also employed, such as fine-grain, single-emulsion screenless radiography and magnification radiography using small focal spot x-ray sources of 6 to 8 μm, typically using 5× geometric magnification. These uncommon radiographic methods served to optimize the radiographic technique, allowing earlier detection of smaller erosions and greater sensitivity overall. Presumably, this also led to more accurate scoring using established scoring systems, such as the Sharp and Larsen scoring systems, which involve counting as well as measuring rheumatoid erosions.[6-12] As such, these optimized planar radiography techniques probably represent a fairer "gold standard" with which to compare the more advanced cross-sectional methods, such as MRI, despite their limited use in practice. It is clear, however, that MRI surpasses the ability of even the most optimal radiographic methods for the detection and characterization of erosions in rheumatoid disease—in fact, it has been firmly established that MRI is the single best modality for the detection and evaluation of erosions in RA, and, further, its use has revealed the existence of pre-erosive antecedent bony changes that are not apparent radiographically. Finally, MRI-based observations have also given substantial support to the prevailing hypothesis that erosive changes in RA are the result of rheumatoid synovitis, rather than there being an unrelated or separate disease process or epiphenomenon.[13,14]

MRI VS. ULTRASONOGRAPHY IN CLINICAL PRACTICE

In comparison with ultrasonography, MRI takes significantly longer to perform, is generally more costly, and as a direct result of time and cost constraints, typically only one site (e.g., the dominant or most symptomatic hand and wrist) can be evaluated at a single session, whereas multiple sites can be readily imaged using ultrasound. With MRI, there is superior tissue contrast resolution and a more favorable signal-to-noise ratio (SNR). Images are visually pleasing and are generally limited to the conventional three anatomic planes. As such, they are more straightforward to interpret by the clinician and are easier to use as adjunctive "visual aids" in discussion with patients. Indeed, many rheumatologists prefer MRI over ultrasound images in practice, because MRI is the preferred modality in the detection of erosions, and there is a high clinical comfort level with the tracking of erosions as an indicator of disease progression in RA,[7,15] and because the images are visually analogous to radiographs in that they depict anatomic structures in familiar ways. As an added advantage of MRI over ultrasonography, the comprehensive regional anatomic overview uniquely provided by MRI can often detect and characterize additional lesions that may have been unexpected or even unrelated to the patient's arthritis in the course of the evaluation.

In addition to these clinical factors driving the utilization of MRI for evaluation of patients with RA, there are also economic inducements that may have a significant impact as well. In the United States and elsewhere, ownership of an MRI system by a physician group may provide significant income to the practice, because third-party payer reimbursement for the technical component of MRI studies can be significant and is much higher than that for radiography or ultrasonography. This has created a significant emerging market for imaging equipment manufacturers, who have responded by producing relatively inexpensive imaging systems with reduced fields of view, tailored for the imaging of small joints. These so-called "niche" magnets, which offer relatively low acquisition costs, high-quality imaging output, ease of use, and low space requirements are ideally suited for an office-based rheumatology practice when there is a large enough patient base to support their use. Such units are heavily marketed to academic and private rheumatology practices, with both their clinical and financial benefits to the practice emphasized by the manufacturer's representatives. It is undeniable that the combination of aggressive marketing of systems by the manufacturers and the substantial financial incentives of the health care marketplace contribute to a greater acceptance of MRI in the practice of rheumatology in the United States relative to ultrasonography.

As was discussed in the previous chapter in some detail, ultrasound has great utility in the evaluation of synovitis in RA[16]; however, MRI with gadopentetate dimeglumine (Gd-DTPA) contrast administration is also capable of this assessment. Indeed, there have been many published studies utilizing MRI primarily for the evaluation of synovitis in RA, although most have been studies of relatively few patients and there has been little comparison in the literature between high- and low-field MRI scanners or in comparative assessment of other technical factors. For the evaluation of synovitis by MRI in clinical practice, it is common to use conventional spin-echo T1-weighted and T2-weighted sequences, usually with spectral fat suppression and Gd-DTPA intravenous contrast, supplemented with the occasional use of short tau inversion recovery (STIR) sequences. Imaging sequences are obtained in coronal and axial planes and typically utilizing a high-resolution extremity surface coil. Because equipment manufacturers are constantly upgrading and improving available MRI systems and technologies, it is likely that future MRI systems will offer additional imaging options and ultimately may significantly outperform results published in the current literature.

RHEUMATOID EROSIONS AND PRE-EROSIVE CHANGES ON MRI

True RA erosions, that is, those involving frank cortical destruction and detected by T1-weighted, spin-echo MRI, can often also be demonstrated on radiographs. Gd-DTPA contrast enhancement may be a common feature of erosions in RA, seen in up to 72% of erosions to some degree.[17] In addition, the use of MRI has also revealed the existence of reversible, "pre-erosive" lesions that are, in fact, seen *only* on MRI (i.e., erosion-like lesions that do *not* correlate with radiographic erosions and that are not visible with ultrasound or on CT) and that may completely vanish in response to effective chemotherapy. Ostergaard and coworkers[4] have suggested that these early bone marrow signal changes seen on fluid-sensitive MRI sequences at the joint margins of patients with RA appear to represent a type of "pre-erosive" osteitis—an inflammatory rather than an erosive process occurring at the typical location of rheumatoid erosions—reflecting the presence of inflammatory or edematous changes in the bone marrow but with the overlying bony cortex still intact. These pre-erosive lesions are indeed distinguishable from true erosions on MR images by their intact cortical margins and internal signal characteristics. On MRI, true erosions show cortical interruption and have well-defined, rounded margins and contain only synovial fluid or synovial tissue signal. In contradistinction, these pre-erosive lesions have free water signal within the medullary space and tend to have somewhat ill-defined margins. Furthermore, unlike true erosions, they may also appear to contain interspersed trabecular bone or even fat.[18]

Of particular note, these nonerosive inflammatory changes have been observed to be at least potentially reversible and heal in some cases, whereas in other cases they progress into true rheumatoid erosions that can be seen on plain films. In essence, then, MRI has demonstrated both the natural history of developing erosions in RA and also the repair or healing of what amounts to early erosion-precursor lesions previously not known to exist. The preponderance of evidence seems to suggest that when a lesion is seen only as a focus of relatively high signal on fluid-sensitive sequences, such as T2-weighted imaging, and is not evident on T1-weighted, spin-echo sequences, such a lesion generally may be thought of as a reversible osteitis or "pre-erosive change" that will not correlate with erosions on the radiograph; to the contrary, low-signal defects on T1-weighted, spin-echo images are generally seen with irreversible bone damage and correlate more completely with radiographically demonstrated rheumatoid erosions. Most importantly, it has been shown that the former often evolves into the latter with time.[18,19]

As noted earlier, the pattern of MRI changes observed across numerous experimental studies using differing techniques supports the view that *synovitis* is the antecedent change in RA, leading to *osteitis* and, in most if not all cases, ultimately producing *bony erosions.* Based on MRI data, some authorities have questioned whether the two (synovitis and erosive disease) occur out of proportion to each other, which would suggest, at the very least, that the linkage between synovitis and bone erosions may be a complex or indirect one.[2] Nevertheless, it is clear that neither the osteitis seen on MRI nor the bony erosions seen by plain film, CT, MRI, or ultrasonography appear to occur in the absence of synovitis. Most experts are convinced of a temporal sequence or natural progression of changes as depicted on MRI, progressing from normal (no erosions or synovitis), to synovitis or tenosynovitis, demonstrable by MRI or ultrasound, to osteitis with signal changes on T2-weighted imaging, to finally frank erosions that appear dark on T1-weighted imaging and are visible on plain radiographs and CT and ultrasound images (Fig. 6-1).[13,20-22]

In adult RA, erosions occur as an early manifestation in the course of disease—usually within the first 6 months of symptom onset. As such, there may be a signifi-

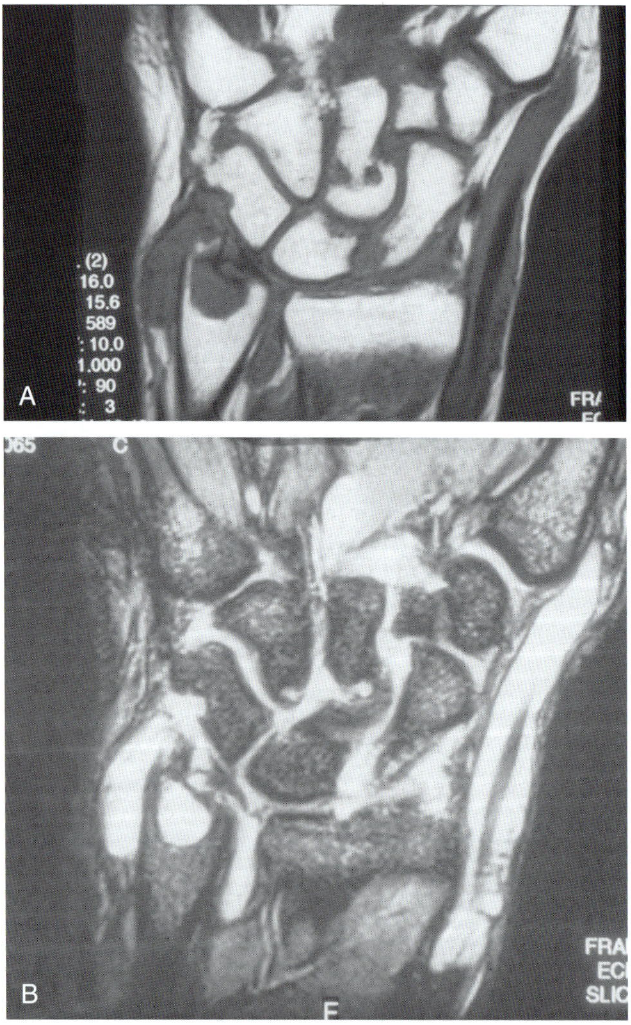

FIGURE 6-1. **A,** T1-weighted, spin-echo MR image of the wrist of a patient with RA. Note the presence of bony erosions and synovial pannus, which appears of medium signal intensity, and synovial thickening/tenosynovitis surrounding the tendons. **B,** T2-weighted, fat-suppressed, spin-echo MR image from the same patient. Synovial pannus and erosions appear bright. (Courtesy of Dr. J. Tehranzadeh, University of California, Irvine.)

cant clinical advantage in their early detection. Because of its high sensitivity and predictive value, McQueen and associates[23,24] have advocated the use of MRI in the patient's dominant wrist in newly diagnosed RA to identify those patients who manifest early erosive and pre-erosive changes, because these patients would more likely benefit from early, aggressive chemotherapy than those who lacked evidence of early erosive (and pre-erosive) change.

MRI may be particularly useful in evaluating the hand and wrist, where the earliest and most frequent erosions are found.[25]

MRI OF SYNOVITIS IN RHEUMATOID ARTHRITIS

The inflamed synovium in RA, as was noted in the previous chapter, is a highly vascularized, complex tissue that is richly cellular and whose overall volume correlates well with clinical disease severity and poor clinical outcome. On conventional spin-echo images, the thickened, inflamed synovium (pannus) in RA is of intermediate signal intensity on T1 weighting, appears bright on T2 weighting, and enhances robustly after intravenous administration of gadolinium-based contrast material. The intense signal change evident within the inflamed synovial tissues in RA patients is not seen to any significant degree in normal volunteers, although occasional minimal synovial enhancement has been reported in normal subjects.[26] The phenomenon of contrast enhancement seen in RA synovitis occurs very quickly on intravenous administration of a contrast agent and thus reflects an unusually rapid increase in the concentration of gadolinium that occurs within the abnormal (but not within normal) synovium. This, in turn, reflects the abnormally increased synovial blood flow, vascularization, and capillary permeability present in active RA synovitis, features that are reversible with effective treatment. In the presence of active disease, the synovium become suffused with Gd-DTPA, which results in substantial T1 shortening within the inflamed synovial tissues—visualized as a bright region of enhancement on T1-weighted images. Indeed, bright and immediate gadolinium-induced T1 signal enhancement is seen fairly homogeneously throughout the inflamed synovium in patients with RA and JRA.

Because MRI is a cross-sectional "volumetric" method, it is possible to derive a quantitative estimate of the volume of the inflamed synovial tissue that is so well delineated by gadolinium. Measurements of this type must be done using fairly rapid imaging, however, because the contrast material diffuses rapidly from the synovium into the surrounding joint fluid, rendering it bright on T1-weighted images (sometimes referred to as an "arthrogram effect" because it mimics the injection of contrast agent directly into the fluid) and thus rendering the margins of the inflamed synovium itself relatively inconspicuous on the images. Diffusion of Gd-DTPA contrast into joint fluid occurs in patients without synovitis, albeit more slowly, and is the basis of the "indirect arthrogram" technique sometimes used to evaluate shoulder and knee tendons and other internal derangements of joints with MRI. The assessment of rheumatoid synovitis by Gd-DTPA–enhanced T1-weighted MRI, therefore, requires a rapid imaging technique that affords dynamic assessments of the rate and degree of signal enhancement in the first few minutes after intravenous gadolinium contrast administration (Fig. 6-2). A rapid-bolus intravenous infusion of Gd-DTPA contrast, combined with a rapid imaging sequence protocol such as FLASH (fast low-angle shot), allows the accurate measurement of signal change as a function of time, generally referred to as time-enhancement or "time-intensity" curves. The slope of the time-intensity enhancement curve has been shown to be quantitatively predictive, at least in its early rising phase, of the severity of the underlying synovitis (Figs. 6-3 and 6-4).

The underlying concept of dynamic contrast enhancement being a useful method for evaluation of synovitis is that temporal changes in the signal intensity, which are measurable immediately after bolus intravenous contrast injection, reflect a rapid increase in the local concentration of the contrast molecules within the affected

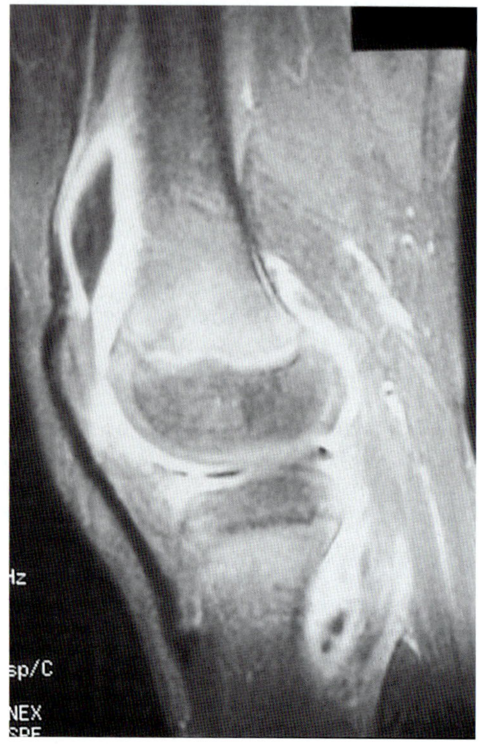

FIGURE 6-2. Fat-suppressed, T1-weighted, spin-echo MR image obtained within minutes of intravenous administration of Gd-DPTA in a patient with JRA. There is intense, bright and uniform synovial enhancement. The joint fluid is still of low signal. (Courtesy of Dr. J. Blebea, University of Pennsylvania, School of Medicine.)

tissues. In turn, the increased gadolinium concentration within the inflamed synovium reflected in the time-intensity curve is believed to be in proportion to the severity of the underlying disease processes—such as capillary permeability, overall tissue perfusion, and increased (abnormal) tissue vascularity. The relative contribution of each of these individual pathophysiologic factors to the overall degree of signal enhancement or to the slope of the rising phase of the time-enhancement curve effect is unknown, which is why some consider MRI contrast enhancement in RA to be a "black box" effect. Because the contrast enhancement time-intensity curve tends to saturate quickly after contrast injection, attention has been focused on analyzing the early, or rising limb of the curve (Fig. 6-5).

Measurement of dynamic enhancement, as recently reviewed by Farrant and associates,[27,28] typically involves investigator selection of a region of interest for analysis, as well as the use of a rapid signal method, such as FLASH, combined with a discrete small-volume contrast bolus injection. While the rate of signal change *immediately after contrast administration* can discriminate between active and inactive synovitis, later enhancement is less of a discriminator, because increased capillary permeability and neovascularization lead to a high degree of overall signal enhancement in nearly all RA patients.[29] As such, for the purpose of evaluation of synovitis, there is a consensus that all imaging should be performed as fast as possible, and ideally within the first 5 minutes after injection.[4,27,28]

A few studies have provided histologic verification of the value of synovial enhancement as a surrogate marker for the severity of synovitis. In a biopsy study of 21 patients, Gaffrey and colleagues[30] showed that the dynamic rate of enhancement in MRI correlates well with histologic features of acute inflammation ($P < .01$) on synovial biopsy, but only poorly with laboratory and rheumatologists' clinical assessments in patients with RA. This reflects the general observation that MRI is more accurate than either clinical examination or laboratory testing in RA, both of which have previously been shown to underestimate the severity of disease.[24]

In addition to using the rate of synovial enhancement as a surrogate marker for disease severity, volumetric assessment of the synovium has also been shown to be

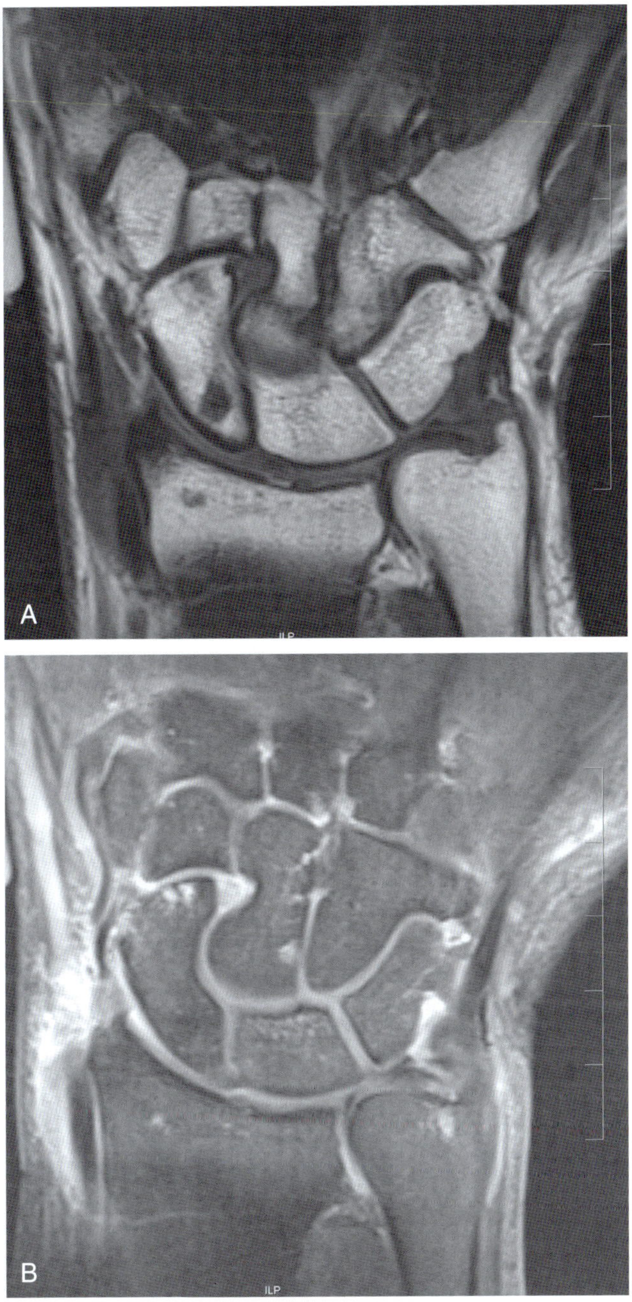

FIGURE 6-3. T1-weighted images of the wrist of a patient with RA obtained at 3.0T. **A,** Note scattered erosions and pannus appearing of intermediate signal intensity on the precontrast image. **B,** This image was obtained after intravenous administration of Gd-DTPA and utilizes fat suppression. Note the bright synovial enhancement, evidence of tenosynovitis, and enhancement within the erosions. (Courtesy of Dr. J. Tehranzadeh, University of California, Irvine.)

a useful quantity to measure in the evaluation of response to treatment. As noted earlier, by delineating the margins of the inflamed synovium immediately after intravenous contrast administration, MRI can readily yield a quantitative estimate of the *volume* of vascularized (i.e., "enhancing") inflamed synovium. In so doing, contrast-enhanced MRI can facilitate quantification and measurement of a distinct and responsive indicator of synovitis in RA.[31] A few relevant observations regarding this phenomenon are consistently observed:

- Synovial volume is significantly increased in active RA.
- Synovial volume decreases with effective treatment.
- Predictive value is greatest when both signal enhancement and synovial volume are studied.

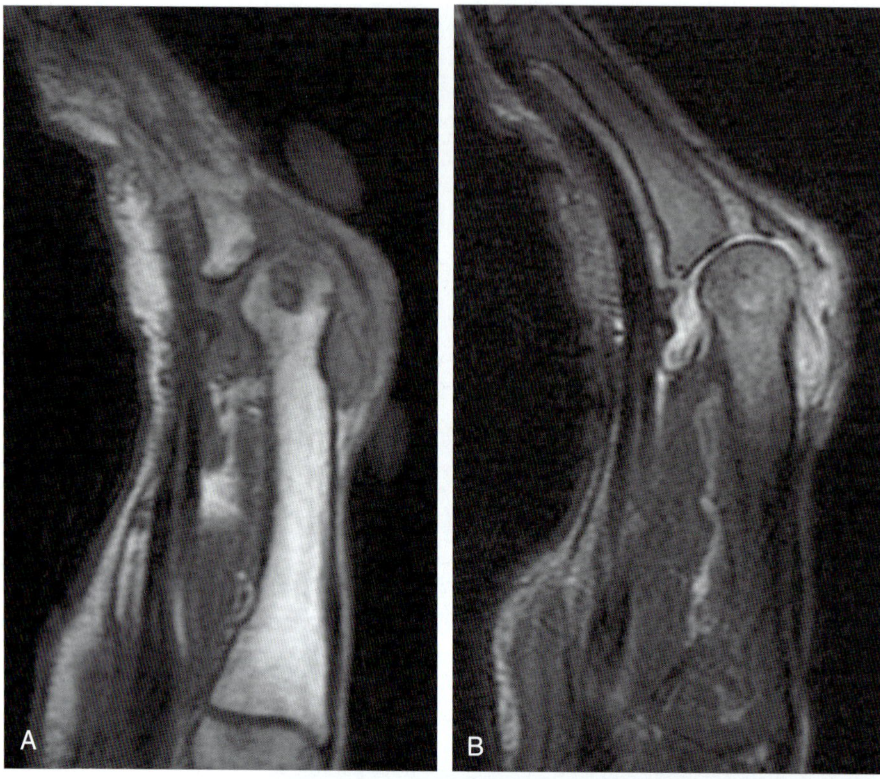

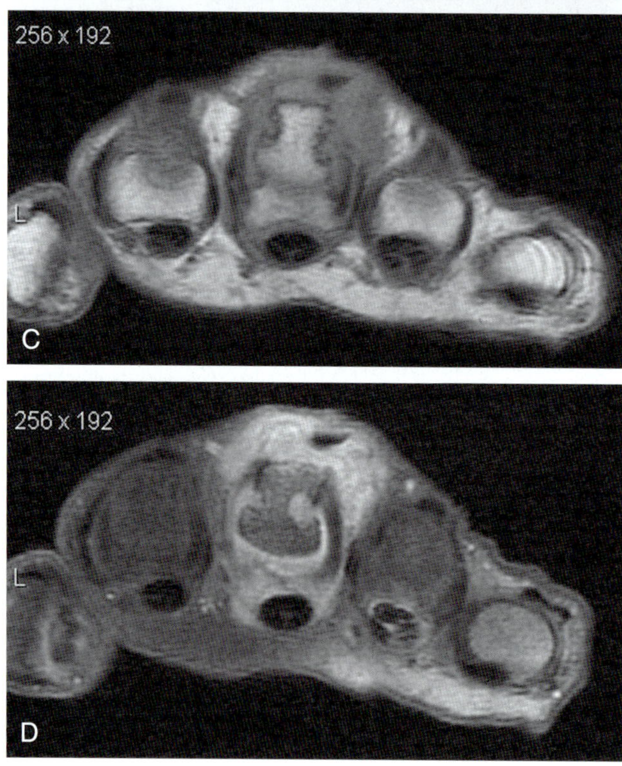

FIGURE 6-4. **A,** T1-weighted sagittal image showing erosions and pannus in RA. **B,** T1-weighted sagittal image obtained with fat suppression and after administration of Gd-DTPA. T1-weighted (**C**) and fat-suppressed T1-weighted images after administration of Gd-DTPA. (**D**) Note extensive, homogeneous bright enhancement within the synovial pannus and both flexor and extensor tendon sheaths, indicating synovitis and tenosynovitis, and enhancement within the articular erosions seen within the third metacarpal head. Findings are characteristic of the MRI appearance of RA. (Courtesy of Dr. J. Tehranzadeh, University of California, Irvine.)

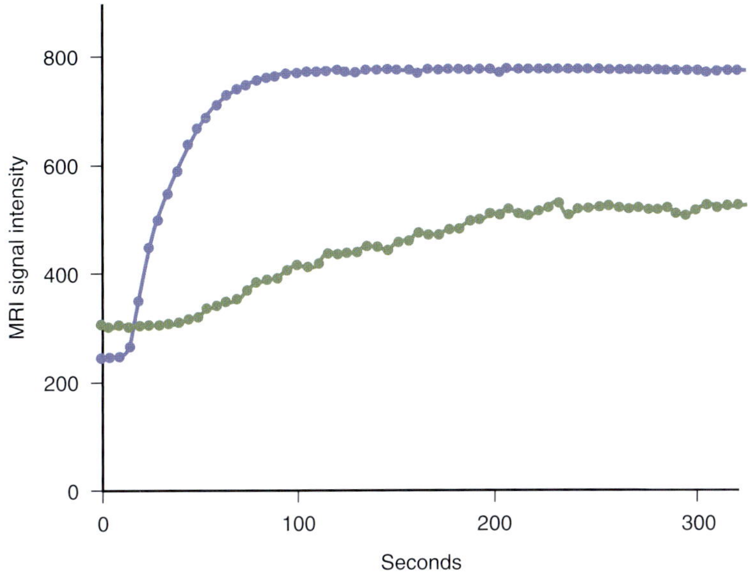

FIGURE 6-5. Typical time-intensity enhancement curve. The graph depicts the rate of change in MR signal within a selected synovial region of interest in a patient with RA, comparing the degree of enhancement in the same patient before and after treatment. Green dots are from a contrast-enhanced MRI study obtained before initiation of treatment with DMARD, and the blue-dotted curve was obtained in the same patient 5 weeks after initiation of clinically effective treatment. Note the striking change in the initial (rising) phase of the curve, as well as the overall degree of enhancement (arbitrary units). (Reprinted with permission from Peterfy CG. MRI of the wrist in rheumatoid arthritis. Semin Muscle Radiol 2001; 5:275-288.)

Huh and associates[32] quantitatively estimated the "inflamed synovial volume" by MRI in a study of 16 patients using hand-drawn regions of interest and demonstrated a significant difference between clinical remission and non-remission groups ($P < .05$) with excellent inter-reader reliability. In this elegant study, contrast-enhanced, fat-suppressed, 3D, spoiled gradient-recalled acquisition (SPGR) with thin slices and high tissue contrast was utilized, showing a brisk decrease in synovial volume after effective treatment with disease-modifying antirheumatic drugs (DMARDs). Typically, the response to effective treatment is evident on MRI within 2 weeks. Both the early dynamic enhancement and synovial volume assessment quantitatively respond to therapy-induced changes.[5,33]

Synovial volume measurements also appear to correlate well with ultrasound assessment of synovitis in RA. Terslev and coworkers[34] published a study comparing MRI measures of RA synovitis with those of ultrasonography in 29 patients. Contrast-enhanced synovial thickness was compared with the Doppler ultrasound resistive index (see Chapter 5), showing a good correlation between estimated synovial volume on MRI and an established ultrasonographic method of evaluating synovitis and its underlying neovascularization.

With regard to quantitative MRI methods, there are, however, significant issues of reproducibility and reliability. The process of manually selecting regions of interest for analysis is time consuming and introduces a component of subjectivity to the assessment. Automation of the process will be needed to make it into a clinically practical tool. It is perhaps because of the subjectivity inherent in the region of interest selection that several studies utilizing these methods have yielded interobserver reliability that is only fair to moderate as shown by κ statistics.[35]

THE OMERACT: TOWARD STANDARDIZATION OF MRI IN RA

As was mentioned in Chapter 5, an informal international research group known as OMERACT (Outcome Measurement in Rheumatoid Arthritis Clinical Trials) is focusing on the development of an international consensus for the standardization of all forms of patient assessment in RA, including development of standardized scoring systems for all modalities of imaging, as well as consensus standards for laboratory values and clinical questionnaires and examination techniques. Within the larger organization there are several focus groups composed of experts in each of the subtopics of interest to the group as a whole. One focus group within OMERACT has been primarily on the application of MRI to RA and to the developing of a standardized scoring system through which MRI data from multiple clinical trials could be pooled. This group has met every 2 years since 1992 and has periodically published papers outlining the current status of the work and future directions.[36-38]

Finding Consensus Outcome Measures in Rheumatology—The "OMERACT Filter"

A unique and extremely practical contribution toward consensus in this field was suggested at the original OMERACT conference in 1992. It was an intellectual discipline that has become known as "The OMERACT filter." The idea is simply that any potential research tool or measurement that is useful for clinical trials in RA will only be acceptable if it can pass the OMERACT filter in its intended setting. The OMERACT filter itself is summarized in three words: *truth, discrimination*, and *feasibility*. Each represents a question to be answered of the proposed new outcome measure in each of its intended settings:

1. *Truth*: Is the measure truthful, that is, does it actually measure what it intends to measure? Is the result unbiased and relevant?
2. *Discrimination*: Does the measure discriminate between situations that are of interest? The situations can be states at one time (for classification or prognosis) or states at different times (to measure change).
3. *Feasibility:* Can the measure be applied easily, given constraints of time, money, and interpretability to a clinical trial?

In 2001, the OMERACT special interest group for MRI published a set of working recommendations for imaging and scoring of MRI studies in RA. These included image acquisition specifications, definitions of lesions to be scored, and an MRI scoring system, which has become known as the RAMRIS.[38] The RAMRIS has already been applied in published studies and is a tool of recognized value. Since the RAMRIS was published, a European organization known as EULAR (European League Against Rheumatism) has combined with the OMERACT interest group to develop an even larger consensus in MRI definitions and standardized MRI methods, including a new standardized reference atlas, known as the EULAR-OMERACT RA MRI reference image atlas. This atlas of standard MR images is based on a standardized "core set" of MR imaging sequences and is itself intended to provide a standardized semiquantitative assessment tool through which patients' images can be compared with standard reference images.[37] Considerable international effort has been expended by experts in the field to the development of this new MR image atlas. The effectiveness of the atlas and visual image comparison being proposed as the basis of clinical trials in RA has yet to be proven, although similar strategies have been successfully applied to other types of image-based assessments in radiology.[39]

The OMERACT Definitions of RA Synovitis and Erosion on MRI

The OMERACT definition of synovitis on MRI is somewhat vague in that it specifies the identification of an area of the synovium that shows "above normal gadolinium enhancement" of a thickness "greater than the width of the normal synovium."[36] Unfortunately, no accepted value exists for the normal synovial thickness! The OMERACT definition of an erosion on MRI is more straightforward. It is "a sharply marginated bone lesion, with the correct juxta-articular location and typical signal characteristics, which is visible in at least two planes and with a cortical break seen in at least one plane."

Although a fully comprehensive consensus on several topics has yet to be achieved by OMERACT in MRI, the major goal stated at the formation of the group has already been realized, namely, to demonstrate the utility of the modality as a powerful assessment tool capable of providing outcomes measures in RA. By achieving further consensus on MRI techniques, including image acquisition protocols and definitions, it should be possible in future years for researchers using MRI methods to pool data on thousands of patients derived from clinical trials performed worldwide.

FUTURE DIRECTIONS FOR MRI IN RHEUMATOID ARTHRITIS

Parametric Imaging

Parametric imaging is a general term that refers to any quantitative technique in which a 2D image or "map" is created that depicts a *measured or derived numerical index,* or quantifiable "parameter," as that parameter is distributed anatomically. As an example, MRI T2 cartilage mapping is an example of parametric imaging used in the study of osteoarthritis that is discussed in Chapter 8. Typically, the parametric index map is of substantially lower spatial resolution than typical medical images. For anatomic correlation, therefore, the parametric map is often displayed as a color overlay onto gray-scale images, creating a composite or "fused" image that contains easily recognized anatomic landmarks as well as displaying the anatomic distribution and value (or range of values) of the measured or derived parameter.

Recently, Kubassova and colleagues at the School of Computing, University of Leeds and the Academic Unit of Medical Physics of the Leeds General Infirmary[40] published a paper describing a new automated parametric imaging approach to dynamic contrast enhancement in RA. This is a contrast MRI method that requires the use of dynamic Gd-DTPA enhancement and generation of time-intensity curves. Preprocessing and postprocessing computational methods are used to determine the values of a set of previously chosen features of the early enhancement kinetics of the inflamed synovium. The method represents a novel type of parametric image mapping—one in which the chosen parameters are not straightforward or even completely understood but instead are examples of so-called *black box* parameters—a term the researchers use to signify that the value of the parameters as related to their underlying physiology and their true relationship to the disease processes that determine their value are strictly unknown or undefined. Rather than attempting to first choose a particular physiologic parameter in RA and then attempt to measure its spatial variations and map it anatomically, these experiments approach the problem from the reverse perspective and study various different parameters to attempt to discover which features of the dataset may (or may not) be *empirically relevant* to the pathophysiology of disease.

In this experiment, time-intensity curves were derived from rapid-sequence SPGR imaging of the joints of patients with active RA after bolus Gd-DTPA administration. Once obtained, the enhancement image data were subjected, voxel-by-voxel, to various mathematical algorithms to determine the value of each of the two parameters of interest: (1) the maximum rate of enhancement, which the authors' abbreviate "ME," and (2) the initial rate of enhancement, abbreviated "IRE." Both of these test parameters are mathematically related to the slope of the early enhancement curve. The parametric maps thus derived are merged with the anatomic MR image of the inflamed joints in RA. Blood vessels, soft tissues outside of the joints, and the central, extra-articular portion of the bones were excluded from the analysis by automated selection of regions of interest. The final images are subsequently assembled that fuse the parametric data to the conventional, anatomic MR images (Fig. 6-6).

The approach was designed to begin to explore which features of the MRI time-intensity curves might ultimately be the most relevant to the evaluation of disease activity assessment, as well as to address the many technical difficulties inherent to such a computationally intense, automated approach. Although the value of the chosen indices, the ME or IRE, in the assessment of disease severity and treatment response remains to be demonstrated, future experience with these or other so-called black box parameters may prove to be of great value, both for clinical application and to further clarify basic features of the disease process.

USPIO Nanoparticle Imaging

It is known that synovial macrophages play a significant role in the inflammatory processes in RA and that the abundance and activity of macrophages within the joint pannus correlate significantly with the clinical severity of RA (see Fig. 6-6).[41] Newly developed nanoparticle contrast media, known as "ultrasmall superparamagnetic iron oxide" (USPIO) particles, have been shown to localize to the synovial macrophages in RA. Within the joints, the nanoparticles provide significant MRI "negative" contrast, with signal loss on T2-weighted imaging due to T2 shortening caused by their magnetic susceptibility. This negative contrast effect is highly localized to the specific areas of macrophage accumulation within affected joints and appears to be

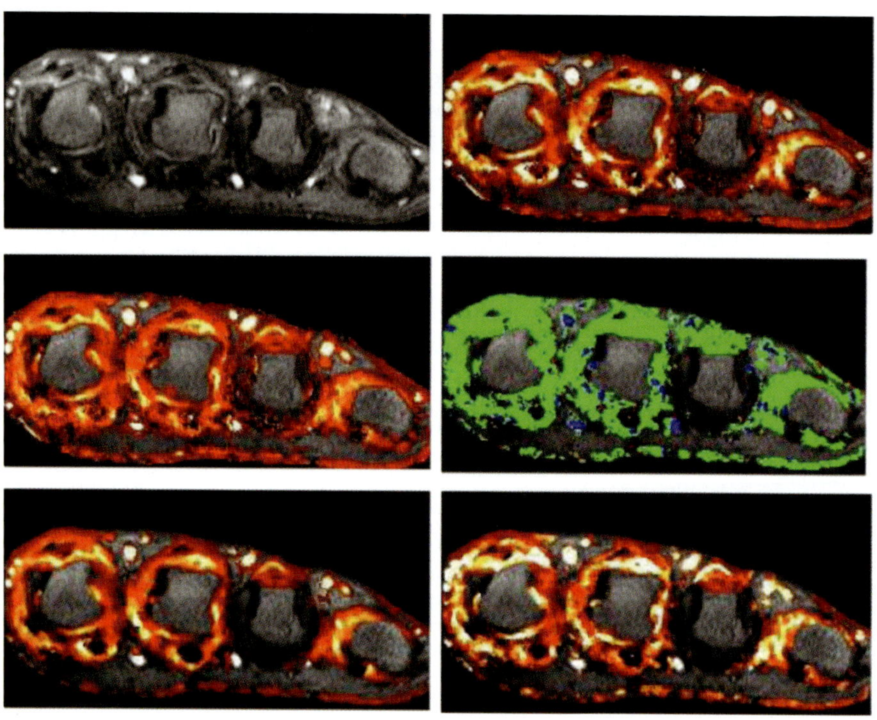

FIGURE 6-6. Parametric maps from contrast-enhanced MRI of the MCP joints in RA. ***Top,*** T1-weighted postcontrast image, parametric map of the "ME" parameter (see text). ***Middle,*** Parametric map of the "IRE" parameter (see text), and overall Gd-DTPA uptake map (*in green*). ***Bottom,*** Parametric maps of "ME" (*left*) and "IRE" (*right*) with additional postprocessing steps added to compensate for motion and other artifacts. The images demonstrate the ability to display dynamic contrast data in ways that may increase diagnostic accuracy. (Reprinted with permission from Kubassova OA, Boyle RD, Radjenovic A. Quantitative analysis of dynamic contrast-enhanced MRI datasets of the metacarpophalangeal joints. Acad Radiol 2007; 14:1189-1200.)

quantitatively measurable. A full discussion of these agents and their various applications in MRI is well beyond the scope of this chapter, but it is noteworthy that a few early studies using animal models of RA have shown promise in the use of this type of cellular-based "contrast" agent.[42,43] Quantitative imaging using USPIO particles in humans is therefore likely to be a fruitful avenue for investigation over the next several years.

SUMMARY

The advantages of MRI in rheumatoid arthritis include:

- Sensitive detection of erosions and pre-erosive changes—and discrimination between the two
- Qualitative and quantitative assessments of synovitis
- Assessment of immediate and delayed responses to treatment
- Evaluation of adjacent soft tissues, including ligaments and tendons, useful for evaluation of comorbidities and prediction of outcomes

Future research is likely to emphasize:

- Refined technical standardization of MRI techniques and improved interobserver reliability in MRI clinical trials
- Greater consensus among scoring systems and outcomes measures
- More predictive parametric imaging methods
- Greater automation of quantitative measures, eliminating human error and unintended biases
- Use of novel contrast agents, such as USPIO particles, for quantification
- Clarification of the relative importance of, and relationship between, joint erosions and the various measures of synovitis

References

1. Wakefield FJ, Gibbon WW, Conaghan PG, et al. The value of sonography in the detection of bone erosions in patients with rheumatoid arthritis: a comparison with conventional radiography. Arthritis Rheum 2000; 43:2762-2770.
2. Backhaus T, Kamradt D, Sandrock D, et al. Arthritis of the finger joints: a comprehensive approach comparing conventional radiography, scintigraphy, ultrasound, and contrast-enhanced magnetic resonance imaging. Arthritis Rheum 1999; 42:1232-1245.
3. Hoving JL, Buchbinder R, Hall S, et al. A comparison of magnetic resonance imaging, sonography and radiography of the hand in patients with early rheumatoid arthritis. J Rheumaol 2004; 31:663-675.
4. Ostergaard M, Hansen M, Stoltenberg M, et al. New radiographic bone erosions in the wrists of patients with rheumatoid arthritis are detectable with magnetic resonance imaging a median of 2 years earlier. Arthritis Rheum 2003; 48:2128-2131.
5. Ostergaard M, Ejbjerg B, Szkudlarek M. Imaging in early rheumatoid arthritis: roles of magnetic resonance imaging, ultrasonography, conventional radiography and computed tomography. Best Pract Res Clin Rheumatol 2005; 19:91-116.
6. Sharp JT, Young DY, Bluhm GB, et al. How many joints in the hands and wrists should be included in a score of radiologic abnormalities used to assess rheumatoid arthritis? Arthritis Rheum 1985; 28:1326-1335.
7. Sharp JT, Wolfe F, Mitchell DM, et al. The progression of erosion and joint space narrowing scores in rheumatoid arthritis during the first twenty-five years of disease. Arthritis Rheum 1991; 34:660-668.
8. Sharp JT. Scoring radiographic abnormalities in rheumatoid arthritis. Radiol Clin North Am 1996; 34:233-241.
9. Genant HK. Methods of assessing radiographic change in rheumatoid arthritis. Am J Med 1983; 5:35-47.
10. Genant HK, Jiang Y, Peterfy C, et al. Assessment of rheumatoid arthritis using a modified scoring method on digitized and original radiographs. Arthritis Rheum 1998; 41:1583-1590.
11. Kaye JJ, Nance EP, Calahan LF, Carroll FE. Observer variation in quantitative assessment of rheumatoid arthritis: II. A simplified scoring system. Invest Radiol 1987; 22:41-46.

12. Pincus T, Larsen A, Brooks RH, et al. Comparison of 3 quantitative measures of hand radiographs in patients with rheumatoid arthritis: Seinbrocker stage, Kaye modified Sharp score and Larsen score. J Rheumat 1997; 24:2106-2112.
13. Kirwan JR. The relationship between synovitis and erosions in rheumatoid arthritis. Br J Rheumatol 1997; 36:225-228.
14. McGonagle D, Conaghan PG, O'Connor P, et al. The relationship between synovitis and bone changes in early untreated rheumatoid arthritis: a controlled magnetic resonance imaging study. Arthritis Rheum 1999; 42:1706-1711.
15. McQueen FM, Benton N, Crabbe J, et al. What is the fate of erosions in early rheumatoid arthritis? Tracking individual lesions using x rays and magnetic resonance imaging over the first two years of disease. Ann Rheum Dis 2001; 60:859-868.
16. Teh J, Stevens K, Williamson L, et al. Power Doppler ultrasound of rheumatoid synovitis: quantification of therapeutic response. Br J Radiol 2003; 76:875-879.
17. Tonolli-Sesubin I, Poet JL, Dufour M, et al. Magnetic resonance imaging of the wrist in rheumatoid arthritis: comparison with other inflammatory joint diseases and control subjects. Clin Rheumatol 1996; 15:137-142.
18. Peterfy CG. MRI of the wrist in rheumatoid arthritis. Semin Musculoskelet Radiol 2001; 5:275-288.
19. Guermazi A, Taouli B, Lynch J, et al. Imaging of bone erosion in rheumatoid arthritis. Semin Musculoskelet Radiol 2004; 98:269-285.
20. Conaghan PG, O'Connor P, McGonagle D, et al. Elucidation of the relationship between synovitis and bone damage: a randomized magnetic resonance imaging study of individual joints in patients with early rheumatoid arthritis. Arthritis Rheum 2003; 48:64-71.
21. Gibbon WW. Applications of ultrasound in arthritis [Review]. Semin Musculoskelet Radiol 2004; 8:313-328.
22. Tehranzadeh J, Ashikyan O, Anavim A, et al. Enhanced MR imaging of tenosynovitis of hand and wrist in inflammatory arthritis. Skeletal Radiol 2006; 35:814-822.
23. McQueen FM, Stewart N, Crabbe J, et al. Magnetic resonance imaging of the wrist in early rheumatoid arthritis reveals a high prevalence of erosions at four months after symptom onset. Ann Rheum Dis 1998; 57:330-336.
24. McQueen FM, Stewart N, Crabbe J, et al. Magnetic Resonance Imaging of the wrist in early rheumatoid arthritis reveals progression of erosions despite clinical improvement. Ann Rheum Dis 1999; 58:156-163.
25. Gasson T, Gandy SJ, Huber CW, et al. MRI of RA in the MCP joints. Skeletal Radiol 2000; 29:324-334.
26. Ejbjerg B, Narvestad E, Rostrup E, et al. Magnetic resonance imaging of wrist and finger joints in healthy subjects occasionally shows changes resembling erosions and synovitis as seen in rheumatoid arthritis. Arthritis Rheum 2004; 50:1097-1106.
27. Farrant JM, O'Connor PJ, Grainger AJ. Advanced imaging in rheumatoid arthritis: I. Synovitis [Review]. Skeletal Radiol 2007; 36:269-279.
28. Farrant JM, Grainger AJ, O'Connor PJ. Advanced imaging in rheumatoid arthritis: II. Erosions [Review]. Skeletal Radiol 2007; 36:381-389.
29. Szkudlarek M, Narvestad E, Klarlund M, et al. Ultrasonography of the metatarsophalangeal joints in rheumatoid arthritis: a comparison with magnetic resonance imaging, conventional radiography, and clinical examination. Arthritis Rheum 2004; 50:2103-2112.
30. Gaffney K, Cookson J, Blake D, et al. Quantification of rheumatoid synovitis by magnetic resonance imaging. Arthritis Rheum 1995; 38:1610-1617.
31. Tehranzadeh J, Ashikyan O, Dascalos J. Magnetic resonance imaging in early detection of rheumatoid arthritis. Semin Musculoskelet Radiol 2003; 7:79-94.
32. Huh YM, Suh JS, Jeong EK, et al. Role of the inflamed synovial volume of the wrist in defining remission of rheumatoid arthritis with gadolinium-enhanced 3D-SPGR MR imaging. J Magn Res Imaging 1999; 10:202-208.
33. Ribbens C, Andrew B, Marcelis S, et al. Rheumatoid hand joint synovitis: gray-scale and power Doppler US quantifications following anti-tumor necrosis factor-α treatment: pilot study. Radiology 2003; 229:562-569.
34. Terslev L, Torp-Pedersen S, Savnik A, et al. Doppler ultrasound and magnetic resonance imaging of synovial inflammation of the hand in rheumatoid arthritis: a comparative study. Arthritis Rheum 2003; 48:2434-2441.
35. Ostergaard M, Hansen M, Stoltenberg M, et al. Quantitative assessment of the synovial membrane in the rheumatoid wrist: an easily obtained MRI score reflects the synovial volume. Br J Rheumatol 1996; 35:965-971.
36. Ostergaard M, Peterfy C, Conghan P, et al. OMERACT rheumatoid arthritis MRI studies core set of MRI acquisitions, joint pathology, definitions, and the OMERACT RA-MRI Scoring System. J Rheumatol 2003; 30:1385-1386.
37. Bird P, Conaghan P, Ejbjerg B, et al. The development of the EULAR-OMERACT rheumatoid arthritis MRI reference image atlas. Ann Rheum Dis 2005; 64(Suppl 1):8–10.
38. Conaghan P, Edmonds J, Emery P, et al. Magnetic resonance imaging in rheumatoid arthritis: summary of OMERACT activities, current status, and plans. J Rheumatol 2001; 28:1158-1162.

39. Bruno MA, Milne ENC, Stanford W, et al. Pulmonary oligemia in aortic valve disease. Radiology 1999; 210:37-45.
40. Kubassova OA, Boyle RD, Radjenovic A. Quantitative analysis of dynamic contrast-enhanced MRI datasets of the metacarpophalangeal joints. Acad Radiol 2007; 14:1189-1200.
41. Kinne RW, Brauer R, Stuhlmuller B, et al. Macrophages in rheumatoid arthritis. Arthritis Res 2000; 2:189-202.
42. Dardzinski BJ, Schmithorst VJ, Holland SK, et al. MR imaging of murine arthritis using ultrasmall superparamagnetic iron oxide particles. J Magn Reson Imaging 2001; 19:1209-1216.
43. Simon GH, von Vopelius-Feldt J, Wendland MF, et al. MRI of arthritis: comparison of ultrasmall superparamagnetic iron oxide vs. Gd-DTPA. J Magn Reson Imaging 2006; 23:720-727.

Chapter 7

NUCLEAR (SCINTIGRAPHIC) METHODS AND FDG-PET IN RHEUMATOID ARTHRITIS AND OSTEOARTHRITIS

Clio Ribbens and Roland Hustinx

Imaging of inflammatory joint diseases remains challenging. The development in recent years of biologic treatments that are highly efficacious as well as expensive has stimulated the research for imaging of inflammation. This has been particularly true for rheumatoid arthritis (RA), which constitutes the most prevalent inflammatory arthritis, affecting 1% of the population. RA is an autoimmune systemic disease characterized by chronic inflammation of the synovium, with a massive leukocyte infiltration, proliferation of the synovial membrane, and neovascularization. The hyperplastic and hypertrophic rheumatoid synovium, termed the *pannus,* if left untreated gradually erodes the adjacent cartilage and bone, leading to joint degradation and marked disability. Although conventional radiography displays joint space narrowing and bone erosions, the hallmark of rheumatoid disease, it does not allow evaluation of the inflammatory component of the disease but only its end-stage irreversible characteristics. MRI can detect bone erosions earlier than conventional radiography and also allows the study of cartilage, tendons, and ligaments, as well as the synovium, especially after the injection of gadolinium. However, in gadolinium-enhanced MRI the uptake of the contrast agent by the inflamed synovium is also due to hypervascularization and capillary permeability. Ultrasonography is noninvasive, allows the study of many joints in one time frame, and when associated with power Doppler imaging can also give information about synovial vascularization. Although these two imaging modalities are of high value in the clinical assessment of arthritis (as discussed more fully in other chapters), they remain purely morphologic and do not provide information about cell metabolism. In this chapter we review the nuclear medicine techniques available for assessing arthritis, with a particular interest in positron emission tomography (PET).

BONE SCINTIGRAPHY

Bone scintigraphy is one of the most commonly performed procedures in nuclear medicine and is a classic imaging technique used for the investigation of bone and joint diseases. The first suitable radionuclides developed for bone scintigraphy in the early 1960s were strontium-85m, strontium-87m, and fluoride-18. Technetium-99m (^{99m}Tc)-labeled diphosphonates were introduced in the 1970s and have been used since then, the most common being ^{99m}Tc-methylene diphosphonate (MDP) and ^{99m}Tc-hydroxymethylene diphosphonate (HDP). The energy of the photon emitted by the ^{99m}Tc nuclide is well adapted to the physics properties of the current gamma cameras. Both MDP and HDP have a high affinity for bone, and approximately 50% of the dose of ^{99m}Tc-diphosphonate is distributed in the skeleton within 3 hours after intravenous administration, the remainder being excreted in the urine.[1] Their uptake in bone is related not only to osteoblastic activity but also to the regional blood flow. Accordingly, an increased uptake is seen in synovitis where there are increased blood flow, expanded blood pool volume, and vascular permeability. The hyperemia involves not only the synovial membrane but also the juxta-articular bones.[2] Therefore, although this technique is very sensitive for the detection of joint and subchondral bone abnormalities, it cannot discriminate accurately between actively inflamed joints and chronically damaged joints[3,4] and does not allow correct evaluation of inflammatory arthritis. Other radiotracers have thus been investigated for the evaluation of arthritis: gallium (^{67}Ga) citrate, indium-111 chloride ($^{111}InCl_3$), ^{99m}Tc-hexamethylpropylene amine oxime (HMPAO)-labeled leukocytes, ^{99m}Tc-liposomes, ^{99m}Tc-polyclonal human immunoglobulin G (IgG) monoclonal antibodies to granulocytes, and ^{99m}Tc-labeled anti-CD4 monoclonal antibodies.[2] Indium and gallium possess a high affinity for iron-binding proteins and probably bind to transferrin receptors abundant in the inflamed synovium, explaining their affinity for the inflammatory site compartment.[5] However, scanning with gallium necessitates a 24-hour delay before imaging, entailing two patient visits, and is associated with a relatively high radiation exposure; in addition, the image quality is limited. Other tracers used for evaluating inflammation include radiolabeled liposomes, which are phagocytosed by macrophages abundant in inflammatory sites, and radiolabeled IgG, which probably leak at the capillary bed and are trapped by Fc receptors of the inflammatory cells, targeting inflammation nonspecifically. These "inflammation-targeted" radiotracers are also used for evaluating infectious diseases and are not specific for any arthritis. The improved understanding of pathophysiologic mechanisms of disease has led to the development of new radiotracers targeting more specific markers of inflammation. Scintigraphy targeting the adhesion molecule E-selectin, expressed by activated endothelial cells in various inflammatory states and, in particular, postcapillary venules of rheumatoid synovium, has been developed and shown to be more specific for targeting active joint inflammation compared with ^{99m}Tc-MDP.[6] On the other hand, ^{99m}Tc-labeled interleukin-8 allows the detection of infection without accumulating in noninfectious inflammatory disorders.[7] Another potential target is the synovial apoptosis, which is shown to be defective in the rheumatoid synovium.[8] During apoptosis, annexin V binds to the cell membrane phospholipid phosphatidylserine, and this binding allows apoptosis imaging. Post and colleagues have shown in collagen-induced arthritis in a mouse model of RA that there is an increased uptake of annexin V in paws of arthritic animals when compared with controls.[9] Treatment with methylprednisolone for 1 week decreased annexin V uptake. Annexin V imaging in human patients with various cancers (Apomate, Theseus Imaging, Boston) has demonstrated the induction of apoptosis in the first 48 hours after chemotherapy. Patients with annexin V uptake at tumor sites had a complete or partial response, in contrast to the progressive disease in those without significant annexin V uptake, thus conferring a prognostic value to annexin V imaging.[10] Apomate could therefore be of use for evaluation of apoptosis in RA patients.

These techniques remain experimental for the time being, and bone scintigraphy with ^{99m}Tc-labeled diphosphonates remains the standard nuclear medicine approach for assessing joint involvement in a whole-body approach. Despite a low specificity and poor resolution, bone scintigraphy reveals the pattern of joint involvement and may therefore be of value, alone or in combination with other techniques, such as

MRI, in the differential diagnosis of undifferentiated arthritis.[11] Recent technologic developments, in particular the advent of gamma cameras with tomographic capabilities combined with a CT scanner (SPECT-CT) may improve the clinical usefulness of bone scintigraphy, but no data are available yet.

POSITRON EMISSION TOMOGRAPHY

Positron emission tomography (PET) is a technique using molecules labeled with isotopes that emit positrons from their nucleus. The most commonly used isotopes are fluoride-18 (^{18}F), oxygen-15 (^{15}O), nitrogen-13 (^{13}N), and carbon-11 (^{11}C). They are created in a cyclotron, a device used to accelerate charged particles to create the relatively short-lived positron-emitting isotopes. The most commonly used tracer is 2-deoxy-2-(^{18}F)fluoro-D-deoxyglucose (FDG) in which one of the hydrogens has been replaced by the ^{18}F radioisotope. After intravenous injection, FDG distributes to the extravascular compartments and is taken up by the cells according to their level of glucose metabolism. Indeed, FDG is transported through the cell membrane via glucose transporters (GLUT) into the cytosol, phosphorylated by the hexokinase, and trapped intracellularly as FDG-6-phosphate. Most tumor cells display highly increased glucose metabolism and FDG uptake, hence the numerous oncologic applications of the technique. Activated leukocytes, through different biologic processes, similarly display increased FDG uptake. The spatial resolution of the most recent clinical PET scanners is 4 to 6 mm. It is a fully tomographic technique, offering 3D visualization of the glucose metabolism. FDG-PET, therefore, presents many advantages over bone scintigraphy. Its uptake by inflammatory cells results in the direct visualization of the inflammatory synovitis rather than the indirect hyperemia detected by bone scintigraphy. Its spatial resolution and count rates are also much improved when compared with planar scintigraphy.[12] Finally, the advent of PET/CT allows for a precise anatomic location of the increased metabolic activity.

Methodologic Aspects of PET

The optimal methodology for performing and interpreting the PET/CT studies is not fully defined. To fully contribute to the diagnostic information, the CT scan should be acquired with the appropriate parameters in terms of dose and collimation, possibly with intravenous contrast agents. Whether such a full diagnostic CT is really needed in addition to the low-dose CT remains an unanswered question. Because inflammatory joint diseases often affect young patients, radiation dose has to be taken into account. By using a low-dose CT and injecting 222 to 370 MBq FDG, we obtain good quality images while keeping the equivalent dose in the 8- to 12-mSv range, which is acceptable.[13]

Although a typical pattern of synovitis is easily recognized on the PET images, quantitative measurements are desired to assess the activity of the disease and its response to treatment. As in oncologic PET, the most appropriate quantitative methods will have to be determined. The simple standard uptake value (SUV) is likely to be the best parameter. The question of which normalization (body weight, body surface area, or lean body mass) should be preferred for calculating the SUV remains to be answered, although there should not be major differences between those methods. There are indications that FDG uptake by inflammatory lesions is more influenced by blood glucose level than cancer cells.[14] In particular, glucose loading decreased the expression of the GLUT-1 transporters in noninfectious inflammatory lesions in a rat model.[15] It may therefore be critical to correct for the patient's blood glucose level.

A well-known limitation of PET stems from its limited spatial and anatomic resolutions. Although this is not a major issue regarding large joints such as the knees, it may be very difficult to identify synovitis in small joints of the hands or feet.

Indeed, these patients often also suffer from inflammation of the tendon sheaths, which may be mistaken for the pannus itself. The same problem may arise when high muscular uptake is observed. In all cases, reading such studies is a tedious and time-consuming process. Nevertheless, the reported intraobserver and extraobserver coefficients of variation are consistently low. The visual identification of the synovitis pattern was obtained with κ values of 0.90 and 0.82 (intraobserver and extraobserver variability, respectively).[16] For measuring the SUVs, the intraobserver coefficient of variation was 3.9%. The extraobserver coefficient was higher, 14.9%, and related to the type of joint, ranging from 0% in the knees to 23% in the metacarpophalangeal joints.[16] These results were obtained with a now outdated PET device, and without the help of the CT information. Palmer and coworkers obtained similarly high inter-observer agreement values.[17] These data indicate that, at least in the context of a prospective study, the metabolic activity of the inflamed synovium may be reproducibly quantified. The added value of PET/CT over PET is likely to be significant but remains to be fully evaluated.

PET in Preclinical Models of Inflammation

Although the uptake of FDG by malignant tumors is the basis for FDG-PET in the evaluation of cancer, false-positive findings have been encountered in inflammatory pathologic processes.[18] Animal models have demonstrated that FDG uptake by tumors is not only due to the tumor cells themselves but also to the inflammatory cells appearing in association with growth or necrosis of the tumor. FDG accumulation was higher in macrophages and young granulation tissues than in the tumor cells in mice transplanted subcutaneously with malignant tumors.[19] Up to 29% of the glucose utilization was derived from nontumor tissue in these lesions.[19] Microautoradiographic studies of transplanted tumors in mice revealed a higher and faster FDG uptake in the newly formed granulation tissue around the tumor and in macrophages than in viable tumor cells, allowing a differentiation between neoplastic and non-neoplastic cells using dynamic analysis of FDG uptake.[20] A turpentine-induced model of inflammation in rats also demonstrated a FDG uptake in the inflammatory tissue, in the zone surrounding the abscess wall consisting of young fibroblasts, endothelial cells, macrophages, and neutrophils.[21] This suggests that macrophages and neutrophils in inflammatory tissue utilize glucose as an energy source for chemotaxis and phagocytosis while fibroblasts also use glucose for proliferation. This glucose utilization by inflammatory cells is made possible by their increased expression of glucose transporters when they are activated.[22,23] In conclusion, these data demonstrate the increased glucose metabolism of many inflammatory cell types and the FDG uptake by inflammatory tissues and are the basis for the use of FDG-PET in the detection and monitoring of chronic inflammatory pathologic processes.[18]

PET in Animal Models

PET can be useful for studying mechanisms of arthritis. Many animal models of RA have been developed and have given an insight into the pathophysiologic mechanisms of arthritis. The K/BxN murine model of RA is characterized by the spontaneous development of a chronic polyarthritis in mice expressing the transgenic KRN T-cell receptor on the nonobese diabetic (NOD) genetic background. The transfer of K/BxN autoantibodies specific for glucose-6-phosphate isomerase (GPI) into naive mice of most strains can induce the acute symptoms of arthritis. This joint selectivity of anti-GPI antibodies is surprising in view of the ubiquitous expression of GPI. By using PET to track the movement and accumulation of GPI-specific antibodies in vivo, Wipke and associates have shown that the autoantibodies localize specifically to distal joints in the front and rear limbs within minutes of intravenous injection, in contrast to control IgG.[24] This joint-specific localization of a ubiquitously expressed self-antigen expands our understanding of autoimmunity; that is, a tissue-specific autoimmune response can be directed against an antigen whose expression is not limited to specific tissues.[24]

PET in Rheumatoid Arthritis

The first reports of accumulation of FDG in inflamed joints were incidental findings in two patients evaluated for cancer screening or follow-up.[25,26] In a patient with thyroid cancer and RA, the FDG uptake was noted not only in the inflamed joints but also in lung rheumatoid nodules devoid of any malignant or infectious process.[26] Palmer and colleagues reported more than 10 years ago the ability of PET to quantify joint inflammation in patients with inflammatory arthritis of the wrist.[17] Nine patients with RA and 3 with psoriatic arthritis exhibiting active disease and observable synovitis of the wrist were evaluated by clinical examination, MRI, and PET. Patients were evaluated after a washout period for nonsteroidal anti-inflammatory drugs, 2 weeks after treatment with a nonsteroidal anti-inflammatory drug or with low-dose steroid (10 mg prednisone daily), and finally 12 to 14 weeks after treatment with low-dose methotrexate (5-10 mg weekly). All baseline PET images demonstrated increased metabolic activity in the wrist, mainly in the radiocarpal and distal radioulnar joints, but also in the different tendon sheaths. The regions of greatest FDG uptake on PET images corresponded to the presence of enhancing pannus on MRI. Quantitative assessments found a significant linear correlation between the volume of enhancing pannus (VEP) measured by MRI and total uptake value (TUV) as well as regional uptake value (RUV) of FDG measured by PET. Clinical measurements of inflammation in the imaged wrist (pain, tenderness, and swelling) were closely correlated with VEP, RUV, and TUV.[17] This correlation between PET evaluation of synovitis and MRI measurement of pannus in an individual joint has been confirmed in knee synovitis by our group.[27] We evaluated knee synovitis in 16 patients with active RA by clinical examination, PET, ultrasonography, and MRI, all being conducted by independent assessors within 4 days. Physical examination determined the presence of swelling and of tenderness. PET acquisition was started 93 minutes on average after intravenous injection of the tracer (4 MBq/kg), and knee positivity was determined by the uptake of FDG in areas presumed to correspond to joint synovium. The metabolic activity was quantified using the maximum pixel value of the SUV normalized for the lean body mass. Ultrasonography was performed using a B-mode 13-MHz transducer, and positivity was defined as a synovitis of 1-mm thickness.[28] Positivity for MRI was visually appreciated, and synovitis was defined as enhancement of thickness greater than the width of the joint capsule after gadolinium injection. Dynamic MRI allowed the measurement of the relative enhancement at 30 seconds after gadolinium injection (RE_{30}) in the external and internal recesses, as well as the rate of early enhancement at 55 seconds after gadolinium injection (REE_{55}), parameters shown to be related to active RA.[29] Knee synovitis was found to be present in 13 of the 16 knees by clinical evaluation, 11 knees by PET (Fig. 7-1), 11 by MRI, and 12 by ultrasonography. Positivity on one imaging technique was significantly associated with positivity on the other two. In comparison with PET-negative knees, PET-positive knees displayed higher SUVs, higher MRI parameters, and higher ultrasound-determined synovial thickness. SUVs were significantly correlated to MRI parameters, synovial thickness, and serum levels of C-reactive protein and matrix metalloproteinase-3, a synovial-derived parameter reflecting joint inflammation.[30] These correlations suggest strong relationships between the size of synovitis measured by ultrasonography, its metabolic activity measured by PET, and also its vascularization and leukocyte infiltration shown to be correlated with the dynamic MRI parameters.[31,32] Roivanen and coworkers[33] have also shown a correlation between MRI assessment of synovitis and PET assessment using not only FDG, a marker of inflammation, but also ^{11}C-choline, an indirect

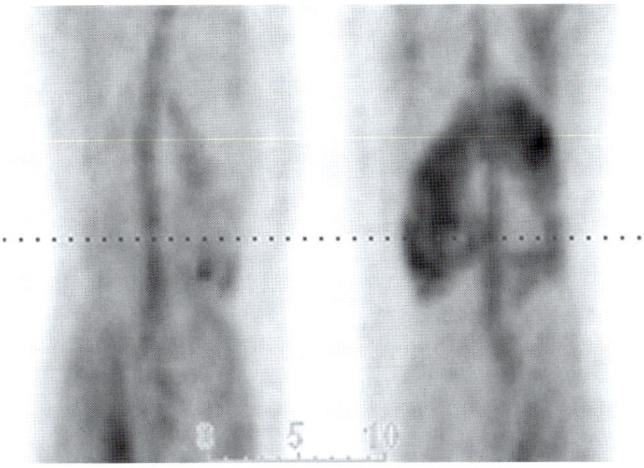

FIGURE 7-1. Three-dimensional projection image of both knees. The highly active synovitis is clearly visualized in the left knee, whereas the right one appears normal.

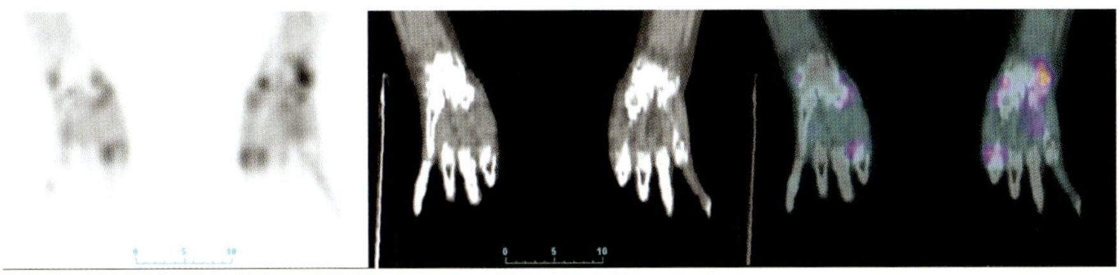

FIGURE 7-2. FDG-PET/CT study in a patient with RA (coronal sections). The PET images (*left*) show various foci of increased FDG uptake in the wrists and in the metacarpophalangeal joints of both hands, which are precisely localized on the CT (*middle*) and fused PET/CT (*right*) images. Note that this patient was unable to completely extend her fingers, thus explaining the incomplete visualization of all fingers in these sectional images.

marker of cellular proliferation. In all 10 patients with clinical symptoms, high uptakes of both ^{11}C-choline and FDG were noted at the site of the arthritic synovium compared with the unaffected joint. The location of the highest uptakes of ^{11}C-choline and FDG corresponded to the presence of proliferating synovium on MR images. PET can therefore assess the metabolic activity of synovitis, not only because the inflammatory cells have an increased uptake of glucose but also because the pannus contains rapidly proliferating cells that contain large amounts of phospholipids, particularly phosphatidylcholine.

Although these studies have demonstrated a correlation between PET evaluation of synovitis and ultrasonographic or MRI measurements of pannus in an individual joint, PET has the advantage over the two other imaging techniques to allow a global evaluation of all joints in a polyarticular disease such as RA. We have shown this in 21 patients suffering from active RA.[16] The patients were studied by clinical joint examination, ultrasonography, and PET, with all examinations being performed in a 48-hour time frame. Knees were evaluated in all patients in addition to either wrists and hands (metacarpophalangeal and proximal interphalangeal joints) or ankles and the first metatarsophalangeal joints according to clinical complaints. Figure 7-2 illustrates the precise identification of wrist and metacarpophalangeal inflammation in a patient. Sixty-three percent of joints were PET positive in the RA patients, in contrast to none in control subjects. PET positivity was closely correlated to positivity by ultrasonography (1-mm synovial thickness) and by clinical examination (tender or swollen joints). The proportion of PET-positive joints increased with the number of abnormal clinical and ultrasonographic parameters: 41% when only one parameter (swelling, tenderness or increased ultrasound synovial thickness) was present, 53% when two were present, and 90% when all three were present. PET positivity was more frequently found in knees with a synovitis (82%) than in knees with only an effusion (37%). The synovial thickness measured by ultrasonography was significantly higher in PET-positive knees (mean, 8.2 mm) than in PET-negative knees (mean, 2.9 mm), and synovial thickness was significantly correlated with SUVs except in the first metatarsophalangeal joints. PET positivity was also more frequently found in joints with a positive Doppler signal (96%) than without (83%). A global RA PET activity index was generated by calculating the number of PET-positive joints per patient as well as the cumulative SUV, that is, the sum of SUVs in PET-positive joints, in patients with knee and hand evaluations. Both parameters were highly correlated to the number of tender and swollen joints, patient's and physician's global assessment scores, biologic parameters of inflammation (erythrocyte sedimentation rate and C-reactive protein levels), ultrasound parameters (number of ultrasound-positive joints and the cumulative synovial thickness), and the composite indices of RA disease activity (DAS_{28} and SDAI).[34,35] PET is therefore a suitable quantitative method for evaluating metabolism of multiple joints in RA patients. A limitation of PET can be the lack of anatomic details when small joints are evaluated. Indeed, based on the metabolic images, it is not possible to ascertain whether the foci of increased activity correspond to the synovitis, tendon sheaths, or even muscle. Such uncertainty is greatly reduced with the newer PET/CT devices, which provide high-quality CT images (millimetric slices) coupled with the corresponding PET images. Although comparative studies have yet to be published, such devices are likely to increase the interobserver agreement, simplify the image interpretation, and possibly improve the diagnostic performances.

PET in Psoriatic Arthritis

The first report of FDG uptake in psoriatic arthritis–affected joints was, as for RA, in a patient undergoing PET for cancer evaluation.[36] A 58-year-old woman with a history of psoriatic arthritis referred for FDG-PET evaluation of lymphoma after chemotherapy reported a recurrence of arthritic pain in her hands and wrists, her methotrexate treatment had been stopped for a year. There was an excellent correlation between the areas of arthritic pain and the regions of increased FDG uptake in her hands, evaluated 130 minutes after injection.[36] We have prospectively assessed knee synovitis in 17 patients with active psoriatic arthritis.[37] A typical pattern of synovitis was identified in 13 joints of 9 patients. Two patterns of FDG uptake were observed, with a maximum activity of the inflamed synovium at 2 minutes after injection in 4 knees and at 16 minutes in 9 knees. In all cases, the SUV_{max} did not significantly vary thereafter, with similar values at 28, 40, and 76 minutes, indicating that the beginning of acquisition may be shortened to 30 minutes when evaluating inflammatory joint disease.[37] Interestingly enough, active cutaneous psoriasis lesions display highly increased glucose metabolism, as shown in Figure 7-3.

PET in Osteoarthritis

Few data are available in the literature concerning the use of PET in osteoarthritis (OA), a disease primarily affecting the articular cartilage, with remodeling of sub-

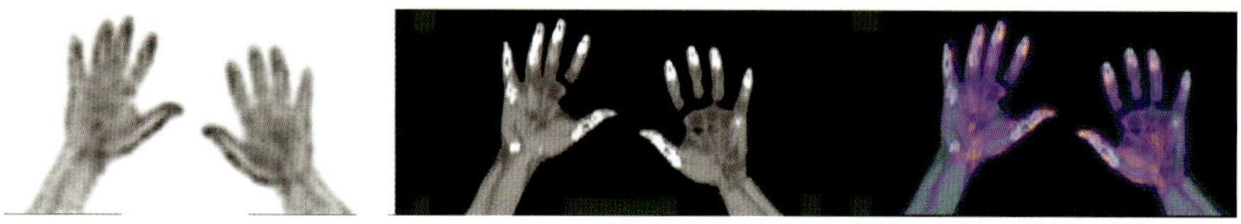

FIGURE 7-3. FDG-PET/CT study in a patient with extensive cutaneous psoriasis. There is no joint involvement in this case; the skin lesions, which cover most of both hands, are highly hypermetabolic on the PET images at left.

chondral bone, secondary new bone formation leading to the typical osteophytes, and, in some cases, a secondary synovitis. Conventional radiography is the standard method for diagnosis and evaluation of the severity of OA, with cartilage degradation being assessed by loss of joint space width. However, this provides an indirect and crude evaluation of the articular cartilage. More refined methods such as MRI have therefore been developed to study the cartilage. MRI can accurately assess cartilage thickness and volume. Because the cartilage matrix is composed of glycosaminoglycan and maintained by the glucose metabolism of chondrocytes, one might expect changes in cartilage metabolism to be detected by PET.[38] Only two reports have focused on OA affecting the shoulder and knee, respectively. The first report was a "random" shoulder evaluation in 24 patients undergoing FDG-PET for oncologic assessment.[38] Patients underwent physical examination for the shoulder and completed a questionnaire assessing the presence and severity of shoulder disease as well as the Disabilities of the Arm, Shoulder, and Hand (DASH) questionnaire. Total-body FDG-PET scans were performed, with patients being positioned with arms down in a neutral (thumbs up) position. No standard radiographs were performed for confirmation of the OA diagnosis. CT or MRI results were available for some patients. Fourteen patients had both history and physical findings consistent with a specific diagnosis and PET abnormalities. These consisted of three recognizable patterns of uptake in 12 of the 14 patients: (1) a circumferential/diffuse uptake in 10 patients, 7 of whom had a clinical diagnosis of OA, 1 with bursitis, 1 with a rotator cuff injury, and 1 with a normal shoulder examination; (2) asymmetrical localized uptake at the greater tuberosity in 4 patients, of which 2 had known rotator cuff injuries, 1 a frozen shoulder, and 1 a normal examination; and (3) a pattern of focal glenoid uptake in 4 patients, 2 with frozen shoulder, 1 with OA, and 1 with a normal examination. The circumferential/diffuse uptake in 7 of the 8 patients with clinical OA of the shoulder was hypothesized to be related to a chronic, nonspecific synovitis. Overall, there was no significant difference in maximum SUV between patients with or without clinical symptoms. There was, however, a statistical significant correlation between the maximum SUV and age.[38] The other recent study focusing on OA is a prospective study of medial knee OA.[39] Fifteen patients of a mean age of 71 years underwent clinical examination, standing radiographs to evaluate the Kellgren/Lawrence grade, MRI, and FDG-PET. FDG commonly accumulated in the periarticular region and was lacking in the articular cartilage. Both mean and peak SUVs were significantly higher in OA than in three young healthy controls. Apart from peripheral uptake, the localization of FDG accumulation was the intercondylar notch in 13 of 15 knees, with an extension of FDG accumulation along the posterior cruciate ligament in 4 knees. Twelve knees had osteophytes, and one half of these showed high accumulation of FDG around them. In 4 cases, FDG accumulated in the subchondral bone of the medial tibial condyle, with MR images suggestive of bone edema. There was no significant difference in maximum nor in mean SUV between patients with or without clinical symptoms (effusion, swelling, rest pain).[39] These studies show an increased FDG uptake in OA joints that could be due to increased metabolic activity in cartilage, bony osteophytes, subchondral bone, or also secondary synovitis. Whether PET will be of clinical use in OA remains to be proved, but it is of potential interest given the burden of this disease in health care.

PET in the Monitoring of Arthritis Treatment

The development of very effective but costly biologic treatments for RA has prompted the interest of new methods for assessing their efficacy, in addition to the crude clinical counts of tender and swollen joints and to the late radiologic measures of erosions. Ultrasonography allows an assessment of the reduction of synovitis after anti–tumor necrosis factor (TNF)-α treatment[28] but remains an observer-dependent method and is time consuming if all the joints are to be evaluated simultaneously. In this regard, PET seems to be an exciting method for evaluating the whole-body joint inflammatory activity. Early studies more than a decade ago showed the ability of PET to monitor the effects of prednisone and methotrexate treatments in patients with inflammatory synovitis of the wrist,[17,40] the decrease in FDG uptake after treatment being correlated to the decrease of the volume of enhancing pannus determined by MRI.[17] The effects of intra-articular glucocorticoid injections were demonstrated in 7 patients with knee arthritis using (N-methyl-^{11}C)-D-deprenyl PET.[41] All patients showed a high uptake of the radiotracer in the para-articular structures of the knee. Reevaluation 6 to 14 days later of the five knees injected showed an approximate 50% reduction in uptake.[41] PET evaluation of joints after anti–TNF-α treatment has been reported in two studies. We have shown in 16 patients with knee synovitis[27] that after 4 weeks of anti–TNF-α treatment, changes in PET parameters (SUVs) were correlated with changes in MRI parameters and with changes in serum levels of metalloproteinase-3, a synovial-derived parameter[30] whose production is known to be induced by TNF-α. Changes in PET parameters were not correlated to changes in ultrasound parameters, probably because metabolic changes are likely to precede morphologic changes and 4 weeks is too short a period to appreciate a reduction in synovial thickness. Figure 7-4 illustrates such a decrease in synovial FDG uptake after anti–TNF-α treatment. Goerres and associates reported a decrease in the FDG-PET global joint score in five responders of 7 RA patients

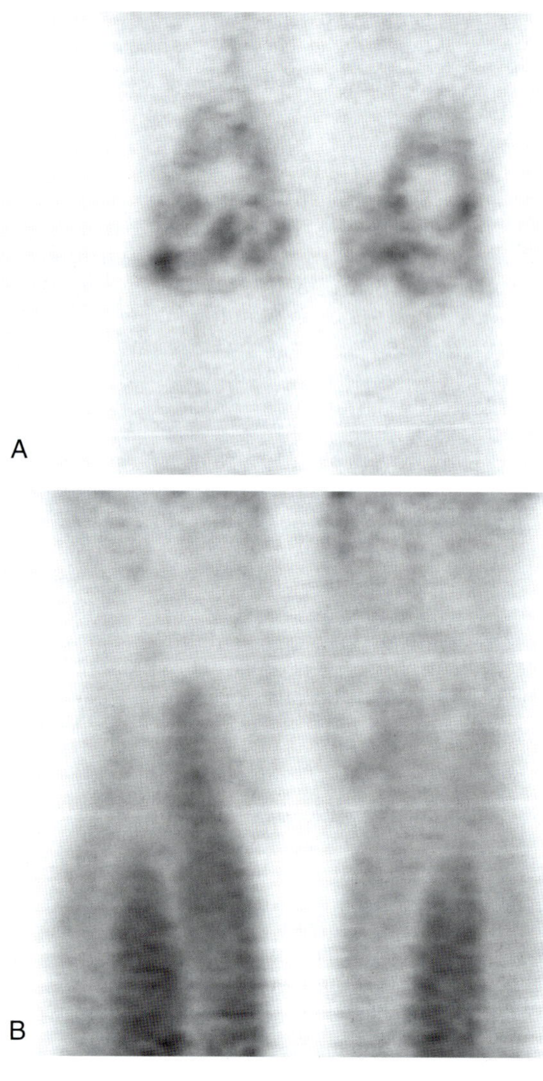

FIGURE 7-4. Synovitis of knees before (**A**) and 4 weeks after (**B**) treatment with anti–TNF-α therapy (infliximab). Note the nonspecific muscular uptake in the post-treatment image.

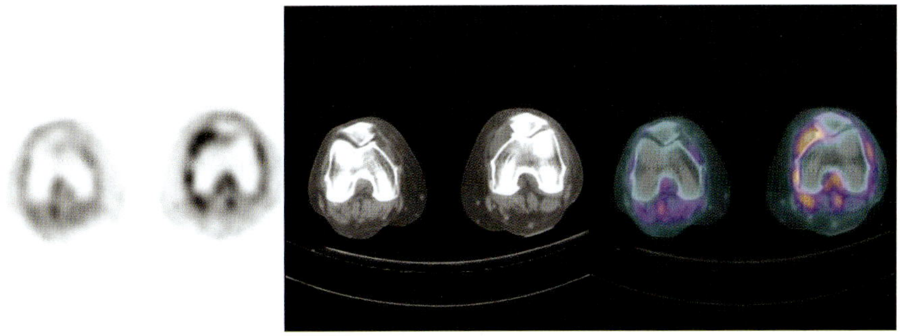

FIGURE 7-5. PET, CT, and fused PET/CT images (transverse sections) of the knees. There is a significant increase FDG uptake in the left knee, corresponding to synovial thickening. In the right knee there is a very faint uptake, with only very limited thickening on the medial aspect of the internal condyle.

treated with infliximab and evaluated after 12 weeks of treatment.[42] Change from baseline was similar in clinical and PET evaluations in 78% of joints (Fig. 7-5). The reduction of FDG uptake was noted not only in joints but also in the bursae of three responders and in tendon sheaths of four responders. This study in a small cohort of patients confirms the use of PET for a whole-body assessment of RA disease activity at baseline as well as after anti–TNF-α treatment. It remains to be proved whether PET metabolic assessment of RA disease activity can distinguish anti–TNF-α responders and nonresponders earlier or in a more sensitive way than clinical assessment. It also remains unknown whether pretherapeutic SUV can be of prognostic value in RA as it is in oncology.[43,44] The underlying hypothesis, that is, that more aggressive tumors are metabolically more active, may also apply to RA.[45] Indeed, the rheumatoid pannus is a highly inflamed synovium with an important neovascularization and is sometimes compared with a tumoral tissue because of its ability to invade cartilage and bone and because of the "transformed" phenotype of the fibroblast-like synoviocytes. Because SUV is increased in joints with a positive Doppler signal,[16] that is, joints with hypervascularization and thus with an aggressive synovitis, it may predict which joints are likely to respond to treatment, and cumulative SUV could be even more predictive than SUVs of single joints.[45] PET may therefore provide information about a potential aggressive course of the rheumatoid disease at an individual patient level, such a prediction of outcome being difficult in this highly heterogeneous disease.

SUMMARY

Bone scintigraphy with technetium-labeled diphosphonates remains the workhorse among nuclear medicine techniques in bone and joint diseases. In inflammatory joint diseases, however, its actual value and impact on patients' management remain fairly limited. Recent data with new technologies combining high-resolution positron imaging and CT with FDG, a tracer that targets activated inflammatory cells, are highly promising. The clinical applications that are most likely to prove useful include prognostic assessment and early evaluation of response to biologic treatments.

References

1. O'Connor MK, Brown ML, Hung JC, Hayostek RJ. The art of bone scintigraphy: technical aspects. J Nucl Med 1991; 32:2332-2341.
2. Rosenthall L. Nuclear medicine techniques in arthritis. Rheum Dis Clin North Am 1991; 17:585-597.

3. Desaulniers M, Fuks A, Hawkins D, et al. Radiotechnetium polyphosphate joint imaging. J Nucl Med 1974; 15:417-423.
4. Helfgott S, Rosenthall L, Esdaile J, Tannenbaum H. Generalized skeletal response to ^{99m}technetium methylene diphosphonate in rheumatoid arthritis. J Rheumatol 1982; 9:939-941.
5. Sewell KL, Ruthazer R, Parker JA. The correlation of indium-111 joint scans with clinical synovitis in rheumatoid arthritis. J Rheumatol 1993; 20: 2015-2019.
6. Jamar F, Houssiau FA, Devogelaer JP, et al. Scintigraphy using a technetium 99m-labelled anti–E-selectin Fab fragment in rheumatoid arthritis. Rheumatology 2002; 41:53-61.
7. Bleeker-Rovers CP, Rennen HJJM, Boerman OC, et al. ^{99m}Tc-labeled interleukin-8 for the scintigraphic detection of infection and inflammation: first clinical evaluation. J Nucl Med 2007; 48:337-343.
8. Firestein GS, Yeo M, Zvaifler NJ. Apoptosis in rheumatoid arthritis synovium. J Clin Invest 1995; 96:1631-1638.
9. Post AM, Katsikis PD, Tait JF, et al. Imaging cell death with radiolabeled Annexin V in an experimental model of rheumatoid arthritis. J Nucl Med 2002; 43:1359-1365.
10. Belhocine T, Steinmetz N, Hustinx R, et al. Increased uptake of the apoptosis-imaging agent (99m)Tc recombinant human Annexin V in human tumors after one course of chemotherapy as a predictor of tumor response and patient prognosis. Clin Cancer Res 2002; 8:2766-2774.
11. Duer A, Østergaard M, Vallo J, Horslev-Petersen K. Magnetic resonance imaging and bone scintigraphy in the differential diagnosis of unclassified arthritis. Ann Rheum Dis 2008; 67:48-51.
12. Hustinx R, Malaise MG. PET imaging of arthritis. PET Clin North Am 2006; 1:131-139.
13. Brix G, Lechel U, Glatting G, et al. Radiation exposure of patients undergoing whole-body dual-modality ^{18}F-FDG PET/CT examinations. J Nucl Med 2005; 46:608-613.
14. Zhao S, Kuge Y, Tsukamoto E, et al. Effects of insulin and glucose loading on FDG uptake in experimental malignant tumours and inflammatory lesions. Eur J Nucl Med 2001; 28:730-735.
15. Zhao S, Kuge Y, Tsukamoto E, et al. Fluorodeoxyglucose uptake and glucose transporter expression in experimental inflammatory lesions and malignant tumours: effects of insulin and glucose loading. Nucl Med Commun 2002; 23:545-550.
16. Beckers C, Ribbens C, Andre B, et al. Assessment of disease activity in rheumatoid arthritis with ^{18}F-FDG PET. J Nucl Med 2004; 45:956-964.
17. Palmer WE, Rosenthal DI, Schoenberg OI, et al. Quantification of inflammation in the wrist with gadolinium-enhanced MR imaging and PET with 2-[F-18]-fluoro-2-deoxy-D-glucose. Radiology 1995; 196:647-655.
18. Zhuang H, Alavi A. 18-Fluorodeoxyglucose positron emission tomographic imaging in the detection and monitoring of infection and inflammation. Semin Nucl Med 2002; 32:47-59.
19. Kubota R, Yamada S, Kubota K, et al. Intratumoral distribution of fluorine-18-fluorodeoxyglucose in vivo: high accumulation in macrophages and granulation tissues studied by autoradiography. J Nucl Med 1992; 33:1972-1980.
20. Kubota R, Kubota K, Yamada S, et al. Microautoradiographic study for the differentiation of intratumoral macrophages, granulation tissues and cancer cells by the dynamics of fluorine-18-fluorodeoxyglucose uptake. J Nucl Med 1994; 35:104-112.
21. Yamada S, Kubota K, Kubota R, et al. High accumulation of fluorine-18-fluorodeoxyglucose in turpentine-induced inflammatory tissue. J Nucl Med 1995; 36:1301-1306.
22. Gamelli RL, Liu H, He LK, Hofmann CA. Augmentations of glucose uptake and glucose transporter-1 in macrophages following thermal injury and sepsis in mice. J Leukoc Biol 1996; 59:639-647.
23. Mochizuki T, Tsukamoto E, Kuge Y, et al. FDG uptake and glucose transporter subtype expressions in experimental tumor and inflammation models. J Nucl Med 2001; 42:1551-1555.
24. Wipke BT, Wang Z, Kim J, et al. Dynamic visualization of a joint-specific autoimmune response through positron emission tomography. Nature Immunol 2002; 3:366-372.
25. Yasuda S, Shohtsu A, Ide M, et al. F-18 FDG accumulation in inflamed joints. Clin Nucl Med 1996; 21:740.
26. Bakheet SMB, Powe J. Fluorine-18-fluorodeoxyglucose uptake in rheumatoid-arthritis–associated lung disease in a patient with thyroid cancer. J Nucl Med 1998; 39:234-236.
27. Beckers C, Jeukens X, Ribbens C, et al. ^{18}F-FDG PET imaging of rheumatoid knee synovitis correlates with dynamic magnetic resonance and sonographic assessments as well as with the serum level of metalloproteinase-3. Eur J Nucl Med Mol Imaging 2006; 33:275-280.
28. Ribbens C, Andre B, Marcelis S, et al. Rheumatoid hand joint synovitis, gray-scale and power Doppler US quantifications following anti-tumor necrosis factor-alpha treatment: pilot study. Radiology 2003; 229:562-569.
29. Cimmino MA, Innocenti S, Livrone F, et al. Dynamic gadolinium-enhanced magnetic resonance imaging of the wrists in patients with rheumatoid arthritis can discriminate active from inactive disease. Arthritis Rheum 2003; 48:1207-1213.
30. Ribbens C, Martin y Porras M, Franchimont N, et al. Increased matrix metalloproteinase-3 serum levels in rheumatic diseases: relationship with synovitis and steroid treatment. Ann Rheum Dis 2002; 61:161-166.
31. ØstergaardM, Stoltenberg M, Lovgreen-Nielsen P, et al. Quantification of synovitis by MRI: correlation between dynamic and static gadolinium-enhanced magnetic resonance imaging and microscopic and macroscopic signs of synovial inflammation. Magn Reson Imaging 1998; 16:753-758.

32. Gaffney K, Cookson J, Blades S, et al. Quantitative assessment of the rheumatoid synovial microvascular bed by gadolinium-DTPA enhanced magnetic resonance imaging. Ann Rheum Dis 1998; 57:152-157.
33. Roivainen A, Parkkola R, Kerttula P, et al. Use of positron emission tomography with methyl-^{11}C-choline and 2-^{18}F-fluoro-2-deoxy-D-glucose in comparison with magnetic resonance imaging for the assessment of inflammatory proliferation of synovium. Arthritis Rheum 2003; 48:3077-3084.
34. Prevoo ML, van't Hof MA, Kuper HH, et al. Modified disease activity scores that include twenty-eight-joint counts: development and validation in a prospective longitudinal study of patients with rheumatoid arthritis. Arthritis Rheum 1995; 38:44-48.
35. Smolen JS, Breedveld FC, Schiff MH, et al. A simplified disease activity index for rheumatoid arthritis for use in clinical practice. Rheumatology 2003; 42:244-257.
36. Yun M, Kim W, Adam L, et al. F-18 FDG uptake in a patient with psoriatic arthritis: imaging correlation with patient symptoms. Clin Nucl Med 2001; 26:692-693.
37. Beckers C, Bernard C, Kaiser MJ, et al. Time-course study of [F-18]-FDG uptake in psoriatic synovitis. J Nucl Med 2005; 46(Suppl 2):183P.
38. Wandler E, Kramer EL, Sherman O, et al. Diffuse FDG shoulder uptake on PET is associated with clinical findings of osteoarthritis. AJR Am J Roentgenol 2005; 185:797-803.
39. Nakamura H, Masuko K, Yudoh K, et al. Positron emission tomography with 18F-FDG in osteoarthritic knee. Osteoarthritis Cartilage 2007; 15:673-681.
40. Polisson RP, Schoenberg OI, Fischman A, et al. Use of magnetic resonance imaging and positron emission tomography in the assessment of synovial volume and glucose metabolism in patients with rheumatoid arthritis. Arthritis Rheum 1995; 38:819-825.
41. Danfors T, Bergström M, Feltelius N, et al. Positron emission tomography with ^{11}C-D-deprenyl in patients with rheumatoid arthritis. Scand J Rheumatol 1997; 26:43-48.
42. Goerres GW, Forster A, Uebelhart D, et al. F-18 FDG whole-body PET for the assessment of disease activity in patients with rheumatoid arthritis. Clin Nucl Med 2006; 31:386-390.
43. Downey RJ, Akhurst T, Gonen M, et al. Preoperative F-18 fluorodeoxyglucose-poistron emission tomography maximal standardized uptake value predicts survival after lung cancer resection. J Clin Oncol 2004; 22:3255-3260.
44. Pandit N, Gonen M, Krug L, Larson SM. Prognostic value of [18F]FDG-PET imaging in small cell lung cancer. Eur J Nucl Med Mol Imaging 2003; 30:78-84.
45. Brenner W. ^{18}F-FDG PET in rheumatoid arthritis: there still is a long way to go. J Nucl Med 2004; 45:927-929.

Part II

The Future of Advanced Imaging in Arthritis

Chapter 8

New MRI Techniques for Osteoarthritis

Cartilage Morphometry and Spoiled Gradient-Recalled-Echo, Driven Equilibrium Fourier Transform, Steady-State, High-Field, Phase-Sensitive, and Forward-Looking/Experimental MRI Methods

Garry E. Gold

Articular cartilage pathology may be the result of degeneration or acute injury. Osteoarthritis is an important cause of disability in our society[1-5] and is primarily a disease of articular cartilage.[6-8] Acute injury to cartilage may be characterized using MRI.[9] Whether the result of degeneration or injury, MRI offers a noninvasive means of assessing the degree of damage to cartilage and adjacent bone and measuring the effectiveness of treatment.

Many imaging methods are available to assess articular cartilage. Conventional radiography can be used to detect gross loss of cartilage, which is evident as narrowing of the distance between the bony components of the joint,[10] but it does not image cartilage directly. Secondary changes such as osteophyte formation can be seen, but conventional radiography is insensitive to early chondral damage. Arthrography, alone or combined with conventional radiography or CT, is also mildly invasive and provides information limited to the contour of the cartilage surface.[11]

MRI, with its excellent soft tissue contrast, is the best technique currently available for assessment of articular cartilage.[12-16] Imaging of regions of cartilage damage has the potential to provide morphologic information about the region, such as fissuring and the presence of partial-or full-thickness cartilage defects. The many tissue parameters that can be measured by MRI techniques have the potential to provide biochemical and physiologic information about cartilage.[13]

An ideal MRI study for cartilage should provide accurate assessment of cartilage thickness and volume, demonstrate morphologic changes of the cartilage surface, demonstrate internal cartilage signal changes, and allow evaluation of the subchondral bone for signal abnormalities. Also desirable would be an evaluation of the underlying cartilage physiology, including the status of the proteoglycan and collagen matrices. Conventional MRI sequences in current clinical use, however, do not provide a comprehensive assessment of cartilage and are lacking in either spatial resolution[17] or specific information about cartilage physiology or require impractically long scan times for such assessments.

CONVENTIONAL MRI METHODS

MRI has emerged as the leading method of imaging soft tissue structures around joints.[18] One of the major advantages of MRI is the ability to manipulate contrast to highlight tissue types. The common contrast mechanisms used in MRI are 2D or multi-slice T1-weighted, proton-density (PD)–weighted, and T2-weighted imaging, with or without fat suppression. Imaging hardware and software have changed considerably over time, including improved gradients and radiofrequency coils, fast or turbo spin-echo imaging, and techniques such as water-only excitation.

Whereas the tissue relaxation times and imaging parameters are the major determinants of contrast between cartilage and fluid, lipid suppression increases contrast between nonlipid and lipid-containing tissues and affects how the MR scanner sets the overall dynamic range of the image. The most common type of lipid suppression is fat saturation, in which fat spins are excited and then dephased before imaging. Another option is spectral-spatial excitation, in which only water spins in a slice are excited.[19] Finally, in areas of magnetic field inhomogeneity, inversion recovery provides a way to suppress lipids at the expense of signal to noise and contrast to noise.

The type of contrast used in cartilage imaging is critical to the visibility of lesions and the signal-to-noise ratio (SNR) of the cartilage itself. Although T2-weighted imaging creates contrast between cartilage and synovial fluid, it does so at the expense of cartilage signal. The high signal from fluid is useful to highlight surface defects such as fibrillation or fissuring, but variation in internal cartilage signal is poorly depicted. These scans also are often done in 2D, leaving a small gap between slices, which may therefore miss small areas of cartilage damage.

Spatial Resolution

MRI of cartilage requires close attention to imaging spatial resolution. To see degenerating cartilage, imaging with resolution on the order of 0.2 to 0.4 mm is required.[17] The ultimate resolution achievable is governed by the SNR possible within a given imaging time and with a given radiofrequency coil. Ultimately, a high-resolution imaging technique that combines morphologic and physiologic information would be ideal in the evaluation of osteoarthritis. Given current techniques, it is likely that a combination of a high-resolution morphologic imaging sequence with a sequence for matrix evaluation will be the most useful.

2D Fast Spin-Echo Imaging

Currently, imaging of the musculoskeletal system with MRI is often limited to 2D multi-slice acquisitions acquired in multiple planes. This is commonly done with turbo or fast spin-echo (FSE) methods. These methods provide excellent signal to noise and contrast between tissues of interest, but the inherently anisotropic voxels in these 2D acquisitions require that multiple planes of data be acquired to minimize partial-volume artifacts. For example, a typical sagittal image may have 0.3 to 0.6 mm in plane resolution but a slice thickness of 3 to 5 mm. FSE techniques show excellent results in the detection of cartilage lesions (Figs. 8-1 and 8-2).[20] These methods provide excellent depiction of structures in the the imaging plane, but evaluation of oblique or small structures across multiple slices can be challenging. For these reasons, 3D acquisitions with thin sections are appealing.

3D Gradient-Recalled-Echo Techniques

Traditional 3D gradient-recalled-echo (GRE) methods have the potential to acquire data with more isotropic voxel sizes but suffer from a lack of contrast compared with

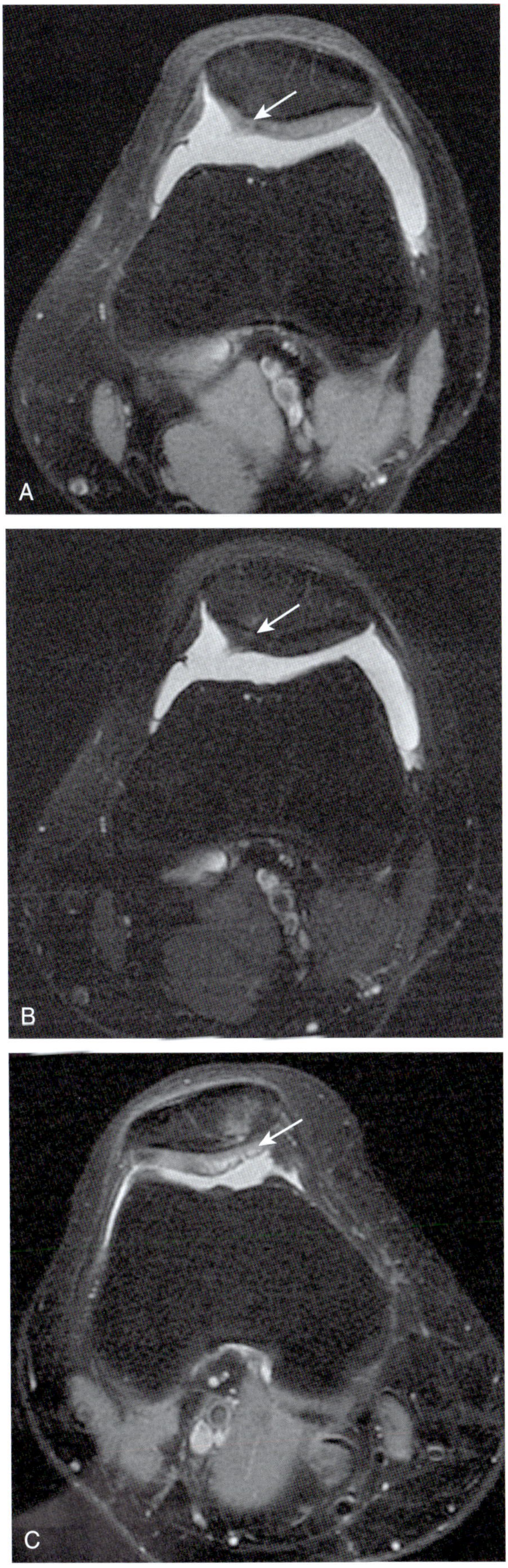

Figure 8-1. Axial images showing degrees of patellar cartilage damage. **A,** Axial intermediate-weighted, fast spin-echo (FSE) image showing superficial fibrillation and signal changes in the patellar cartilage (*arrow*). **B,** Axial T2-weighted FSE image showing marrow edema at the same location (*arrow*). **C,** Axial intermediate-weighted FSE image showing fissuring involving approximately 50% of the thickness of the cartilage (*arrow*). **D,** Axial intermediate-weighted FSE image showing a full thickness cartilage fissure in the patella (*arrow*).

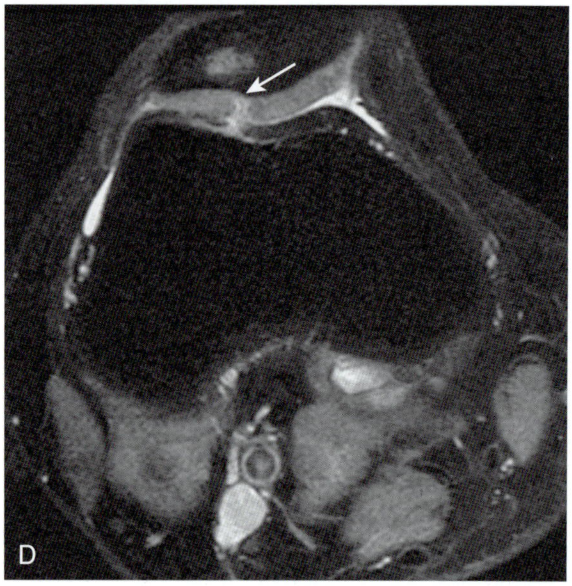

FIGURE 8-1, cont'd

spin-echo approaches. High accuracy for cartilage lesions has been shown with 3D-SPGR (spoiled gradient-recalled-echo) imaging.[21-23] There are two main disadvantages to this approach: lack of reliable contrast between cartilage and fluid that outlines surface defects and long imaging times (approximately 8 minutes). In addition, SPGR imaging uses gradient and radiofrequency spoiling to reduce artifacts and achieve near T1 weighting. This reduces the overall signal compared with steady-state techniques.[24-26] Despite these limitations, 3D-SPGR is considered the standard for morphologic imaging of cartilage.[24,27]

Both SPGR and GRE techniques produce excellent quality images with high resolution ($0.3 \times 0.6 \times 1.5$ mm).[28] The SPGR method suppresses signal from joint fluid, whereas the GRE method accentuates it. Compared with balanced steady-state free precession (SSFP), which is described later in greater detail, these methods are less SNR efficient but also less sensitive to magnetic field inhomogeneity. Therefore, an ideal 3D cartilage imaging sequence that provides an optimal combination of resolution, SNR efficiency, and minimal artifacts has yet to be established. As such, a number of newer techniques have been established to improve cartilage imaging.

NEW MRI METHODS

DESS Imaging

Dual-echo steady-state imaging (DESS) has proved useful for evaluation of cartilage morphology.[29-32] This technique acquires two gradient echoes separated by a refocusing pulse and then combines both echoes into the image. This results in an image with higher T2* weighting, which has bright cartilage signal and bright synovial fluid.

DEFT Imaging

Driven equilibrium Fourier transform (DEFT) has been used in the past as a method of signal enhancement in spectroscopy.[33] The sequence uses a 90-degree pulse to return magnetization to the z-axis, increasing signal from tissue with long T1 relax-

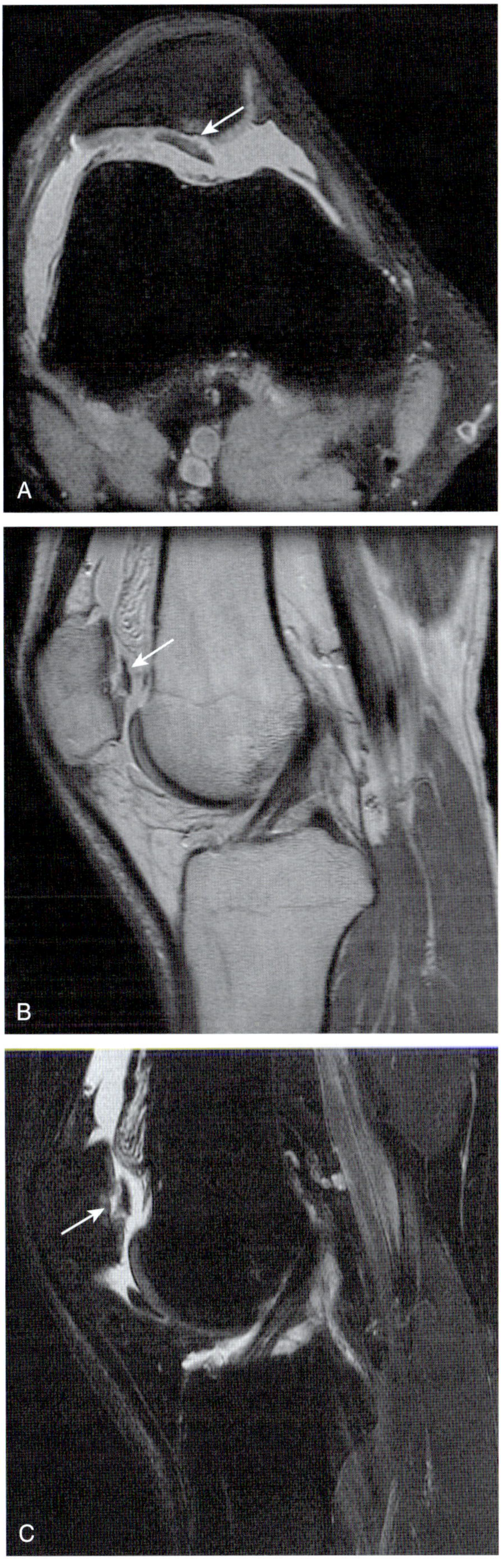

FIGURE 8-2. Fast spin-echo images of a cartilage fragment from the patellar cartilage with full-thickness loss (*arrows*). **A,** Axial intermediate-weighted FSE image showing the cartilage fragment. **B,** Sagittal intermediate-weighted image without fat suppression. **C,** Sagittal T2-weighted image with fat suppression showing edema in the patella and the fragment (*arrow*).

ation times such as synovial fluid. Unlike conventional T1- or T2-weighted MRI, the contrast in DEFT is dependent on the ratio of the T1/T2 of a given tissue.

For musculoskeletal imaging, DEFT produces contrast by enhancing the signal from synovial fluid rather than attenuation of cartilage signal as in T2-weighted sequences. This results in bright synovial fluid at short repetition times (TR). At short TR, DEFT shows much greater cartilage to fluid contrast than SPGR, PD-FSE, or T2-weighted FSE.[34]

DEFT imaging has been combined with a 3D echoplanar readout to make it an efficient 3D cartilage imaging technique. In DEFT there is no blurring of high spatial frequencies such as in PD-FSE.[35] Unlike T2-weighted FSE, cartilage signal is preserved owing to the short echo time (TE). A high-resolution 3D dataset of the entire knee using a 512 × 192 matrix, a 14-cm field of view (FOV), and 3-mm slices can be acquired in about 6 minutes. Initial studies of cartilage morphology have been done using DEFT imaging,[36,37] but this technique has not been conclusively proved superior to 2D approaches. A sequence similar to DEFT that has been used in musculoskeletal imaging is FSE with driven equilibrium pulses, referred to as DRIVE.[38]

Balanced Steady-State Free Precession Imaging

Balanced steady-state free precession (SSFP) MRI is an efficient, high-signal method for obtaining 3D MR images.[39] Depending on the manufacturer of the MRI scanner, this method has also been called True-FISP (Siemens), FIESTA (General Electric), or balanced FFE imaging (Phillips).[40] With recent advances in MR gradient hardware, it is now possible to use balanced SSFP without suffering from the banding or off-resonance artifacts that were previously a problem with this method. However, banding artifacts due to off resonance are still an issue as TR increases, or at 3.0T. Hence, TR is usually kept below 10 ms with these techniques, which limits overall image resolution. Multiple acquisition SSFP can be used to achieve higher resolution[41,42] at the cost of additional scan time.

Fat Suppression in Balanced SSFP Imaging

Many methods have been proposed to provide fat suppression with SSFP imaging. If the repetition time is sufficiently short and the magnetic field homogeneous, conventional fat suppression or water excitation pulses can be used.[43] Linear combinations of SSFP[44] and fluctuating equilibrium MRI (FEMR)[45] use the frequency difference between fat and water and multiple acquisitions to separate fat and water. Intermittent fat suppression[46] uses transient suppression methods to provide intermittent fat saturation pulses and suppress lipid signal. Iterative decomposition of water and fat with echo asymmetry and least-squares estimation (IDEAL) uses multiple acquisitions to separate fat and water but does not depend on the fat-water frequency difference to constrain the repetition time.[47] Rapid separation of water and fat can be achieved with phase detection.[48,49] Fat and water separation has also been achieved with phase detection and a radial acquisition method using multiple echoes.[50,51]

FEMR Imaging

Fluctuating equilibrium MRI (FEMR) is a variant of SSFP that may be useful in imaging cartilage.[45] Similar to DEFT, FEMR and other SSFP-based sequences produce contrast based on the ratio of T1/T2 in tissues. With appropriate choice of flip angle, this results in bright fluid signal while preserving cartilage signal. In scanning the entire knee, FEMR can produce 3D images with a 2-mm slice thickness using a 512 × 256 matrix over a 16-cm FOV in about 2 minutes and 30 seconds.[52] The TR was set at 6.6 ms at 1.5 T, which can be used for fat/water separation with careful shimming to minimize artifacts. An example water image using high-resolution FEMR is shown in Figure 8-3, compared with a 3D-SPGR image that took almost 9 minutes to acquire.

Linear Combinations of Balanced SSFP and Fat-Suppressed SSFP

Other SSFP approaches may provide more reliable fat suppression at high resolution than FEMR. These methods include linear combination balanced steady-state free precession (LC-SSFP),[44] which uses multiple acquisitions to create fat and water images. Fat-suppressed SSFP uses intermittent fat saturation pulses with preparation pulses that allow transitions in and out of the steady state.[53]

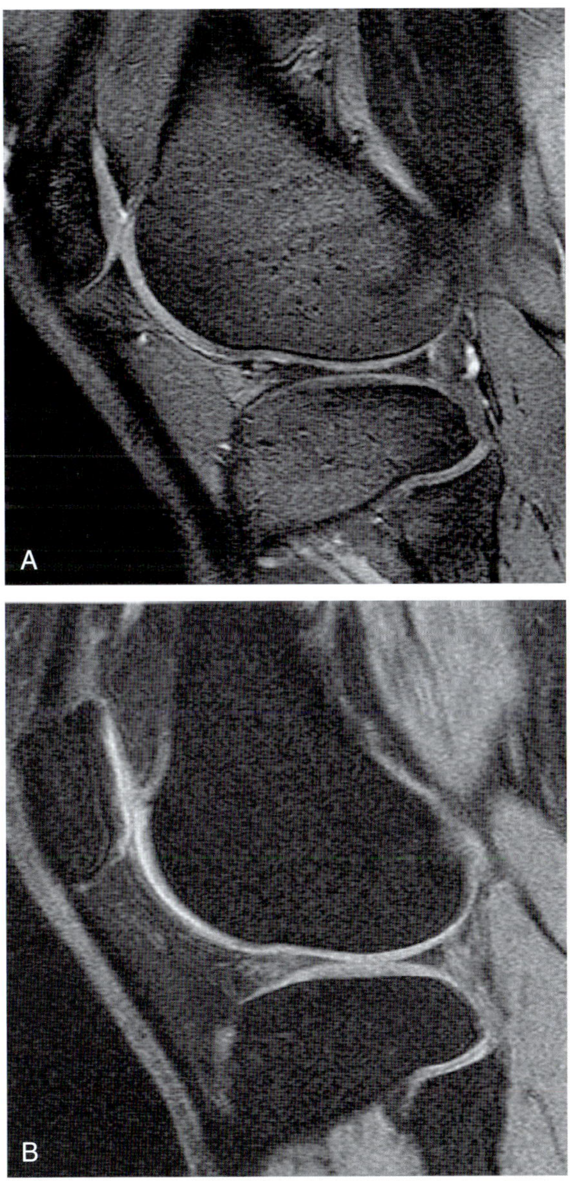

FIGURE 8-3. Two sagittal images from the knee of a normal volunteer. **A,** Fluctuating equilibrium MR (FEMR): scan time 2:43 min. **B,** Spoiled gradient-recalled-echo (SPGR) imaging: scan time 8:56 min. Both scans were done at the same spatial resolution (512 × 256, 2-mm slice thickness) and have similar signal-to-noise ratios (SNR). The higher SNR efficiency of FEMR allows a similar morphologic scan to be acquired in a much shorter time. (Reproduced with permission from Gold GE, Hargreaves B, Vasanawala SS, et al. MR imaging of articular cartilage of the knee using fluctuating equilibrium MR [FEMR]—initial experience in healthy volunteers. Radiology 2006; 238:719-724.)

IDEAL SSFP

Another approach to fat/water separation that is relatively insensitive to field variations combines IDEAL with SSFP.[54] Example knee images using this technique are shown in Figure 8-4. Excellent separation of fat and water is seen, with little off-resonance artifact.[55] This method works at both 1.5T and 3.0T.

Phase-Sensitive SSFP Imaging

Phase-sensitive (PS) SSFP employs an SSFP sequence with the TE restricted to be one half of the TR. The spectral response of the signal with respect to resonance frequency is periodic. The periodicity decreases with decreasing TR, resulting in less field inhomogeneity sensitivity.[48] Voxels are assigned to water or fat to form two

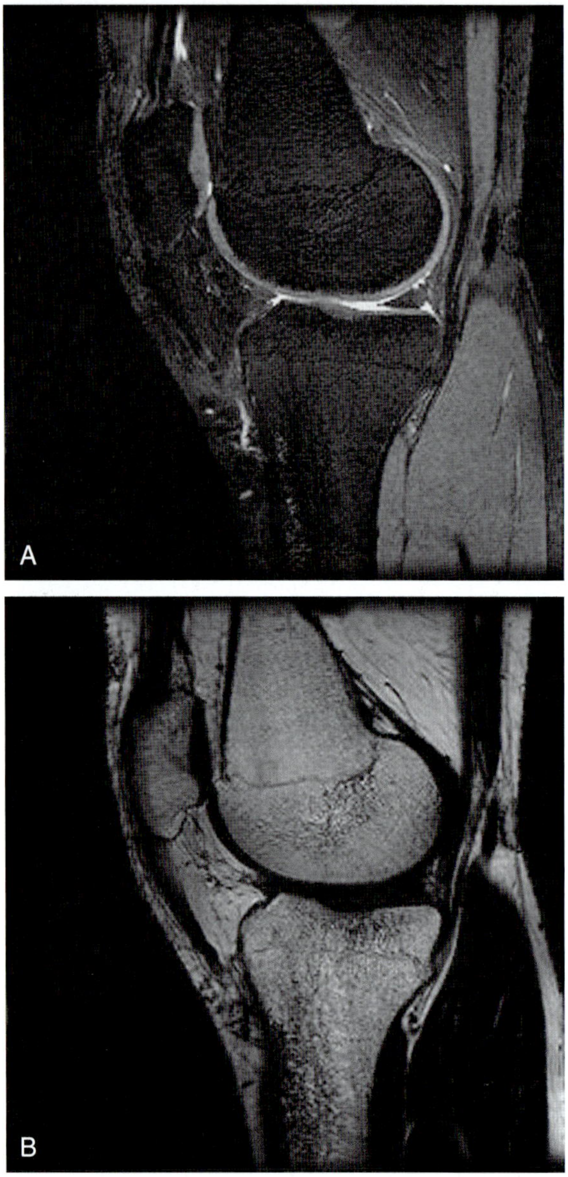

FIGURE 8-4. Balanced steady-state free precession images of the knee of a normal volunteer acquired using iterative decomposition of water and fat with echo asymmetry and least squares (IDEAL) steady-state free precession (SSFP). **A,** Water image. **B,** Fat image. Note that joint fluid is bright in **A** using this SSFP technique. **C** and **D,** Cartilage thickness maps of the femoral cartilage using segmentation of the MRI data.

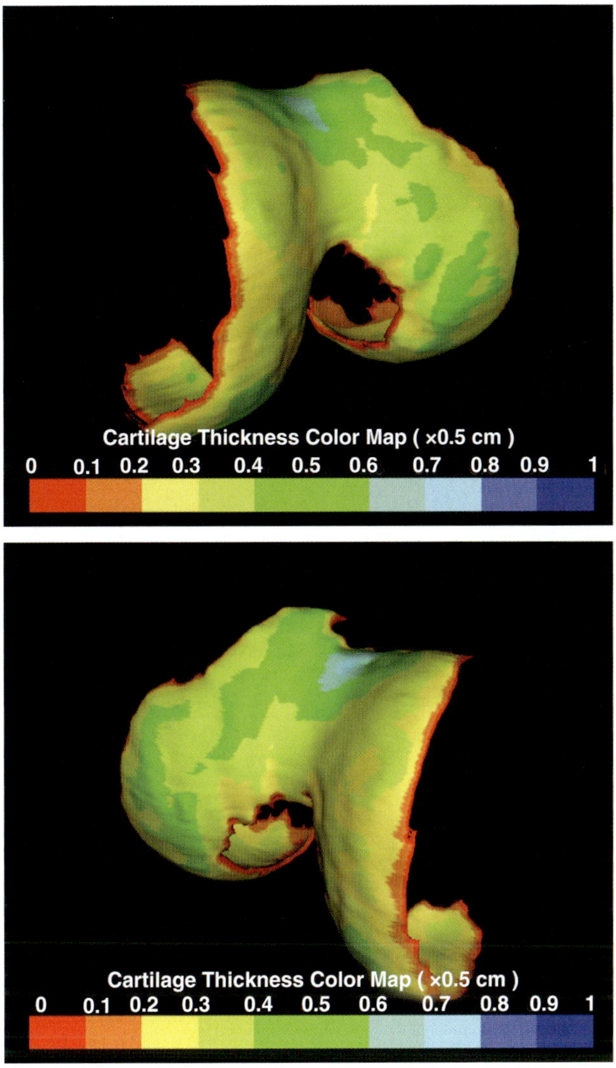

FIGURE 8-4, cont'd

separate images. This method is a rapid means of fat water separation using SSFP and does not require additional acquisitions or saturation pulses.[49] One drawback to this approach is partial volume artifact, because pixels are assigned as either fat or water, so high resolution is required. Example images of this method are shown in Figure 8-5. These images show a 3D, fat-suppressed dataset of an entire knee that can be acquired with 0.625 × 0.625 × 2 mm resolution in about 90 seconds. In a recent limited study, PS-SSFP was sensitive to marrow edema and meniscal tears in a similar manner to FSE imaging.[49]

Vastly Interpolated Projection Reconstruction Imaging

Imaging of the knee with a combination of a 3D radial k-space acquisition and SSFP has several advantages. The 3D radial acquisitions are often undersampled in sparse, high-contrast imaging environments such as contrast-enhanced MR angiography (CE-MRA) to decrease imaging time. Vastly interpolated projection reconstruction (VIPR), first developed for time-resolved CE-MRA,[50] was later adapted for SSFP imaging of the musculoskeletal system. Instead of using the radial trajectory to

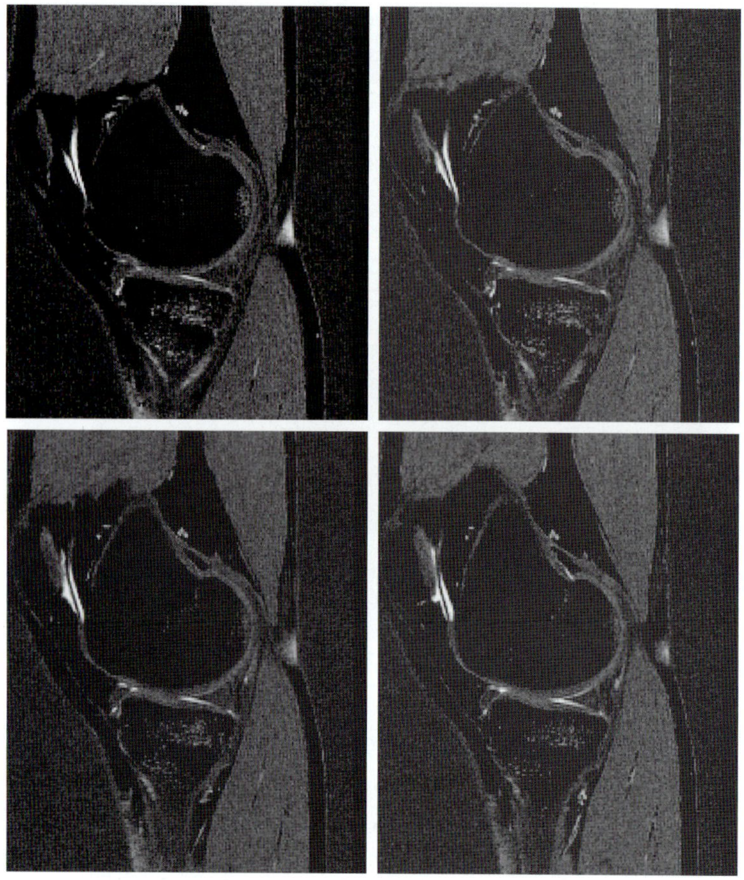

FIGURE 8-5. Phase-sensitive balanced steady-state free precession images from the knee of a normal volunteer. This is from a 3D dataset acquired with fat and water separation with 0.625 × 0.625 × 2-mm resolution in 90 seconds.

undersample in musculoskeletal imaging, the radial acquisition allows for a very efficient k-space trajectory that collects two radial lines each TR without wasting time on frequency dephasing and rephasing gradients. One radial line begins at the k-space origin, while the other is acquired along a different return path to the origin, allowing acquisition to occur during nearly the entire TR. The optimal TR needed for the most efficient implementation of linear combinations of SSFP at 1.5T (2.4 ms) can be met while still having time for adequate spatial encoding.

Application of VIPR to the knee provides isotropic 0.5- to 0.7-mm 3D imaging that allows for reformatted images in arbitrary planes. Because this method is based on SSFP, joint fluid is bright, providing excellent contrast for the diagnosis of meniscal tears, ligament injuries, and cartilage damage.[56] Contrast between the cartilage and bone is generated by separating fat and water with linear combinations of SSFP, as shown in Figure 8-6. Scan time for the isotropic acquisition was only 5 minutes. An alternative single-pass method separates fat and water by exploiting the different phase progression of fat and water spins between the two echoes acquired each TR.[51] At 3T, fat and water separation is achieved by using an alternative fat stopband with a TR of 3.6 ms. Here the multi-echo acquisition allows for the removal of the unwanted passband between the water and fat resonance frequencies at the longer TR.[57]

3D FSE Imaging

Recent advances in parallel imaging technology have enabled 3D FSE imaging with reasonable imaging times. These methods also commonly employ a method of flip

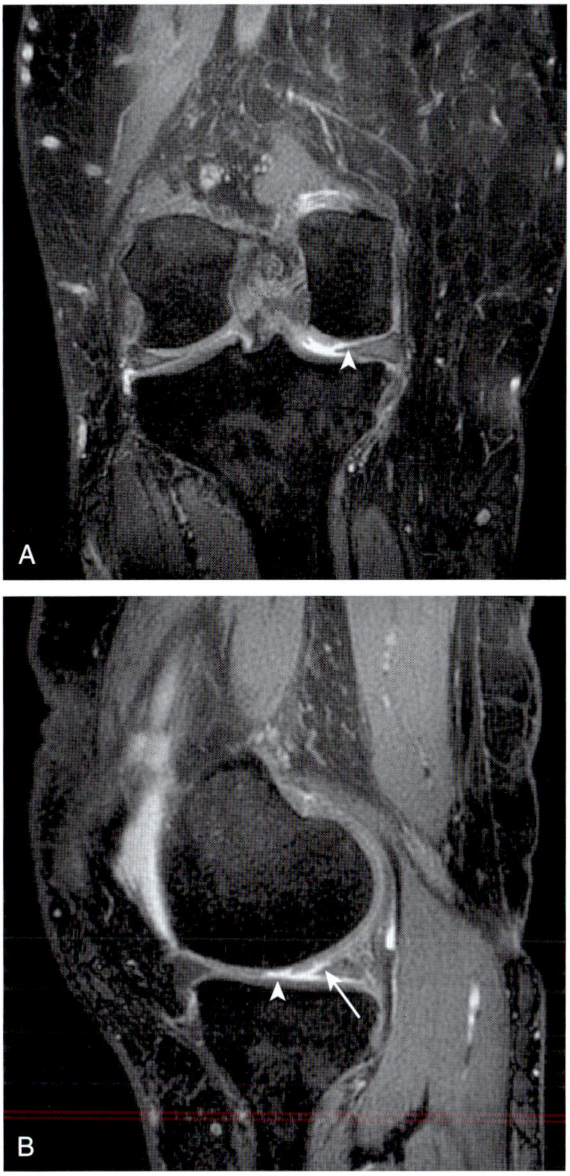

FIGURE 8-6. Vastly interpolated projection reconstruction (VIPR) balanced steady-state free precession (SSFP) imaging of the knee at 1.5T. This SSFP-based technique produces isotropic 0.7-mm resolution across the knee, allowing reformatted images in any plane. Scan time was only 5 minutes. **A,** Coronal image with cartilage defect (*arrowhead*). **B,** Sagittal reformatted image showing cartilage defect (*arrowhead*) and the meniscus (*arrow*). (Courtesy of R. Kijowski and W. Block, University of Wisconsin, Madison.)

angle modulation along the echo train to reduce the effects of blurring. When combined with multi-channel coils, isotropic resolution on the order of 0.6 mm can be achieved in an imaging time of 5 to 8 minutes.[58] This enables one to obtain reformatted images of articular cartilage as well as be able to evaluate ligaments, menisci, and other important joint structures. An example of using 3D FSE imaging for articular cartilage in the knee is shown in Figure 8-7.

High-Field MRI

High-field MRI may enable the acquisition of morphologic images at spatial resolutions that cannot be achieved in a reasonable scan time at 1.5T. Currently, 3.0T MRI units are available that, theoretically, have twice the signal to noise of 1.5T scanners. In addition, the increased chemical shift allows for shorter fat suppression or water

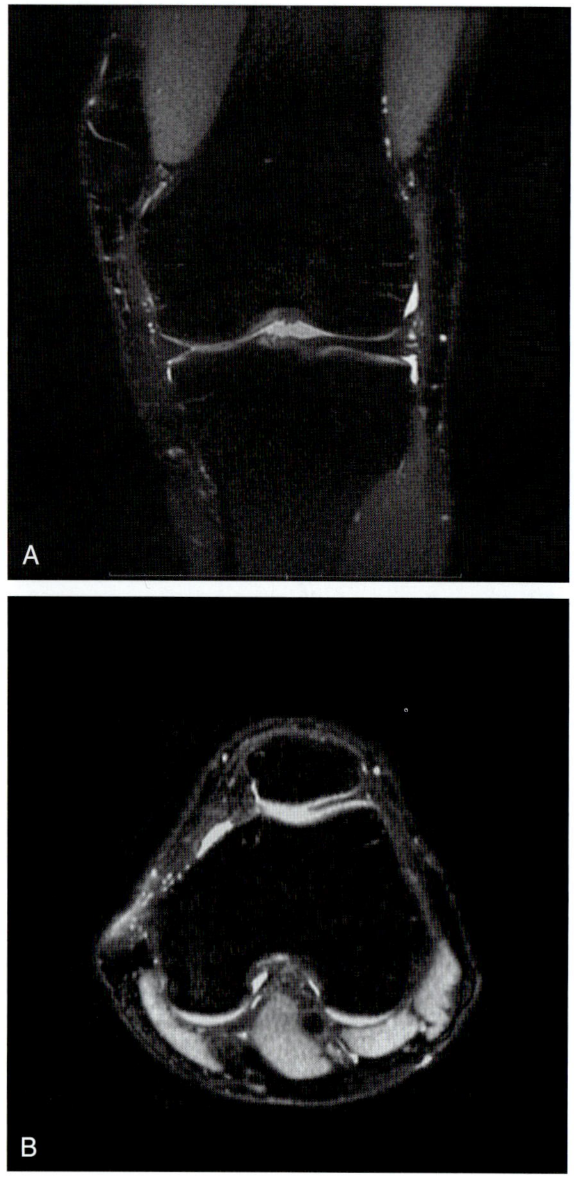

FIGURE 8-7. 3D fast spin-echo imaging done with flip angle modulation and parallel imaging at 1.5T. Conventional fat suppression was used with an isotropic resolution of 0.7 mm. **A,** Coronal source image. **B,** Axial reformatted image from the same dataset.

excitation pulses, improving the speed of 3D-SPGR and 3D-GRE scans. IDEAL fat/water separation is also available at 3.0T,[59,60] with both SPGR and GRE imaging, as shown in Figure 8-8. Also available are fat, water, and combined images that are corrected for chemical shift.[61] This method could be used to measure subchondral bone thickness. Other fat suppression methods for balanced SSFP imaging, such as FEMR and LC-SSFP, are less applicable to high-field MRI because the shortest TR during which the relative phase of fat and water changes by π is only 1.1 ms. This TR is too short to create any meaningful spatial encoding, and the radiofrequency power deposition would be high.

Sodium MRI

Atoms with an odd number of protons and/or neutrons possess a nuclear spin momentum and therefore exhibit the MR phenomenon. Sodium-23 (^{23}Na) is an

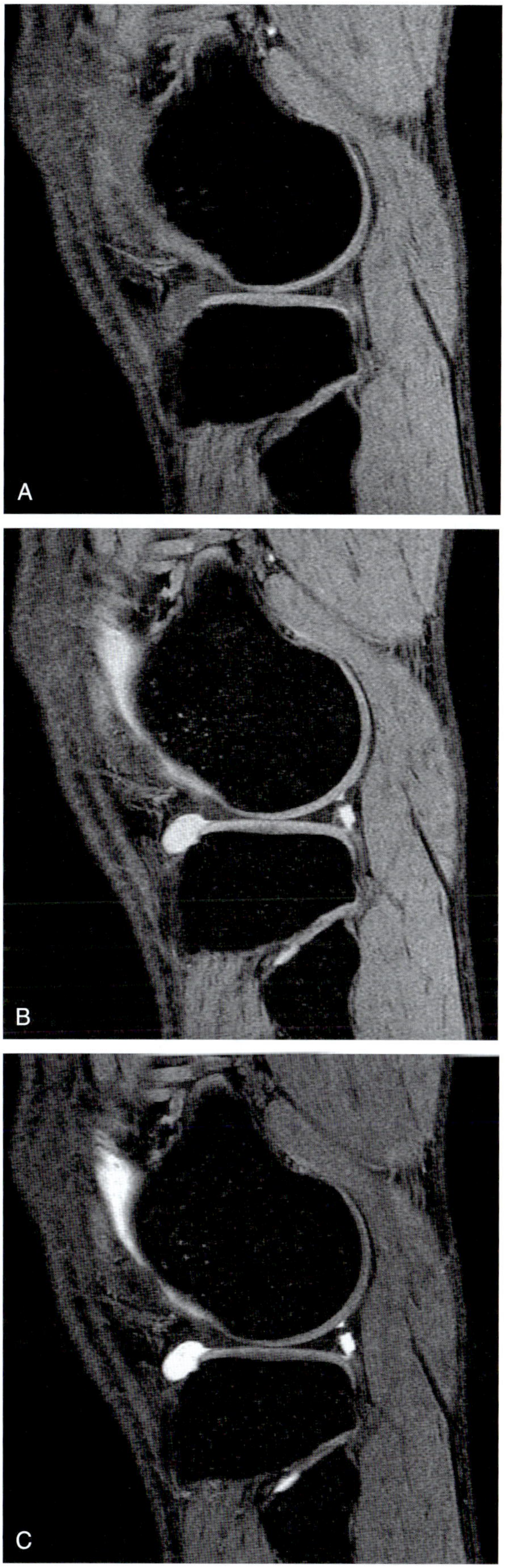

FIGURE 8-8 Iterative decomposition of water and fat with echo asymmetry and least squares (IDEAL) spoiled gradient-echo (SPGR) and gradient-echo (GRE) images at 3.0T. **A,** IDEAL SPGR image. **B,** IDEAL GRE image, with flip angle of 14 degrees. **C,** IDEAL GRE image, with flip angle of 25 degrees. Increasing the flip angle increases the contrast between synovial fluid and articular cartilage.

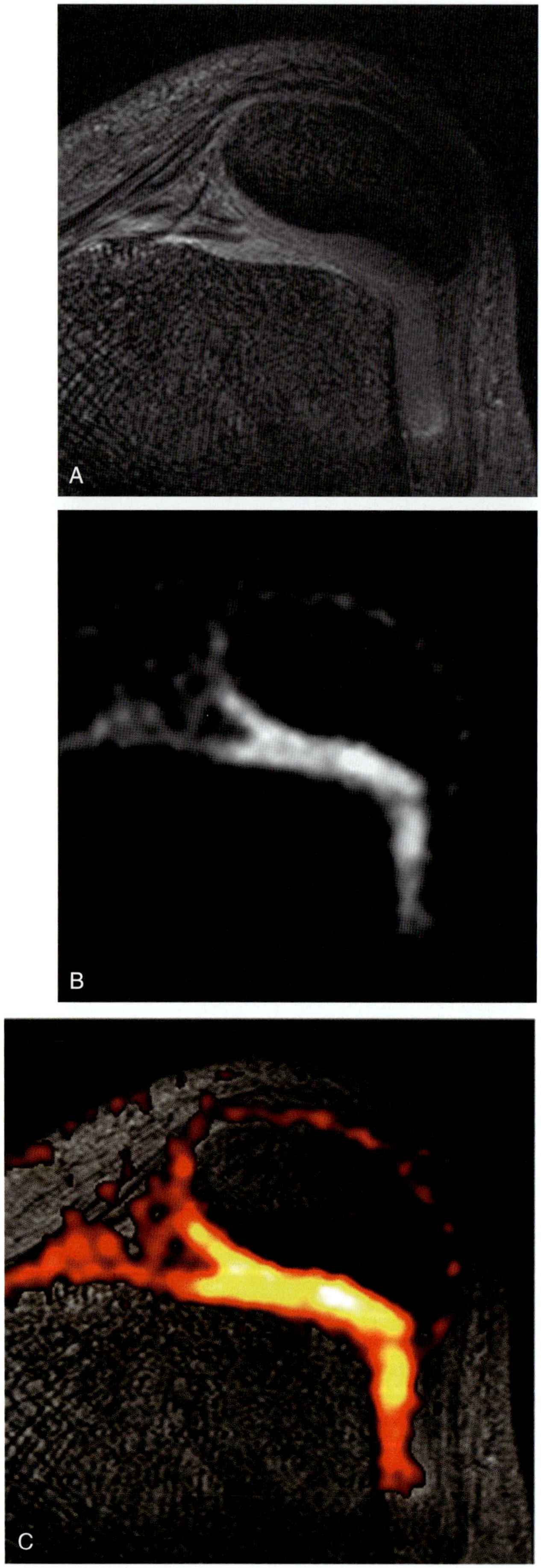

FIGURE 8-9. Sodium images acquired at 7.0T. **A,** Axial fat-suppressed gradient-echo proton image. **B,** Axial sodium image, showing high signal from the patella cartilage. **C,** Registered axial hydrogen/sodium image, with the sodium signal shown as a heat scale. High sodium concentrations in healthy articular cartilage make this a promising biomarker for early cartilage degeneration.

example of a nucleus other than hydrogen-1 (^{1}H) that is useful in cartilage imaging. The Larmor frequency of ^{23}Na is 11.262 MHz/T, compared with ^{1}H at 42.575 MHz/T. This means that at 1.5T the resonant frequency of ^{23}Na is 16.9 MHz, whereas it is 63 MHz for ^{1}H. The concentration of ^{23}Na in normal human cartilage is about 320 μM, with T2 relaxation times of between 2 and 10 ms.[62] The combination of lower resonant frequency, lower concentration, and shorter T2 relaxation times than ^{1}H make in-vivo imaging of ^{23}Na challenging. Sodium imaging requires the use of special transmit and receive coils, as well as relatively long imaging times to achieve adequate signal to noise.

Sodium MRI has shown some promising results in the imaging of articular cartilage. This is based on the ability of sodium imaging to depict regions of proteoglycan depletion.[63] ^{23}Na atoms are associated with the high fixed-charge density present in proteoglycan sulfate and carboxylate groups. Some spatial variation in ^{23}Na concentration is present within normal cartilage.[62] Figure 8-9 shows an example of a sodium image through the patellar cartilage of a healthy volunteer done with a twisted-projection technique at 7.0T.[64] High sodium concentration is seen throughout the normal cartilage. In cartilage samples, sodium imaging has been shown to be sensitive to small changes in proteoglycan concentration.[65,66] This method shows promise in being sensitive to early decreases in proteoglycan concentration in osteoarthritis. It is also possible to do triple quantum-filtered imaging of sodium in cartilage, which may be even more sensitive to early changes.[67]

SUMMARY

MRI provides a powerful tool for the imaging and understanding of cartilage. Improvements have been made in morphologic imaging of cartilage, in terms of contrast, resolution, and acquisition time. This allows detailed maps of the cartilage surface to be developed, quantifying both thickness and volume. Much progress has been made in the understanding of cartilage physiology and the ability to detect changes in proteoglycan content and collagen ultrastructure.

The choice of a particular protocol for imaging articular cartilage depends greatly on patient factors. For many patients with internal derangement, imaging with standard FSE and/or 3D-SPGR sequences may suffice. For patients being considered for surgical or pharmacologic therapy, however, a more detailed evaluation may be required. For example, fast morphologic imaging along with evaluation of cartilage physiology may allow for noninvasive evaluation of cartilage implants at different time points.

The fundamental tradeoff between image resolution and SNR still limits our ability to image cartilage in vivo with high resolution in an efficient manner. Patient motion may ultimately limit the resolution achievable at 1.5T; so higher field systems may be required. New techniques based on SSFP may shorten imaging time, allowing the application of other sequences to explore important questions about cartilage physiology and biochemistry. Ideally, the combination of these techniques will lead to an MRI examination for cartilage that is brief and well tolerated but contains important morphologic and physiologic data.

References

1. Felson DT. Clinical practice: osteoarthritis of the knee. N Engl J Med 2006; 354:841-848.
2. Felson DT, Nevitt MC. Epidemiologic studies for osteoarthritis: new versus conventional study design approaches. Rheum Dis Clin North Am 2004; 30:783-797, vii.
3. Peyron JG. Epidemiological aspects of osteoarthritis. Scand J Rheumatol Suppl 1988; 77:29-33.
4. Swedberg JA, Steinbauer JR. Osteoarthritis. Am Fam Physician 1992; 45:557-568.
5. Brandt KD. Osteoarthritis. Clin Geriatr Med 1988; 4:279-293.
6. Poole AR. An introduction to the pathophysiology of osteoarthritis. Front Biosci 1999; 4:D662-D670.

7. Roos H, Adalberth T, Dahlberg L, Lohmander LS. Osteoarthritis of the knee after injury to the anterior cruciate ligament or meniscus: the influence of time and age. Osteoarthritis Cartilage 1995; 3:261-267.
8. van den Berg WB. Pathophysiology of osteoarthritis. Joint Bone Spine 2000; 67:555-556.
9. Gold GE, Thedens DR, Pauly JM, et al. MR imaging of articular cartilage of the knee: new methods using ultrashort TEs. AJR Am J Roentgenol 1998; 170:1223-1226.
10. Boegard T, Rudling O, Petersson IF, Jonsson K. Correlation between radiographically diagnosed osteophytes and magnetic resonance detected cartilage defects in the tibiofemoral joint. Ann Rheum Dis 1998; 57:401-407.
11. Coumas JM, Palmer WE. Knee arthrography: evolution and current status. Radiol Clin North Am 1998; 36:703-728.
12. Disler DG, McCauley TR. Clinical magnetic resonance imaging of articular cartilage. Top Magn Reson Imaging 1998; 9:360-376.
13. Gold GE, McCauley TR, Gray ML, Disler DG. What's new in cartilage? Radio Graphics 2003; 23:1227-1242.
14. Hodler J, Resnick D. Current status of imaging of articular cartilage. Skeletal Radiol 1996; 25:703-709.
15. McCauley TR, Disler DG. Magnetic resonance imaging of articular cartilage of the knee. J Am Acad Orthop Surg 2001; 9:2-8.
16. Recht MP, Resnick D. Magnetic resonance imaging of articular cartilage: an overview. Top Magn Reson Imaging 1998; 9:328-336.
17. Rubenstein JD, Li JG, Majumdar S, Henkelman RM. Image resolution and signal-to-noise ratio requirements for MR imaging of degenerative cartilage. AJR Am J Roentgenol 1997; 169:1089-1096.
18. Resnick D, Kang H. Internal Derangements of Joints. New York, WB Saunders, 1997.
19. Meyer CH, Pauly JM, Macovski A, Nishimura DG. Simultaneous spatial and spectral selective excitation. Magn Reson Med 1990; 15:287-304.
20. Bredella MA, Tirman PF, Peterfy CG, et al. Accuracy of T2-weighted fast spin-echo MR imaging with fat saturation in detecting cartilage defects in the knee: comparison with arthroscopy in 130 patients. AJR Am J Roentgenol 1999; 172:1073-1080.
21. Disler DG. Fat-suppressed three-dimensional spoiled gradient-recalled MR imaging: assessment of articular and physeal hyaline cartilage. AJR Am J Roentgenol 1997; 169:1117-1123.
22. Recht MP, Piraino DW, Paletta GA, et al. Accuracy of fat-suppressed three-dimensional spoiled gradient-echo FLASH MR imaging in the detection of patellofemoral articular cartilage abnormalities. Radiology 1996; 198:209-212.
23. Wang SF, Cheng HC, Chang CY. Fat-suppressed three-dimensional fast spoiled gradient-recalled echo imaging: a modified FS 3D SPGR technique for assessment of patellofemoral joint chondromalacia. Clin Imaging 1999; 23:177-180.
24. Cicuttini F, Forbes A, Asbeutah A, et al. Comparison and reproducibility of fast and conventional spoiled gradient-echo magnetic resonance sequences in the determination of knee cartilage volume. J Orthop Res 2000; 18:580-584.
25. Eckstein F, Schnier M, Haubner M, et al. Accuracy of cartilage volume and thickness measurements with magnetic resonance imaging. Clin Orthop 1998; (352):137-148.
26. Eckstein F, Winzheimer M, Westhoff J, et al. Quantitative relationships of normal cartilage volumes of the human knee joint—assessment by magnetic resonance imaging. Anat Embryol (Berl) 1998; 197:383-390.
27. Eckstein F, Westhoff J, Sittek H, et al. In vivo reproducibility of three-dimensional cartilage volume and thickness measurements with MR imaging. AJR Am J Roentgenol 1998; 170:593-597.
28. Reeder SB, Hargreaves BA, Yu H, Brittain JH. Homodyne reconstruction and IDEAL water-fat decomposition. Magn Reson Med 2005; 54:586-593.
29. Eckstein F, Hudelmaier M, Wirth W, et al. Double echo steady state (DESS) magnetic resonance imaging of knee articular cartilage at 3 Tesla—a pilot study for the Osteoarthritis Initiative. Ann Rheum Dis 2006; 65:433-441.
30. Hardy PA, Recht MP, Piraino D, Thomasson D. Optimization of a dual echo in the steady state (DESS) free-precession sequence for imaging cartilage. J Magn Reson Imaging 1996; 6:329-335.
31. Ruehm S, Zanetti M, Romero J, Hodler J. MRI of patellar articular cartilage: evaluation of an optimized gradient echo sequence (3D-DESS). J Magn Reson Imaging 1998; 8:1246-1251.
32. Woertler K, Strothmann M, Tombach B, Reimer P. Detection of articular cartilage lesions: experimental evaluation of low- and high-field-strength MR imaging at 0.18 and 1.0 T. J Magn Reson Imaging 2000; 11:678-685.
33. Becker ED, Farrar TC. Driven equilibrium Fourier transform spectroscopy: a new method for nuclear magnetic resonance signal enhancement. J Am Chem Soc 1969; 91:7784-7785.
34. Hargreaves BA, Gold GE, Lang PK, et al. MR imaging of articular cartilage using driven equilibrium. Magn Reson Med 1999; 42:695-703.
35. Escobedo EM, Hunter JC, Zink-Brody GC, et al. Usefulness of turbo spin-echo MR imaging in the evaluation of meniscal tears: comparison with a conventional spin-echo sequence. AJR Am J Roentgenol 1996; 167:1223-1227.
36. Gold GE, Fuller SE, Hargreaves BA, et al. Driven equilibrium magnetic resonance imaging of articular cartilage: initial clinical experience. J Magn Reson Imaging 2005; 21:476-481.

37. Yoshioka H, Stevens K, Hargreaves BA, et al. Magnetic resonance imaging of articular cartilage of the knee: comparison between fat-suppressed three-dimensional SPGR imaging, fat-suppressed FSE imaging, and fat-suppressed three-dimensional DEFT imaging, and correlation with arthroscopy. J Magn Reson Imaging 2004; 20:857-864.
38. Woertler K, Rummeny EJ, Settles M. A fast high-resolution multi-slice T1-weighted turbo spin-echo (TSE) sequence with a DRIVen equilibrium (DRIVE) pulse for native arthrographic contrast. AJR Am J Roentgenol 2005; 185:1468-1470.
39. Menick BJ, Bobman SA, Listerud J, Atlas SW. Thin-section, three-dimensional Fourier transform, steady-state free precession MR imaging of the brain. Radiology 1992; 183:369-377.
40. Duerk JL, Lewin JS, Wendt M, Petersilge C. Remember true FISP? A high SNR, near 1-second imaging method for T2-like contrast in interventional MRI at .2 T. J Magn Reson Imaging 1998; 8:203-208.
41. Bangerter NK, Hargreaves BA, Vasanawala SS, et al. Analysis of multiple-acquisition SSFP. Magn Reson Med 2004; 51:1038-1047.
42. Zur Y, Wood ML, Neuringer LJ. Motion-insensitive, steady-state free precession imaging. Magn Reson Med 1990; 16:444-459.
43. Kornaat PR, Doornbos J, van der Molen AJ, et al. Magnetic resonance imaging of knee cartilage using a water selective balanced steady-state free precession sequence. J Magn Reson Imaging 2004; 20:850-856.
44. Vasanawala SS, Pauly JM, Nishimura DG. Linear combination steady-state free precession MRI. Magn Reson Med 2000; 43:82-90.
45. Vasanawala SS, Pauly JM, Nishimura DG. Fluctuating equilibrium MRI. Magn Reson Med 1999; 42:876-883.
46. Scheffler K, Heid O, Hennig J. Magnetization preparation during the steady state: fat-saturated 3D TrueFISP. Magn Reson Med 2001; 45:1075-1080.
47. Reeder SB, Pineda AR, Wen Z, et al. Iterative decomposition of water and fat with echo asymmetry and least-squares estimation (IDEAL): Application with fast spin-echo imaging. Magn Reson Med 2005; 54:636-644.
48. Hargreaves BA, Vasanawala SS, Nayak KS, et al. Fat-suppressed steady-state free precession imaging using phase detection. Magn Reson Med 2003; 50:210-213.
49. Vasanawala SS, Hargreaves BA, Pauly JM, et al. Rapid musculoskeletal MRI with phase-sensitive steady-state free precession: comparison with routine knee MRI. AJR Am J Roentgenol 2005; 184:1450-1455.
50. Du J, Carroll TJ, Brodsky E, et al. Contrast-enhanced peripheral magnetic resonance angiography using time-resolved vastly undersampled isotropic projection reconstruction. J Magn Reson Imaging 2004; 20:894-900.
51. Lu A, Grist TM, Block WF. Fat/water separation in single excitation steady-state free precession using multiple radial trajectories. Magn Reson Med 2005; 54:1051-1057.
52. Gold GE, Hargreaves B, Vasanawala SS, et al. MR imaging of articular cartilage of the knee using fluctuating equilibrium MR (FEMR)—initial experience in healthy volunteers. Radiology 2006; 238:719-724.
53. Hargreaves BA, Vasanawala SS, Pauly JM, Nishimura DG. Characterization and reduction of the transient response in steady-state MR imaging. Magn Reson Med 2001; 46:149-158.
54. Reeder SB, Pelc NJ, Alley MT, Gold GE. Rapid MR imaging of articular cartilage with steady-state free precession and multipoint fat-water separation. AJR Am J Roentgenol 2003; 180:357-362.
55. Kornaat PR, Reeder SB, Koo S, et al. MR imaging of articular cartilage at 1.5T and 3.0T: comparison of SPGR and SSFP sequences. Osteoarthritis Cartilage 2005; 13:338-344.
56. Kijowski R, Lu A, Block WF, Grist TM. Evaluation of articular cartilage in the knee joint with vastly undersampled isotropic projection reconstruction steady-state free precession (VIPR-SSFP). J Magn Reson Imaging 2006; 24:168-175.
57. Jashnani Y, Lu A, Jung Y, et al. Linear combination SSFP at 3T: improved spectral response using multiple echoes. Presented before the ISMRM 14th annual meeting, Seattle, 2006.
58. Gold GE, Busse RF, Beehler C, et al. Isotropic MRI of the knee with 3D fast spin-echo extended echo-train acquisition (XETA): initial experience. AJR Am J Roentgenol 2007; 188:1287-1293.
59. Reeder SB, Pineda AR, Yu H, et al. Water-fat separation with IDEAL-SPGR. Presented before the 13th annual meeting of the ISMRM, Miami, 2005.
60. Reeder SB, Wen Z, Yu H, et al. Multicoil Dixon chemical species separation with an iterative least-squares estimation method. Magn Reson Med 2004; 51:35-45.
61. Yu H, Reeder SB, Shimakawa A, et al. Implementation and noise analysis of chemical shift correction for fast spin-echo "Dixon" imaging. Presented before the 12th annual meeting of the ISMRM, Kyoto, 2004.
62. Shapiro EM, Borthakur A, Gougoutas A, Reddy R. ^{23}Na MRI accurately measures fixed charge density in articular cartilage. Magn Reson Med 2002; 47:284-291.
63. Reddy R, Insko EK, Noyszewski EA, et al. Sodium MRI of human articular cartilage in vivo. Magn Reson Med 1998; 39:697-701.
64. Boada FE, Shen GX, Chang SY, Thulborn KR. Spectrally weighted twisted projection imaging: reducing T2 signal attenuation effects in fast three-dimensional sodium imaging. Magn Reson Med 1997; 38:1022-1028.

65. Borthakur A, Hancu I, Boada FE, et al. In vivo triple quantum filtered twisted projection sodium MRI of human articular cartilage. J Magn Reson 1999; 141:286-290.
66. Borthakur A, Shapiro EM, Beers J, et al. Sensitivity of MRI to proteoglycan depletion in cartilage: comparison of sodium and proton MRI. Osteoarthritis Cartilage 2000; 8:288-293.
67. Hancu I, Boada FE, Shen GX. Three-dimensional triple-quantum-filtered (23)Na imaging of in vivo human brain. Magn Reson Med 1999; 42:1146-1154.

Biochemical and Functional Techniques for Cartilage Imaging

Timothy J. Mosher

A prevailing but yet unproved hypothesis in the treatment of osteoarthritis (OA) is that early diagnosis of cartilage injury is necessary to improve patient outcome.[1-4] Visible changes of cartilage damage such as surface fibrillation and erosion represent relatively late manifestations of OA. These morphologic changes are preceded by biochemical and structural changes in the extracellular matrix that alter the biomechanical properties of the tissue. The sensitivity of the MRI signal to the macromolecular environment of tissue water provides the potential to use measurements of MRI relaxation parameters to detect and monitor these early changes in cartilage in the intact human joint. Potential MRI parameters that have been proposed for the study of cartilage are summarized in Table 8-1. Initial results indicate MRI parametric mapping techniques are sensitive, and in some cases specific, for alterations in the cartilage matrix relevant to the study of early OA. In many cases these techniques have been limited to proof of concept studies in excised osteochondral specimens. Other techniques such as delayed gadolinium-enhanced MRI of cartilage (dGEMRIC) and cartilage T2 mapping have been validated and applied to human studies.

TABLE 8-1. Potential MRI Markers for Biochemical and Functional Assessment of Articular Cartilage

Cartilage Property	MRI Parameter
Water Content	Proton density T1 T2
Proteoglycan content	Sodium MRI T1rho dGEMRIC
Collagen content	MT T2
Collagen orientation	T2 Diffusion tensor imaging
Water mobility	Diffusion T2
Regional cartilage Compressibility	MRI tagging MR elastography T2 mapping

dGEMRIC, delayed gadolinium-enhanced MRI of cartilage.

PROTEOGLYCAN-SENSITIVE TECHNIQUES

Depletion of proteoglycan from cartilage is one of the earliest findings in OA and is strongly correlated with changes in biomechanical properties. MRI methods to measure regional proteoglycan concentration consist of sodium MRI, T1rho imaging, and dGEMRIC.[4] Recently, a novel approach has been proposed for measuring proteoglycan concentration by selective saturation transfer of the exchangeable protons on the glycosaminoglycan (GAG) termed chemical exchange-dependent saturation transfer.[5] Additional studies are needed to determine the possibility of using this technique in the intact joint.

Sodium MRI

Although current clinical MRI is derived from signal generated by the proton, any nucleus with an odd number of protons and/or neutrons possesses a nuclear magnetic moment and is capable of generating a MRI signal. The ^{23}Na nucleus is one such nucleus; however, the signal generated by the ^{23}Na nucleus has less than one half the energy of the signal generated by the proton. In addition, the relatively low concentration of sodium in cartilage (~320 μM) compared with water, and the very short T2 time of the sodium signal, make in-vivo ^{23}Na MRI challenging. Sodium imaging requires the use of specific transmit and receive coils that are not readily available for clinical systems. With the growth of ultra-high field human 7.0T MRI systems, sodium imaging with spatial resolution similar to that currently observed with proton MRI is possible (Fig. 8-10).

In cartilage, sodium ions are associated with the negatively charged keratan sulfate and chondroitin sulfate side chains of the GAG and are the primary component of the fixed charged density in the extracellular matrix.[6,7] Preliminary studies in excised tissue samples have shown sodium MRI is sensitive to small changes in sodium concentration with enzymatic depletion of GAG.[8-12] Techniques have been proposed for obtaining quantitative measures of sodium concentration in cartilage[13,14] and for selectively obtaining the signal from sodium bound to macromolecules in the extracellular matrix.[15-22] Although in-vivo human images have been demonstrated,[11,15] clinical research application of sodium MRI has been limited to proof of concept and feasibility studies.

T1rho Imaging

Although differences in T1 relaxation between tissues is a primary source of image contrast in clinical MRI, T1rho contrast has received limited attention. The relaxation constant T1 refers to the spin lattice relaxation time constant in the presence of a static magnetic field (B0). In contrast, the relaxation time constant T1rho refers to spin lattice relaxation in the presence of the radiofrequency (RF) magnetic field (B1). By varying the magnitude of the B1 field it is possible to selectively sensitize the T1rho relaxation to different water-macromolecular interactions. In the case of normal cartilage and early cartilage degeneration, T1rho appears to be sensitive primarily to the interaction of water protons with GAG.[23] However, with further GAG depletion there also appears to be contribution from collagen water interaction similar to that seen with magnetization transfer (MT) and T2 relaxation maps.[24-26] Several validation studies have been published. Regatte and coworkers have demonstrated a strong correlation between T1rho in tissue and spectrophotometric assays of cartilage proteoglycan content.[27,28] In isolated tissue specimens, T1rho increases with proteoglycan depletion using trypsin digestion[29-31] but not with collagenase treatment. A study using interleukin-1 depletion of proteoglycan in a rabbit model indicates promise for using T1rho to monitor in-vivo changes in proteoglycan content.[32] T1rho elevation is correlated with biochemical measures of proteoglycan

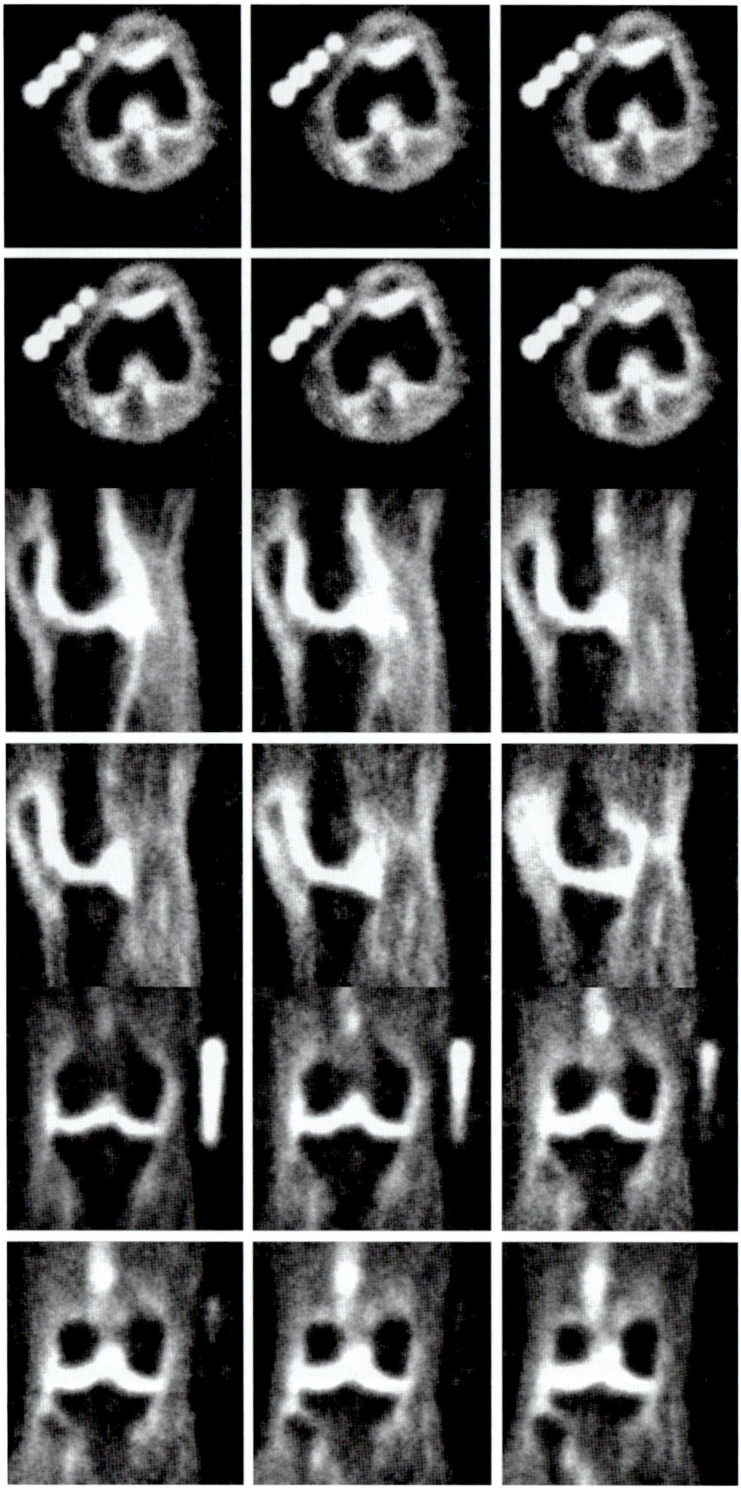

FIGURE 8-10. In-vivo 3D 7.0T ^{23}Na radial imaging of the knee of a healthy volunteer. Total image acquisition time was less than 14 minutes with an isotropic resolution of 1.5 mm. High signal is generated from sodium in synovial fluid and articular cartilage. Representative slices from axial, sagittal, and coronal planes are shown. (Courtesy of Ravinder Regatte, PhD, New York University Medical Center.)

depletion and associated changes in biomechanical properties.[33] There is a strong correlation between T1rho and fixed charge density as assessed using sodium MRI.[34] Analysis of resected cartilage specimens from eight subjects undergoing total knee replacement suggested T1rho had greater responsiveness to tissue degeneration than cartilage T2 mapping.[35]

Although several studies have evaluated T1rho in animal and isolated human cartilage specimens, there have been relatively few in-vivo studies of T1rho in human subjects or clinical trials. An initial feasibility study demonstrated elevated T1rho values in cartilage of symptomatic OA subjects.[36] A case report of two subjects has shown elevation in T1rho at sites of focal traumatic cartilage injury.[37] Recent studies of 16 mild OA subjects demonstrated elevation of T1rho and T2 compared with asymptomatic subjects[38] and correlated changes in subchondral trabecular bone remodeling with elevation of T1rho and cartilage T2.[38,39] Additional studies are needed to confirm reliability and responsiveness of T1rho imaging in a multicenter trial.

Initial application of T1rho in humans was limited to single-slice acquisition,[40] although more recently, multi-slice[41] and 3D acquisitions[36,42-44] have been developed (Fig. 8-11). A potential limitation of the T1rho technique is the relatively large amount of RF power that is applied during the spin-locking preparation pulse, which can result in tissue heating; however, newer versions of the technique suggest this is not a significant limitation at current clinical field strengths of up to 3.0T. Implementation of parallel imaging techniques has reduced imaging times, with acquisition times now in the range of 5 to 10 minutes (Fig. 8-11).[45,46] The recent implementation of T1rho imaging on clinical MRI scanners should expand application of this potentially valuable technique to human research.

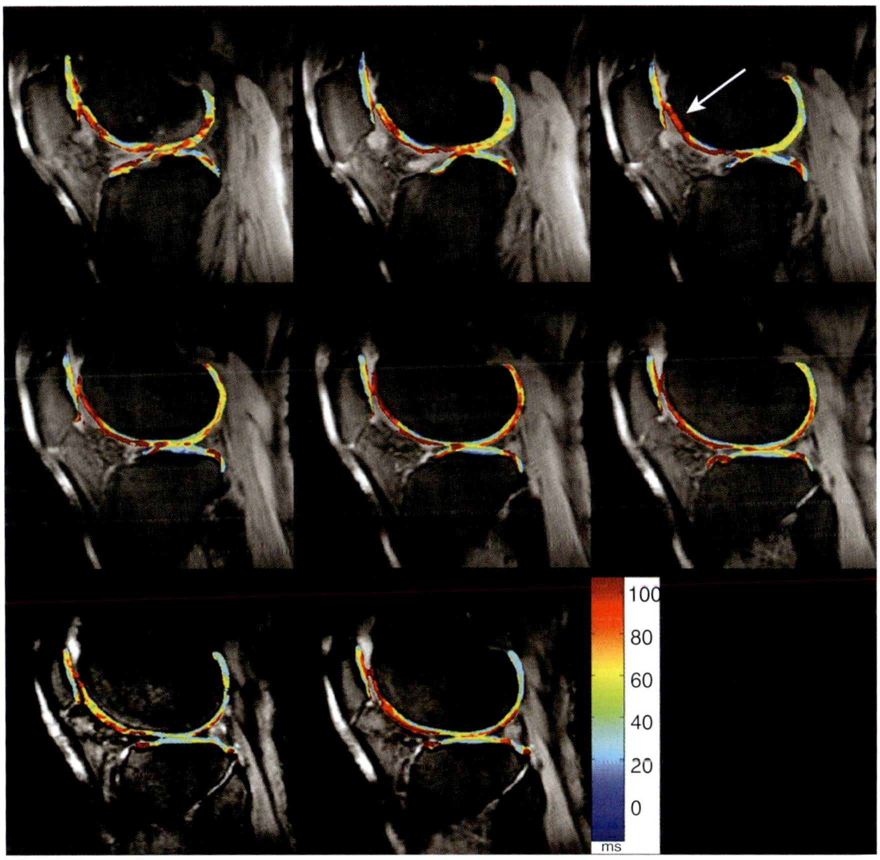

FIGURE 8-11. Representative 3D T1rho maps obtained from a 60-year-old patient with osteoarthritis. 3D T1rho–weighted imaging with parallel imaging (GRAPPA acceleration factor [AF] = 2) was performed with a T1rho preparation pulse cluster and 3D-FLASH as a readout sequence: TR/TE = 175/2.04 ms, spin-lock frequency = 300 Hz, number of slices = 20, time of spin-lock (TSL) = 2/10/20/30 ms, slice thickness = 3 mm, matrix = 256 × 128, FOV = 15 cm, flip angle = 250, bandwidth = 260 Hz. The color bar scale represents the T1rho values in milliseconds. (Courtesy of Ravinder Regatte, PhD, New York University Medical Center.)

Delayed Gadolinium-Enhanced MRI of Cartilage

Unlike sodium MRI, which measures the fixed charge density using the intrinsic sodium ion, the dGEMRIC technique uses a negatively charged contrast agent to indirectly measure regional GAG content in articular cartilage[47,48] and, more recently, as a potential measure of meniscal degeneration.[49] After intravenous injection, the MRI contrast agent gadopentetate dimeglumine (Gd-DTPA; Magnevist) slowly diffuses into synovial fluid and over time will equilibrate with articular cartilage. Because of the steric hindrance and electrostatic repulsion of Gd-DTPA, partitioning of the contrast agent within cartilage is inversely proportional to the distribution of GAG.[50,51] As illustrated in Figure 8-12, areas of low GAG will contain a higher content of contrast agent, which results in more rapid T1 relaxation of adjacent water protons. After obtaining a series of images with differing degrees of T1 weighting, a T1 map can be calculated that provides a regional assessment of relative Gd-DTPA concentration that is inversely proportional to regional GAG content.[52] The acquisition of a single T1 map after administration of Gd-DTPA has been termed a *dGEMRIC index* and has been shown to be similar at 1.5T and 3.0T field strengths.[53] An alternative to T1 mapping has been suggested in which pharmacokinetic modeling of cartilage enhancement has been used to estimate cartilage permeability and extracellular matrix water as measures of cartilage damage.[54] A CT-based form of dGEMRIC has been suggested using anionic radiographic contrast agents.[55]

Technical issues related to optimization of the dGEMRIC technique for human clinical applications have been reviewed.[56] The compound Gd-DTPA has been approved for clinical use as an MRI contrast agent; however, the dGEMRIC technique represents an off-label application. The standard clinical dose is 0.1 mM/kg, but a dose of up to 0.3 mM/kg has been used in clinical neuroimaging applications. There is a dose-dependent response of T1 relaxation in cartilage over the range of 0.1 to 0.3 mM/kg.[57,58] The recommended dose for dGEMRIC studies is 0.2 mM/kg, or twice the recommended clinical dose, but this should be corrected for body mass index because higher plasma levels of Gd-DTPA occur in obese subjects owing to the lower extracellular water content of adipose tissue.[58] Reproducibility of the technique using a test-retest paradigm was slightly better using a double dose of Gd-DTPA and was in the range of plus or minus 15% for regional T1 measurements.[56] Some authors have advocated using a triple dose to improve sensitivity to small changes in GAG.[57] To increase uptake in synovial fluid, it is recommended that subjects exercise the joint for 10 minutes after intravenous injection, and it is neces-

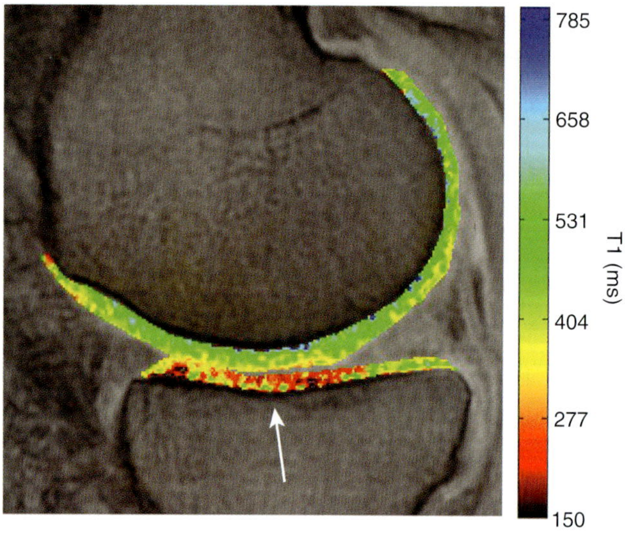

FIGURE 8-12. Delayed gadolinium-enhanced MRI of cartilage (dGEMRIC) demonstrating focal glycosaminoglycan depletion in the tibial plateau (*arrow*). Increased uptake of Gd-DTPA contrast in sites of low glycosaminoglycan content results in shortening of cartilage T1 denoted by the red pixels in the quantitative T1 map. Normal content is indicated by longer T1 values and is measured in the femoral cartilage. (Courtesy of Deborah Burstein, PhD, Harvard Medical School, Beth Israel Deaconess Medical Center.)

sary to wait 2 hours before obtaining T1 maps to allow penetration into thicker patellar cartilage.[57] For thinner cartilage, such as the hip, the interval after injection can be reduced to 90 minutes.[56] Further decreasing the delay period to 30 minutes has been shown to provide better differentiation of individuals with hip OA, however, with lower reproducibility.[59]

Additional safety precautions must be considered when administering gadolinium-based contrast agents. Gadolinium-based MRI contrast media has been linked to nephrogenic systemic fibrosis, a highly debilitating condition resembling scleroderma that occurs in patients with moderate to severe renal impairment.[60-65] Although the pathogenesis of nephrogenic systemic fibrosis is still under investigation, the prevailing theory is that renal impairment leads to prolonged circulating life times of gadolinium contrast, promoting dechelation and accumulation of free Gd^{3+} in tissue.[61] At present there is no cure for nephrogenic systemic fibrosis, although some improvement has been observed after renal transplantation. The risk of this potentially fatal condition necessitates appropriate precautions and screening procedures for all subjects receiving gadolinium contrast such as Gd-DTPA.

Logistical barriers to widespread research application of the dGEMRIC technique are the delay period between injection and imaging and the long imaging time needed to acquire the series of T1-weighted images used to calculate the T1 maps. Using standard spin-echo imaging techniques, total imaging time approaches 1 hour and has limited spatial coverage. The long imaging interval makes it necessary to correct for patient motion that may occur between acquisitions. More recently, techniques have been developed for rapid 3D T1 mapping of tissue that can reduce acquisition times to several minutes with improved spatial coverage.[58,66-68] These techniques are currently undergoing validation.

Several validation studies have shown a strong correlation between GAG content determined using the dGEMRIC technique and biochemical or histologic measures.[50,52,69-72] In isolated cartilage samples the correlation between GAG content determined using dGEMRIC and histologic measurement of GAG is better in superficial cartilage than in deeper layers where MRI can overestimate GAG.[72] Differences between observers in the selection and calculation of regional T1 have been shown not to be a significant source of variation.[73]

Several groups are exploring clinical research application of dGEMRIC in evaluation of OA. Increased uptake of Gd-DTPA was observed in compartments with fibrillation and softening identified arthroscopically.[74] Similar findings have been observed with subjects with patellar chondrosis.[75] Joint space narrowing and malalignment are associated with femoral/tibial compartment differences in dGEMRIC indices.[76] Several studies have used dGEMRIC to evaluate cartilage in the setting of acute or chronic soft tissue derangements of the knee. Areas of increased contrast uptake are associated with sites of meniscal or ligamentous injuries.[77,78] In patients with acute (<3 weeks) tears of the anterior cruciate ligament, increased uptake of contrast was observed in cartilage of the medial compartment as well as in the lateral compartment adjacent to sites of subchondral marrow contusion.[79] There is the potential for dGEMRIC to provide novel information to guide clinical management of patients. Greater uptake of Gd-DTPA has been seen in subjects with acetabular dysplasia and correlated well with both pain and degree of dysplasia.[80] A low dGEMRIC index indicative of GAG depletion was predictive of poor outcomes in patients undergoing periacetabular osteotomy for treatment of acetabular dysplasia.[81]

Another potential clinical application of dGEMRIC is assessment of tissue maturation after cartilage repair.[82-85] Most studies have demonstrated heterogeneous uptake in the repair tissue that persists over time. In this setting, the baseline T1 of the tissue as well as uptake of Gd-DTPA is influenced by regional differences in water content and permeability of the tissue, in addition to GAG content. Because these properties change concurrently as the repair tissue matures, longitudinal changes in the dGEMRIC index may not be a specific measure of GAG content. In the setting of cartilage repair tissue it is necessary to measure T1 both before and after contrast administration to accurately assess GAG content and correct for baseline variability in repair tissue T1.[67,86]

Results of dGEMRIC have demonstrated a high level of responsiveness to changes in cartilage GAG. The dGEMRIC technique has been used to monitor GAG repletion after interleukin-1–induced depletion.[87] Several studies have shown that changes observed with dGEMRIC are closely associated with the biomechanical properties of adult cartilage but are less predictive in skeletally immature cartilage.[88] Increased uptake of Gd-DTPA indicative of low GAG content is associated with increased cartilage compressibility.[89-92] Preliminary findings in osteochondral allografts demonstrate a similar association between indentation stiffness and low GAG as determined using dGEMRIC.[93]

Animal studies have shown that dGEMRIC is sensitive to changes in proteoglycan content of cartilage that occur in response to loading conditions of the joint.[94] A potential research application of MRI is to study habitation of cartilage in response to changes in exercise. A recent study of 37 subjects suggests dGEMRIC may be useful to monitor the adaptive response of cartilage to exercise.[95] Using the dGEMRIC technique, baseline T1 values correlated strongly with level of physical activity with the longest T1 values (high GAG) observed in elite runners and the lowest T1 values in sedentary individuals. This study supports previous work in animals, suggesting load-bearing exercise can increase GAG content in cartilage.[96] These intriguing results illustrate future translational research opportunities to understand the important role of joint biomechanics in cartilage physiology and the role of exercise in the development of OA.

COLLAGEN-SENSITIVE TECHNIQUES

Along with the large aggregating proteoglycan aggrecan, type II collagen is the other major macromolecule present in the extracellular cartilage matrix. It is the confining properties of collagen in response to the swelling properties of aggrecan that provide cartilage with the high interstitial pressure and ability to restrain water movement needed to achieve the normal response to physiologic stress.[97,98] In addition, the collagen fibrils are an essential component for normal cartilage response to shear stress.[99,100] As discussed in Chapter 2, routine clinical TSE imaging is sensitive to regional variations in the organization and content of the type II collagen matrix of cartilage.[101] Two MRI parameters, in particular MT and T2 of cartilage, have demonstrated sensitivity to changes in cartilage collagen. Although both techniques are sensitive to collagen content in cartilage, T2 is also sensitive to the anisotropic organization and orientation of collagen fibrils in the extracellular matrix.

Magnetization Transfer

Substantial MT has been demonstrated in articular cartilage,[102,103] and is greatest in the radial zone near the bone/cartilage interface.[104] The potential for MT is present in any multi-slice MRI technique. It is particularly prominent in TSE techniques because of the rapid application of multiple off-resonance RF pulses. For standard clinical imaging, substantial incidental MT leading to lower signal intensity from cartilage occurs with multi-slice TSE sequences[105,106] and can lead to errors in other quantitative parametric mapping techniques such as T1 or T2 mapping using multi-slice TSE.[107,108] Because GRE techniques do not have a 180-degree refocusing RF pulse and use less energy for the excitation RF pulse there is substantially less MT in GRE images. By applying an off-resonance RF prepulse immediately before the GRE sequence it is possible to impart MT contrast to the image. After subtracting images with MT preparation from control images obtained without the prepulse it is possible to isolate the contribution from MT.[109]

Variability from multiple factors such as RF power, pulse profile, and offset frequency limit quantification of MT, making it difficult to implement as a parametric mapping technique.[110,111] Because calculation of MT is derived from a subtraction of two image sets, the resulting signal to noise is very poor and is prone to artifact from any motion occurring between the two acquisitions. The higher SNR available at 3.0T may improve image quality of MT maps.[112] For human studies, the additional RF power needed for MT is limited by safety guidelines for specific absorption rate in place to limit RF heating. As a result, most MT applications have been nonquantitative, with few demonstrations of quantitative MT techniques in humans.[113-116]

The primary application of MT in the evaluation of articular cartilage has been to improve contrast resolution between cartilage and the overlying synovial fluid,[117,118] which has been shown to increase accuracy of focal cartilage lesion detection.[113,119,120] Studies in excised tissue samples,[115,121-124] bioengineered cartilage tissue,[125] and animal models[126-128] have shown that collagen/water interaction is the major contributor to this effect with little variation in MT occurring with removal of proteoglycan. A few studies have questioned whether proteoglycan depletion contributes to increased MT.[122,129]

Cartilage T2 Mapping

The spin-spin or transverse relaxation time (T2) is an MRI time constant sensitive to the slow molecular motions of protons as they move through the macromolecular environment. Early in development of biologic nuclear magnetic resonance it was recognized that changes in tissue T2 provide a sensitive marker of disease. In cartilage, T2 is sensitive to changes in water content,[130-134] collagen content,[25,26,135-138] and orientation of the highly organized anisotropic arrangement of collagen fibrils in the extracellular cartilage matrix.[103,110,139-149] As illustrated in Figure 8-13, increased water content and damage to the type II collagen matrix prolong cartilage T2. The orientation dependence of T2 is a result of residual quadripolar relaxation mechanisms that are present in cartilage as a result of the anisotropic arrangement of collagen

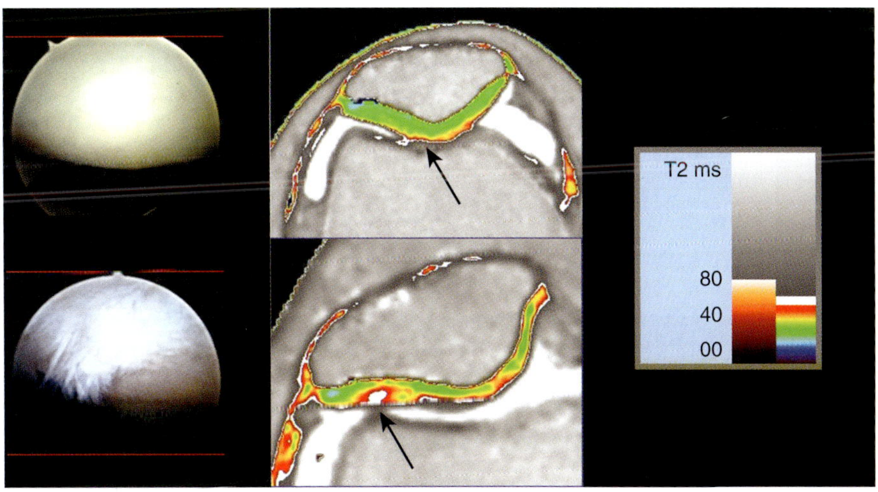

FIGURE 8-13. Quantitative cartilage T2 mapping and corresponding arthroscopy. **Top left, center,** Normal cartilage in a 24-year-old woman undergoing arthroscopic anterior cruciate ligament repair demonstrates a normal depth-dependent variation in T2 with low values indicated in *green* observed in the radial zone near the bone/cartilage interface and longer T2 values indicated in orange (*arrow*) near the articular surface. **Bottom left, center,** Focal chondral erosion and fibrillation observed at arthroscopy results in focally elevated cartilage T2 (*arrow*) in a 54-year-old woman undergoing arthroscopic surgery for a medial meniscal tear.

fibrils[21,25,150-155] and is most pronounced in the radial zone of cartilage where there is a preferential orientation of fibers perpendicular to bone.[140,141,148,156] In addition to orientational variation of collagen fibers with respect to depth from the articular surface, the preferential orientation of the collagen matrix varies regionally within the joint.[157] This regional variation correlates well with the orientation predicted from the collagen remodeling algorithm of Driessen and associates[158] developed for type I collagen remodeling in cardiovascular tissues.[159] There is growing recognition that the orientation of the collagen matrix has a strong influence on the biomechanical properties of cartilage and health of the chondrocyte.[160-164]

Correlation studies in tissue samples have demonstrated a strong inverse correlation between cartilage T2 and optical methods of assessing collagen fiber anisotropy.[139,147,165-167] Most studies have observed a negligible effect on T2 after enzymatic depletion of proteoglycan from cartilage,[24,27,124,168] as well as poor regional correlation between T2 and histologic staining for proteoglycan.[135] A few studies suggest proteoglycan depletion may lead to an increase in cartilage T2.[138,169,170] A study on cartilage with genetic mutation leading to lack of aggrecan in the extracellular matrix suggests that depletion of the large aggregating proteoglycan does not substantially change the mean T2 value but substantially increases the range of distribution of T2, likely owing to increased availability of additional water binding sites and thereby increasing the heterogeneity of the macromolecular environment.[171] As demonstrated in Figure 8-14, genetic defects in *COL2A1,* the gene that encodes for type II collagen, result in marked elevation of cartilage T2 values and loss of the normal spatial dependency of T2 with respect to depth from the articular surface.

Sensitivity to structural changes in the cartilage collagen matrix and the concurrent changes that occur with respect to changes in water content make cartilage T2 mapping a useful probe for study of early OA.[172] Changes in collagen fibril organization are observed during the process of cartilage development,[137,173-176] during aging,[177-180] and in early OA.[181-184] Whereas a decrease in collagen content is a relatively late manifestation of OA, loss of collagen matrix anisotropy occurs early and can be detected with quantitative T2 measurement.[185] Weakening of the collagen fibril meshwork decreases the constraining forces on the hydrated proteoglycan, leading to an increase in water content and increased permeability of cartilage.[97,186] Compressibility and permeability of cartilage are highly correlated with water content, which also contributes to T2 elevation in damaged cartilage. As water content increases, the matrix of the tissue becomes more compressible[98] and a greater portion of the load is carried by the solid components of the extracellular matrix.[187] This subsequently leads to increased stress, structural fatigue, fragmentation of the solid extracellular matrix, and, ultimately, visible changes such as cartilage fibrillation and ulceration.

Several studies have demonstrated a strong association with T2 and histologic measures of OA in both tissue samples[24,91,188] and animal models of OA.[189-191] Using

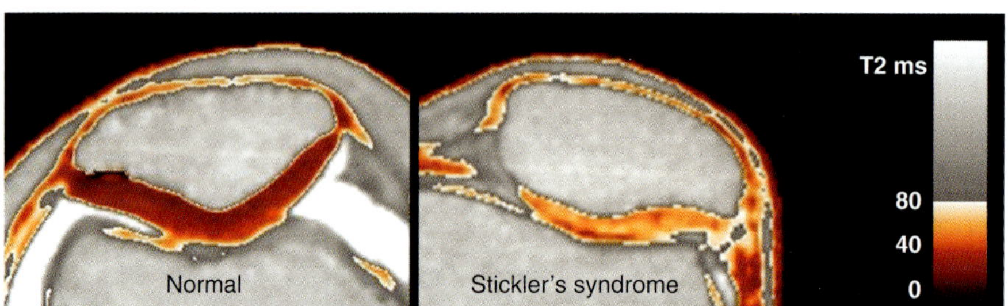

FIGURE 8-14. A 27-year-old man presented with Stickler's syndrome due to a genetic mutation of the type II collagen gene. Note the diffusely elevated cartilage T2 consistent with disorganization of the type II collagen matrix. For comparison, the quantitative cartilage T2 map of an asymptomatic 27-year-old man is shown on the left.

MRI microscopy, cartilage T2 mapping has been used to follow chondral repair in a rat model.[138,192] Although elevated T2 is most frequently associated with cartilage damage, areas of low T2-weighted signal intensity are not infrequently observed in adjacent cartilage in the setting of subacute or chronic cartilage injury. The etiology of this finding is unclear but may be related to fragmentation of collagen fibrils exposing additional hydrophilic sites that could lead to more efficient T2 relaxation and greater MT. Low T2 values can be associated with focal areas of increased collagen deposition[193] and chondrocalcinosis.[194]

Although most validation studies have been performed using high field MRI microscopy scanners on excised tissue, in-vivo human cartilage T2 maps have been obtained from the adult[195-197] and pediatric femoral tibial joint,[198] patellofemoral joint,[199] ankle,[200] hip,[201,202] and the proximal interphalangeal joint of the hand.[203] Technical considerations for human cartilage T2 mapping have been reviewed.[3,204,205] Quantitative T2 maps are derived from multi-echo imaging sequences by fitting the signal intensity of each pixel to a single exponential decay. The calculated cartilage T2 is dependent on both acquisition parameters[206] and the algorithm used in curve fitting routine.[207] Bias in calculation of T2 can occur through the development of stimulated echoes produced by B1 inhomogeneity as well as MT when multi-slice T2 maps are obtained.[107,108] Error from stimulated echoes can be reduced by excluding the initial echo from the T2 calculation. With current multi-slice multi-echo techniques, image acquisition times range from 5 to 10 minutes, depending on spatial resolution. To effectively demonstrate the depth dependent spatial variation in cartilage T2 it is necessary to obtain high-resolution T2 maps. For practical purposes the resolution should be high enough to provide a minimum of 6 pixels across the cartilage plate but ideally would be in the range of 2% of total cartilage thickness for each pixel.[208] With current technology, in-vivo T2 maps with this level of resolution are not feasible. To decrease image acquisition time, parallel imaging,[45] rapid T2 mapping sequences,[197] hybrid gradient-echo/spin-echo,[209] and gradient echo T2* mapping techniques have been explored but to date have not been validated for routine use.

High-resolution T2 mapping studies in humans have demonstrated a spatial variation in T2 similar to that observed with MR microscopy of tissue samples.[149] Shorter T2 values in the range of 30 to 40 ms are observed in subchondral bone, increasing to 50 ms near the articular surface. Based on correlation studies in tissue samples, this spatial dependency is a result of regional differences in the organization of the collagen matrix. Age appears to alter the magnitude of this spatial dependency.[210] Preliminary results in a pediatric population demonstrate a spatial variation in T2 similar to that observed in young adults.[198] However, beginning around age 45 there is a statistically significant increase in T2 of the superficial layer of cartilage compared with individuals younger than age 45 years.[204,211] For individuals older than age 65, statistically significant elevation in T2 is observed throughout the entire thickness of cartilage.[204] This pattern differs from focal T2 elevation that has been described in symptomatic individuals.[211] The results support the hypothesis that aging is associated with degeneration or reorganization of the collagen matrix beginning at the articular surface and progressing to deeper layers. In contrast to age, gender does not appear to have a significant influence on cartilage T2.[212]

Although subjective interpretation of changes in T2 contrast is a standard tool in the clinical evaluation of cartilage damage, there has been limited application of quantitative T2 mapping in evaluating arthritis. In a study of young females with juvenile rheumatoid arthritis there was a diffuse elevation in cartilage T2 compared with healthy age-matched controls; however, the spatial dependency of T2 was similar between the two groups.[213] As illustrated by the case presented in Figure 8-15, elevated quantitative cartilage T2 values are observed in subjects with radiographic knee OA.[35,188,214] Dunn and associates have shown elevation in cartilage T2 in patients with mild radiographic knee OA; however, there was no significant difference between groups with mild and moderate OA.[215] Cartilage T2 elevation in early OA has been correlated with structural remodeling in the subchondral bone plate.[39] A

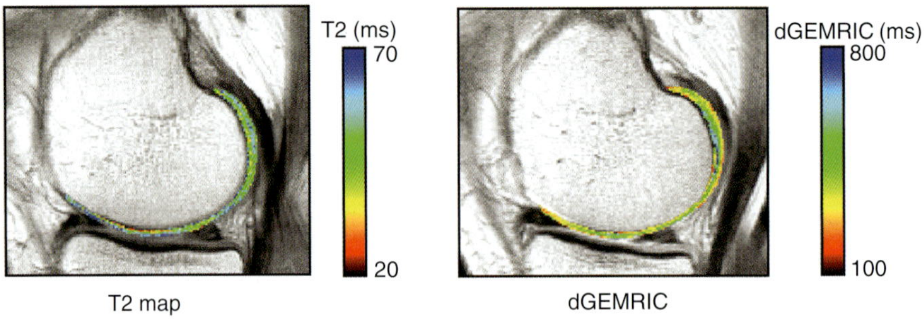

FIGURE 8-15. dGEMRIC and quantitative T2 mapping in the femoral cartilage of a patient with knee osteoarthritis (Kellgren-Lawrence grade 2). Cartilage T2 values are globally elevated with loss of normal depth-dependent variation in T2, indicative of damage to the type II collagen matrix. Cartilage dGEMRIC T1 values are decreased, indicative of diffuse depletion of glycosaminoglycans. (Courtesy of Miika Nieminen, PhD, Oulu University Hospital, Finland.)

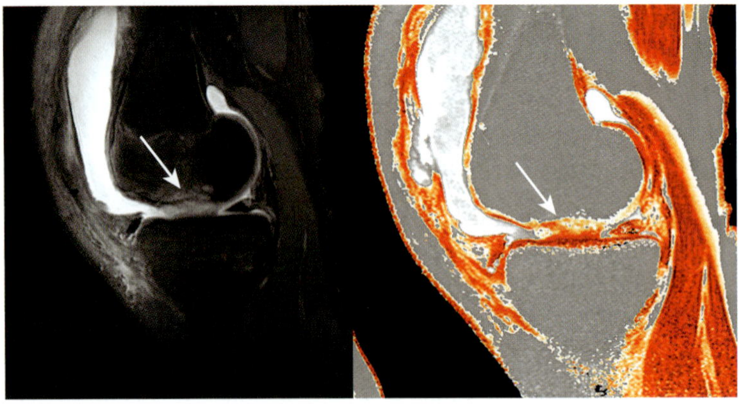

FIGURE 8-16. Sagittal fat-suppressed, proton density–weighted, turbo spin-echo image (*left*) of a 24-year-old woman 3 months after autologous chondrocyte implantation repair of a femoral chondral defect demonstrates a heterogeneously bright signal within the repair site consistent with early healing (*arrows*). Quantitative cartilage T2 mapping (*right*) demonstrated heterogeneous elevation of cartilage T2 with lack of the normal T2 depth dependency observed in normal cartilage.

recent study has demonstrated a strong association between the serum biomarker Col 2-3/4long mono, a collagenase derived neoepitope of type II collagen and knee cartilage T2.[216] This same study found an association between serum cartilage oligomeric matrix protein (COMP) and cartilage volume. This study illustrates the potential for using serum biomarkers in combination with selective image markers to identify specific degenerative pathways in cartilage. It appears cartilage T2 has a nonlinear response to collagen degeneration. It is likely that early degenerative change in organization of the collagen matrix prolongs T2; however, further degeneration does not lead to further elevation in T2. In the future, longitudinal studies are needed to determine the significance of isolated T2 changes. It is unknown if changes associated with T2 elevation invariably progress to morphologic sites of damage or if they can be modified through intervention.

Several studies have applied quantitative cartilage T2 mapping in evaluation of cartilage repair tissue in humans[84,217-220] and animal models.[138,192,221,222] White and coworkers have shown that repair tissue from osteochondral transplantation that has hyaline cartilage histology retains the normal spatial dependency of T2, whereas this variation is absent in repair tissue derived from autologous chondrocyte implantation (ACI) or microfracture techniques.[221] As illustrated in Figure 8-16, early assessment of repair tissue after ACI demonstrates heterogeneously elevated T2 consistent with increased water content and lack of a structural type II collagen matrix. As illustrated in Figure 8-17, repair tissue after ACI can demonstrate dGEMRIC T1 values similar to those of normal cartilage, despite having elevated cartilage T2. The T2 of repair tissue after ACI or microfracture decreases over time and is generally associated with fibrocartilage histology. These results suggest

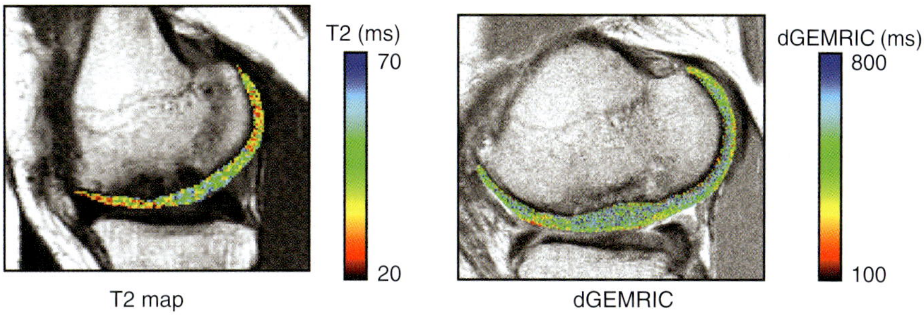

FIGURE 8-17. Quantitative cartilage mapping in the assessment of autologous chondrocyte implantation repair tissue. T2 shows prolonged values indicative of a disorganized collagen structure, whereas dGEMRIC shows relatively normal values suggestive of proteoglycan replenishment. (Courtesy of Miika Nieminen, PhD, Oulu University Hospital, Finland.)

cartilage T2 mapping has the potential to noninvasively assess the composition of chondral repair tissue.

FUNCTIONAL CARTILAGE IMAGING

A relatively new research application of MRI is the study of cartilage biomechanics. Several studies have used quantitative MRI to measure changes in cartilage thickness in response to compressive loading. Initial studies with osteochondral plugs used MRI to monitor real-time change in cartilage thickness during compression creep experiments performed with an MRI-compatible compression device.[223,224] These ex-vivo applications have been extended to studies in intact human joints, including the knee[225] and more recently the ankle.[226,227] Patellar cartilage volume was observed to decrease 6% in young males immediately after performing 50 deep knee bends.[228] The degree of deformation was less (3%) in an elderly cohort.[229] Differences in the degree of patellar cartilage change were observed between static loading (squatting) and dynamic loading (deep knee bends) of the patellofemoral joint.[230] Differences in patellar cartilage deformation have been observed with different exercise. The greatest change occurs after performing deep knee bends (−5.9%), whereas the least occurs after walking (−2.8%).[231] Patellar cartilage deformation after deep knee bends was similar for elite weight lifters, runners, and sedentary controls, suggesting prior training did not significantly alter patellar cartilage response to compressive load. In a study of experienced marathoners by Kessler and coworkers, a transient decrease in cartilage volume of 7% was observed in the patella, and 5% in the tibia occurred after running 20 km, with near-complete recovery after 1 hour of rest.[232] This study also observed a decrease in meniscal volume after running that persisted after rest. A study by Kersting also observed greater cartilage deformation in the patella, femur, and lateral tibial cartilage in trained runners after 1 hour of exercise.[233] In this study, changes in cartilage volume were strongly correlated with changes in serum COMP concentration, which has been suggested to be a short-term indicator of cartilage loading.

Studies using MRI have thus far demonstrated that, while cartilage thinning occurs with decreased compressive load resulting from prolonged immobility, there is limited capacity for cartilage morphology to adapt to increases in biomechanical strain.[234] Greater patellar cartilage thickness and surface area have been observed in professional weightlifters and sprinters compared with controls, but not for femoral tibial cartilage.[235] Similarly, changes in compressive loading either after recovery after prolonged immobilization[236] or as a result of altered joint loading after spinal cord injury[237] suggest cartilage is less adaptive to changes in loading conditions than muscle or bone.

Functional cartilage imaging may be useful in evaluating changes in joint biomechanics after joint injury or surgery. As predicted from models of joint biomechanics, MRI has demonstrated greater cartilage deformation in the central medial tibial cartilage and less in the periphery of the cartilage end plate in patients undergoing medial menisectomy.[238]

Although bulk properties of cartilage biomechanics can be evaluated with standard biomaterial testing techniques, specialized techniques using confocal microscopy have shown significant differences in the biomechanical properties of cartilage in relation to depth from the articular surface.[239,240] When compressed, the superficial layer of cartilage develops large compressive and tensile strain, resulting in significant tissue consolidation and high fluid flow. Little compressive strain occurs in the deep radial zone. Tensile strain develops at the surfaces of cartilage, both at the articular surface and the bone/cartilage interface. Understanding the heterogeneous response of cartilage to physiologic loads will likely improve understanding of the role of biomechanics in OA. A potential application of MRI in evaluation of cartilage biomechanics is the ability to nondestructively evaluate regional properties of cartilage in intact tissue specimens.[241,242] Using double-quantum filtered deuterium nuclear magnetic resonance of cartilage plugs, Shinar and associates were able to demonstrate a loss of collagen fiber anisotropy of the deep radial zone in cartilage placed under static compression.[150] Loss of anisotropy occurs when cartilage is cleaved from bone, indicating fibers anchored in the tidemark zone are essential to maintain normal fibril orientation and suggesting an intact bone/cartilage interface is essential for evaluating cartilage biomechanics.[151] Recently, regional changes in cartilage biomechanics have been explored using MRI tagging techniques to place MRI visible fiducial markers or "tags" within the cartilage that can be tracked with MRI microscopy techniques.[243-245] Similar regional biomechanics have been explored using MR elastography to visualize propagation of pressure waves through cartilage[246-249] and with diffusion tensor imaging to visualize changes in collagen fibril orientation in response to static compressive load.[250-253]

In addition to evaluating cartilage deformation, it is possible to study cartilage biomechanics by monitoring changes in signal intensity during compression.[254] An early study by Rubenstein and associates[110] demonstrated a decrease in cartilage signal intensity when osteochondral plugs were placed under compressive load. This signal change was attributed to extrusion of cartilage water and alteration in orientation of collagen fibers leading to a decrease in cartilage T2. The important role of fiber anisotropy in evaluating regional biomechanical response was confirmed by a strong association between changes in collagen fiber orientation and T2 when cartilage plugs are placed under a static compressive load.[242,255] Interestingly, alteration in collagen fiber orientation appears to be different between static and cyclic loading conditions.[256] Greater deformation of collagen fibers with static loading is observed in deeper layers of cartilage, whereas fiber deformation in cyclic loading is limited to the superficial region. In initial feasibility studies, a decrease in cartilage T2 of the femoral tibial joint was measured when static compression was applied to the leg within the magnet[257] and in patellar cartilage after deep knee bends.[131] More recently, using quantitative T2 mapping of cartilage plugs, zone-specific changes in cartilage T2 were observed during compressive loading.[166] These observations indicate changes in T2 anisotropy may be a potential method for obtaining regional information on cartilage deformation. In an initial study using quantitative T2 mapping in humans, localized decreases in cartilage T2 were observed in the superficial 30% of femoral cartilage immediately after 30 minutes of running exercise (Fig. 8-18).[258] These in-vivo results in humans are consistent with prior studies in excised samples indicating greater compressibility of superficial cartilage[240] and changes in superficial collagen orientation with cyclic loading.[256] The ability to study human cartilage response to physiologic loads provides an opportunity for new translational research for understanding the role of cartilage biomechanics in cartilage physiology and pathogenesis of OA.

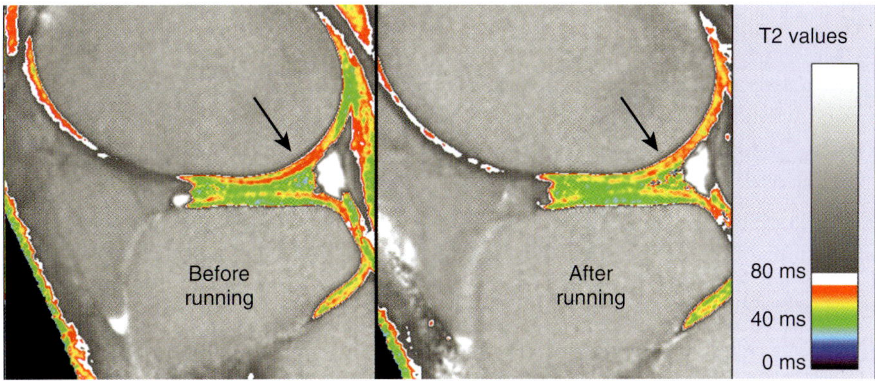

FIGURE 8-18. Quantitative cartilage T2 maps obtained before and after 30 minutes of running demonstrate focal decrease in T2 of the femoral cartilage secondary to focal extrusion of cartilage water and altered orientation of the collagen matrix occurring with cartilage compression.

References

1. Link TM, Stahl R, Woertler K. Cartilage imaging: motivation, techniques, current and future significance. Eur Radiol 2007; 17:1135-1146.
2. Burstein D, Gray ML. Is MRI fulfilling its promise for molecular imaging of cartilage in arthritis? Osteoarthritis Cartilage 2006; 14:1087-1090.
3. Glaser C. New techniques for cartilage imaging: T2 relaxation time and diffusion-weighted MR imaging. Radiol Clin North Am 2005; 43:641-653, vii.
4. Gray ML, Burstein D, Kim YJ, Maroudas A. 2007 Elizabeth Winston Lanier Award Winner. Magnetic resonance imaging of cartilage glycosaminoglycan: basic principles, imaging technique, and clinical applications. J Orthop Res 2008; 26:281-291.
5. Ling W, Regatte RR, Navon G, Jerschow A. Assessment of glycosaminoglycan concentration in vivo by chemical exchange-dependent saturation transfer (gagCEST). Proc Natl Acad Sci U S A 2008; 105:2266-2270.
6. Venn M, Maroudas A. Chemical composition and swelling of normal and osteoarthrotic femoral head cartilage. I. Chemical composition. Ann Rheum Dis 1977; 36:121-129.
7. Maroudas A, Muir H, Wingham J. The correlation of fixed negative charge with glycosaminoglycan content of human articular cartilage. Biochim Biophys Acta 1969; 177:492-500.
8. Borthakur A, Shapiro EM, Akella SV, et al. Quantifying sodium in the human wrist in vivo by using MR imaging. Radiology 2002; 224:598-602.
9. Borthakur A, Shapiro EM, Beers J, et al. Sensitivity of MRI to proteoglycan depletion in cartilage: comparison of sodium and proton MRI. Osteoarthritis Cartilage 2000; 8:288-293.
10. Insko EK, Kaufman JH, Leigh JS, Reddy R. Sodium NMR evaluation of articular cartilage degradation. Magn Reson Med 1999; 41:30-34.
11. Reddy R, Insko EK, Noyszewski EA, et al. Sodium MRI of human articular cartilage in vivo. Magn Reson Med 1998; 39:697-701.
12. Wheaton AJ, Borthakur A, Dodge GR, et al. Sodium magnetic resonance imaging of proteoglycan depletion in an in vivo model of osteoarthritis. Acad Radiol 2004; 11:21-28.
13. Shapiro EM, Borthakur A, Gougoutas A, Reddy R. ^{23}Na MRI accurately measures fixed charge density in articular cartilage. Magn Reson Med 2002; 47:284-291.
14. Shapiro EM, Borthakur A, Dandora R, et al. Sodium visibility and quantitation in intact bovine articular cartilage using high field (23)Na MRI and MRS. J Magn Reson 2000; 142:24-31.
15. Borthakur A, Hancu I, Boada FE, et al. In-vivo triple quantum filtered twisted projection sodium MRI of human articular cartilage. J Magn Reson 1999; 141:286-290.
16. Borthakur A, Mellon E, Niyogi S, et al. Sodium and T1rho MRI for molecular and diagnostic imaging of articular cartilage. NMR Biomed 2006; 19:781-821.
17. Choy J, Ling W, Jerschow A. Selective detection of ordered sodium signals via the central transition. J Magn Reson 2006; 180:105-109.
18. Hancu I, van der Maarel JR, Boada FE. A model for the dynamics of spins 3/2 in biological media: signal loss during radiofrequency excitation in triple-quantum-filtered sodium MRI. J Magn Reson 2000; 147:179-191.
19. Ling W, Jerschow A. Selecting ordered environments in NMR of spin 3/2 nuclei via frequency-sweep pulses. J Magn Reson 2005; 176:234-238.
20. Ling W, Regatte RR, Schweitzer ME, Jerschow A. Behavior of ordered sodium in enzymatically depleted cartilage tissue. Magn Reson Med 2006; 56:1151-1155.

21. Navon G, Shinar H, Eliav U, Seo Y. Multiquantum filters and order in tissues. NMR Biomed 2001; 14:112-132.
22. Shinar H, Navon G. Multinuclear NMR and microscopic MRI studies of the articular cartilage nanostructure. NMR Biomed 2006; 19:877-893.
23. Duvvuri U, Charagundla SR, Kudchodkar SB, et al. Human knee: in vivo T1(rho)-weighted MR imaging at 1.5 T—preliminary experience. Radiology 2001; 220:822-826.
24. Mlynarik V, Trattnig S, Huber M, et al. The role of relaxation times in monitoring proteoglycan depletion in articular cartilage. J Magn Reson Imaging 1999; 10:497-502.
25. Mlynarik V, Szomolanyi P, Toffanin R, et al. Transverse relaxation mechanisms in articular cartilage. J Magn Reson 2004; 169:300-307.
26. Menezes NM, Gray ML, Hartke JR, Burstein D. T2 and T1rho MRI in articular cartilage systems. Magn Reson Med 2004; 51:503-509.
27. Regatte RR, Akella SV, Borthakur A, et al. Proteoglycan depletion-induced changes in transverse relaxation maps of cartilage: comparison of T2 and T1rho. Acad Radiol 2002; 9:1388-1394.
28. Regatte RR, Akella SV, Borthakur A, Reddy R. Proton spin-lock ratio imaging for quantitation of glycosaminoglycans in articular cartilage. J Magn Reson Imaging 2003; 17:114-121.
29. Duvvuri U, Kudchodkar S, Reddy R, Leigh JS. T(1rho) relaxation can assess longitudinal proteoglycan loss from articular cartilage in vitro. Osteoarthritis Cartilage 2002; 10:838-844.
30. Duvvuri U, Reddy R, Patel SD, et al. T1rho-relaxation in articular cartilage: effects of enzymatic degradation. Magn Reson Med 1997; 38:863-867.
31. Akella SV, Regatte RR, Gougoutas AJ, et al. Proteoglycan-induced changes in T1rho-relaxation of articular cartilage at 4T. Magn Reson Med 2001; 46:419-423.
32. Wheaton AJ, Dodge GR, Borthakur A, et al. Detection of changes in articular cartilage proteoglycan by T(1rho) magnetic resonance imaging. J Orthop Res 2005; 23:102-108.
33. Wheaton AJ, Dodge GR, Elliott DM, et al. Quantification of cartilage biomechanical and biochemical properties via T1rho magnetic resonance imaging. Magn Reson Med 2005; 54:1087-1093.
34. Wheaton AJ, Casey FL, Gougoutas AJ, et al. Correlation of T1rho with fixed charge density in cartilage. J Magn Reson Imaging 2004; 20:519-525.
35. Regatte RR, Akella SV, Lonner JH, et al. T1rho relaxation mapping in human osteoarthritis (OA) cartilage: comparison of T1rho with T2. J Magn Reson Imaging 2006; 23:547-553.
36. Regatte RR, Akella SV, Wheaton AJ, et al. 3D-T1rho-relaxation mapping of articular cartilage: in vivo assessment of early degenerative changes in symptomatic osteoarthritic subjects. Acad Radiol 2004; 11:741-749.
37. Lozano J, Li X, Link TM, et al. Detection of posttraumatic cartilage injury using quantitative T1rho magnetic resonance imaging: a report of two cases with arthroscopic findings. J Bone Joint Surg Am 2006; 88:1349-1352.
38. Li X, Benjamin Ma C, Link TM, et al. In vivo T(1rho) and T(2) mapping of articular cartilage in osteoarthritis of the knee using 3 T MRI. Osteoarthritis Cartilage 2007; 15:789-797.
39. Bolbos RI, Zuo J, Banerjee S, et al. Relationship between trabecular bone structure and articular cartilage morphology and relaxation times in early OA of the knee joint using parallel MRI at 3T. Osteoarthritis Cartilage 2008; 16:1150-1159.
40. Akella SV, Regatte RR, Borthakur A, et al. T1rho MR imaging of the human wrist in vivo. Acad Radiol 2003; 10:614-619.
41. Wheaton AJ, Borthakur A, Kneeland JB, et al. Reddy R. In vivo quantification of T1rho using a multislice spin-lock pulse sequence. Magn Reson Med 2004; 52:1453-1458.
42. Pakin SK, Schweitzer ME, Regatte RR. 3D-T1rho quantitation of patellar cartilage at 3.0T. J Magn Reson Imaging 2006; 24:1357-1363.
43. Regatte RR, Akella SV, Borthakur A, et al. In vivo proton MR three-dimensional T1rho mapping of human articular cartilage: initial experience. Radiology 2003; 229:269-274.
44. Borthakur A, Wheaton A, Charagundla SR, et al. Three-dimensional T1rho-weighted MRI at 1.5 Tesla. J Magn Reson Imaging 2003; 17:730-736.
45. Zuo J, Li X, Banerjee S, Han E, Majumdar S. Parallel imaging of knee cartilage at 3 Tesla. J Magn Reson Imaging 2007; 26:1001-1009.
46. Pakin SK, Xu J, Schweitzer ME, Regatte RR. Rapid 3D-T1rho mapping of the knee joint at 3.0T with parallel imaging. Magn Reson Med 2006; 56:563-571.
47. Gray ML, Burstein D, Xia Y. Biochemical (and functional) imaging of articular cartilage. Semin Musculoskelet Radiol 2001; 5:329-343.
48. Gray ML, Burstein D. Molecular (and functional) imaging of articular cartilage. J Musculoskelet Neuronal Interact 2004; 4:365-368.
49. Krishnan N, Shetty SK, Williams A, et al. Delayed gadolinium-enhanced magnetic resonance imaging of the meniscus: an index of meniscal tissue degeneration? Arthritis Rheum 2007; 56:1507-1511.
50. Bashir A, Gray ML, Boutin RD, Burstein D. Glycosaminoglycan in articular cartilage: in vivo assessment with delayed Gd(DTPA)(2−)-enhanced MR imaging. Radiology 1997; 205:551-558.
51. Wiener E, Woertler K, Weirich G, et al. Contrast enhanced cartilage imaging: comparison of ionic and non-ionic contrast agents. Eur J Radiol 2007; 63:110-119.
52. Bashir A, Gray ML, Hartke J, Burstein D. Nondestructive imaging of human cartilage glycosaminoglycan concentration by MRI. Magn Reson Med 1999; 41:857-865.

53. Williams A, Mikulis B, Krishnan N, et al. Suitability of T(1Gd) as the dGEMRIC index at 1.5T and 3.0T. Magn Reson Med 2007; 58:830-834.
54. Sanz R, Marti-Bonmati L, Rodrigo JL, Moratal D. MR pharmacokinetic modeling of the patellar cartilage differentiates normal from pathological conditions. J Magn Reson Imaging 2008; 27:171-177.
55. Kallioniemi AS, Jurvelin JS, Nieminen MT, et al. Contrast agent enhanced pQCT of articular cartilage. Phys Med Biol 2007; 52:1209-1219.
56. Burstein D, Velyvis J, Scott KT, et al. Protocol issues for delayed Gd(DTPA)(2−)-enhanced MRI (dGEMRIC) for clinical evaluation of articular cartilage. Magn Reson Med 2001; 45:36-41.
57. Tiderius CJ, Olsson LE, de Verdier H, et al. Gd-DTPA(2−)-enhanced MRI of femoral knee cartilage: a dose-response study in healthy volunteers. Magn Reson Med 2001; 46:1067-1071.
58. McKenzie CA, Williams A, Prasad PV, Burstein D. Three-dimensional delayed gadolinium-enhanced MRI of cartilage (dGEMRIC) at 1.5T and 3.0T. J Magn Reson Imaging 2006; 24:928-933.
59. Tiderius CJ, Jessel R, Kim YJ, Burstein D. Hip dGEMRIC in asymptomatic volunteers and patients with early osteoarthritis: the influence of timing after contrast injection. Magn Reson Med 2007; 57:803-805.
60. Bellin MF, Van Der Molen AJ. Extracellular gadolinium-based contrast media: an overview. Eur J Radiol 2008; 66:160-167.
61. Idee JM, Port M, Medina C, et al. Possible involvement of gadolinium chelates in the pathophysiology of nephrogenic systemic fibrosis: a critical review. Toxicology 2008; 248:77-88.
62. Kallen AJ, Jhung MA, Cheng S, et al. Gadolinium-containing magnetic resonance imaging contrast and nephrogenic systemic fibrosis: a case-control study. Am J Kidney Dis 2008; 51:966-975.
63. Marckmann P, Skov L, Rossen K, et al. Nephrogenic systemic fibrosis: suspected causative role of gadodiamide used for contrast-enhanced magnetic resonance imaging. J Am Soc Nephrol 2006; 17:2359-2362.
64. Nainani N, Panesar M. Nephrogenic systemic fibrosis. Am J Nephrol 2008; 29:1-9.
65. Wiginton CD, Kelly B, Oto A, et al. Gadolinium-based contrast exposure, nephrogenic systemic fibrosis, and gadolinium detection in tissue. AJR Am J Roentgenol 2008; 190:1060-1068.
66. Li W, Scheidegger R, Wu Y, et al. Accuracy of T1 measurement with 3-D Look-Locker technique for dGEMRIC. J Magn Reson Imaging 2008; 27:678-682.
67. Trattnig S, Marlovits S, Gebetsroither S, et al. Three-dimensional delayed gadolinium-enhanced MRI of cartilage (dGEMRIC) for in vivo evaluation of reparative cartilage after matrix-associated autologous chondrocyte transplantation at 3.0T: preliminary results. J Magn Reson Imaging 2007; 26:974-982.
68. Kimelman T, Vu A, Storey P, et al. Three-dimensional T1 mapping for dGEMRIC at 3.0 T using the Look Locker method. Invest Radiol 2006; 41:198-203.
69. Bashir A, Gray ML, Burstein D. Gd-DTPA2− as a measure of cartilage degradation. Magn Reson Med 1996; 36:665-673.
70. Gillis A, Gray M, Burstein D. Relaxivity and diffusion of gadolinium agents in cartilage. Magn Reson Med 2002; 48:1068-1071.
71. Trattnig S, Mlynarik V, Breitenseher M, et al. MRI visualization of proteoglycan depletion in articular cartilage via intravenous administration of Gd-DTPA. Magn Reson Imaging 1999; 17:577-583.
72. Nieminen MT, Rieppo J, Silvennoinen J, et al. Spatial assessment of articular cartilage proteoglycans with Gd-DTPA-enhanced T1 imaging. Magn Reson Med 2002; 48:640-648.
73. Tiderius CJ, Tjornstrand J, Akeson P, et al. Delayed gadolinium-enhanced MRI of cartilage (dGEMRIC): intra- and interobserver variability in standardized drawing of regions of interest. Acta Radiol 2004; 45:628-634.
74. Tiderius CJ, Olsson LE, Leander P, et al. Delayed gadolinium-enhanced MRI of cartilage (dGEMRIC) in early knee osteoarthritis. Magn Reson Med 2003; 49:488-492.
75. Nojiri T, Watanabe N, Namura T, et al. Utility of delayed gadolinium-enhanced MRI (dGEMRIC) for qualitative evaluation of articular cartilage of patellofemoral joint. Knee Surg Sports Traumatol Arthrosc 2006; 14:718-723.
76. Williams A, Sharma L, McKenzie CA, et al. Delayed gadolinium-enhanced magnetic resonance imaging of cartilage in knee osteoarthritis: findings at different radiographic stages of disease and relationship to malalignment. Arthritis Rheum 2005; 52:3528-3535.
77. Williams A, Gillis A, McKenzie C, et al. Glycosaminoglycan distribution in cartilage as determined by delayed gadolinium-enhanced MRI of cartilage (dGEMRIC): potential clinical applications. AJR Am J Roentgenol 2004; 182:167-172.
78. Young AA, Stanwell P, Williams A, et al. Glycosaminoglycan content of knee cartilage following posterior cruciate ligament rupture demonstrated by delayed gadolinium-enhanced magnetic resonance imaging of cartilage (dGEMRIC): a case report. J Bone Joint Surg Am 2005; 87:2763-2767.
79. Tiderius CJ, Olsson LE, Nyquist F, Dahlberg L. Cartilage glycosaminoglycan loss in the acute phase after an anterior cruciate ligament injury: delayed gadolinium-enhanced magnetic resonance imaging of cartilage and synovial fluid analysis. Arthritis Rheum 2005; 52:120-127.

80. Kim YJ, Jaramillo D, Millis MB, et al. Assessment of early osteoarthritis in hip dysplasia with delayed gadolinium-enhanced magnetic resonance imaging of cartilage. J Bone Joint Surg Am 2003; 85:1987-1992.
81. Cunningham T, Jessel R, Zurakowski D, et al. Delayed gadolinium-enhanced magnetic resonance imaging of cartilage to predict early failure of Bernese periacetabular osteotomy for hip dysplasia. J Bone Joint Surg Am 2006; 88:1540-1548.
82. Gillis A, Bashir A, McKeon B, et al. Magnetic resonance imaging of relative glycosaminoglycan distribution in patients with autologous chondrocyte transplants. Invest Radiol 2001; 36:743-748.
83. Trattnig S, Mamisch TC, Pinker K, et al. Differentiating normal hyaline cartilage from post-surgical repair tissue using fast gradient echo imaging in delayed gadolinium-enhanced MRI (dGEMRIC) at 3 Tesla. Eur Radiol 2008; 18:1251-1259.
84. Kurkijarvi JE, Mattila L, Ojala RO, et al. Evaluation of cartilage repair in the distal femur after autologous chondrocyte transplantation using T2 relaxation time and dGEMRIC. Osteoarthritis Cartilage 2007; 15:372-378.
85. Miyata S, Homma K, Numano T, et al. Assessment of fixed charge density in regenerated cartilage by Gd-DTPA-enhanced MRI. Magn Reson Med Sci 2006; 5:73-78.
86. Watanabe A, Wada Y, Obata T, et al. Delayed gadolinium-enhanced MR to determine glycosaminoglycan concentration in reparative cartilage after autologous chondrocyte implantation: preliminary results. Radiology 2006; 239:201-208.
87. Williams A, Oppenheimer RA, Gray ML, Burstein D. Differential recovery of glycosaminoglycan after IL-1-induced degradation of bovine articular cartilage depends on degree of degradation. Arthritis Res Ther 2003; 5:R97-105.
88. Nissi MJ, Rieppo J, Toyras J, et al. Estimation of mechanical properties of articular cartilage with MRI—dGEMRIC, T2 and T1 imaging in different species with variable stages of maturation. Osteoarthritis Cartilage 2007; 15:1141-1148.
89. Baldassarri M, Goodwin JS, Farley ML, et al. Relationship between cartilage stiffness and dGEMRIC index: correlation and prediction. J Orthop Res 2007; 25:904-912.
90. Kurkijarvi JE, Nissi MJ, Kiviranta I, et al. Delayed gadolinium-enhanced MRI of cartilage (dGEMRIC) and T2 characteristics of human knee articular cartilage: topographical variation and relationships to mechanical properties. Magn Reson Med 2004; 52:41-46.
91. Nissi MJ, Toyras J, Laasanen MS, et al. Proteoglycan and collagen sensitive MRI evaluation of normal and degenerated articular cartilage. J Orthop Res 2004; 22:557-564.
92. Samosky JT, Burstein D, Eric Grimson W, et al. Spatially-localized correlation of dGEMRIC-measured GAG distribution and mechanical stiffness in the human tibial plateau. J Orthop Res 2005; 23:93-101.
93. Vasara AI, Nieminen MT, Jurvelin JS, et al. Indentation stiffness of repair tissue after autologous chondrocyte transplantation. Clin Orthop Relat Res 2005; (433):233-242.
94. Sawamura C, Takahashi M, McCarthy KJ, et al. Effect of in ovo immobilization on development of chick hind-limb articular cartilage: an evaluation using micro-MRI measurement of delayed gadolinium uptake. Magn Reson Med 2006; 56:1235-1241.
95. Tiderius CJ, Svensson J, Leander P, et al. dGEMRIC (delayed gadolinium-enhanced MRI of cartilage) indicates adaptive capacity of human knee cartilage. Magn Reson Med 2004; 51:286-290.
96. Arokoski JP, Jurvelin JS, Vaatainen U, Helminen HJ. Normal and pathological adaptations of articular cartilage to joint loading. Scand J Med Sci Sports 2000; 10:186-198.
97. Maroudas AI. Balance between swelling pressure and collagen tension in normal and degenerate cartilage. Nature 1976; 260:808-809.
98. Armstrong CG, Mow VC. Variations in the intrinsic mechanical properties of human articular cartilage with age, degeneration, and water content. J Bone Joint Surg Am 1982; 64:88-94.
99. Akizuki S, Mow VC, Muller F, et al. Tensile properties of human knee joint cartilage: I. Influence of ionic conditions, weight bearing, and fibrillation on the tensile modulus. J Orthop Res 1986; 4:379-392.
100. Guilak F, Ratcliffe A, Lane N, et al. Mechanical and biochemical changes in the superficial zone of articular cartilage in canine experimental osteoarthritis. J Orthop Res 1994; 12:474-484.
101. Jeffery AK, Blunn GW, Archer CW, Bentley G. Three-dimensional collagen architecture in bovine articular cartilage. J Bone Joint Surg Br 1991; 73:795-801.
102. Koskinen SK, Komu ME. Low-field strength magnetization transfer contrast imaging of the patellar cartilage. Acta Radiol 1993; 34:124-126.
103. Henkelman RM, Stanisz GJ, Kim JK, Bronskill MJ. Anisotropy of NMR properties of tissues. Magn Reson Med 1994; 32:592-601.
104. Regatte RR, Akella SV, Reddy R. Depth-dependent proton magnetization transfer in articular cartilage. J Magn Reson Imaging 2005; 22:318-323.
105. Yao L, Gentili A, Thomas A. Incidental magnetization transfer contrast in fast spin-echo imaging of cartilage. J Magn Reson Imaging 1996; 6:180-184.
106. Dixon WT, Engels H, Castillo M, Sardashti M. Incidental magnetization transfer contrast in standard multislice imaging. Magn Reson Imaging 1990; 8:417-422.
107. Maier CF, Tan SG, Hariharan H, Potter HG. T2 quantitation of articular cartilage at 1.5 T. J Magn Reson Imaging 2003; 17:358-364.

108. Watanabe A, Boesch C, Obata T, Anderson SE. Effect of multislice acquisition on T1 and T2 measurements of articular cartilage at 3T. J Magn Reson Imaging 2007; 26:109-117.
109. Schick F. Pulsed magnetization transfer contrast MRI by a sequence with water selective excitation. J Comput Assist Tomogr 1996; 20:73-79.
110. Rubenstein JD, Kim JK, Morova-Protzner I, et al. Effects of collagen orientation on MR imaging characteristics of bovine articular cartilage. Radiology 1993; 188:219-226.
111. Vahlensieck M, Traber F, Giesecke J, Schild H. [Magnetization transfer contrast (MTC): optimizing off-resonance and on-resonance frequency MTC methods at 0.5 and 1.5 T]. Biomed Tech (Berl) 2001; 46:10-17.
112. Martirosian P, Boss A, Deimling M, et al. Systematic variation of off-resonance prepulses for clinical magnetization transfer contrast imaging at 0.2, 1.5, and 3.0 Tesla. Invest Radiol 2008; 43:16-26.
113. Peterfy CG, van Dijke CF, Janzen DL, et al. Quantification of articular cartilage in the knee with pulsed saturation transfer subtraction and fat-suppressed MR imaging: optimization and validation. Radiology 1994; 192:485-491.
114. Hohe J, Faber S, Stammberger T, et al. A technique for 3D in vivo quantification of proton density and magnetization transfer coefficients of knee joint cartilage. Osteoarthritis Cartilage 2000; 8:426-433.
115. Vahlensieck M, Dombrowski F, Leutner C, et al. Magnetization transfer contrast (MTC) and MTC-subtraction: enhancement of cartilage lesions and intracartilaginous degeneration in vitro. Skeletal Radiol 1994; 23:535-539.
116. Palmieri F, De Keyzer F, Maes F, Van Breuseghem I. Magnetization transfer analysis of cartilage repair tissue: a preliminary study. Skeletal Radiol 2006; 35:903-908.
117. Wolff SD, Chesnick S, Frank JA, et al. Magnetization transfer contrast: MR imaging of the knee. Radiology 1991; 179:623-628.
118. Niitsu M, Hirohata H, Yoshioka H, et al. Magnetization transfer contrast on gradient echo MR imaging of the temporomandibular joint. Acta Radiol 1995; 36:295-299.
119. Peterfy CG, Majumdar S, Lang P, et al. MR imaging of the arthritic knee: improved discrimination of cartilage, synovium, and effusion with pulsed saturation transfer and fat-suppressed T1-weighted sequences. Radiology 1994; 191:413-419.
120. Mori R, Ochi M, Sakai Y, et al. Clinical significance of magnetic resonance imaging (MRI) for focal chondral lesions. Magn Reson Imaging 1999; 17:1135-1140.
121. Kim DK, Ceckler TL, Hascall VC, et al. Analysis of water-macromolecule proton magnetization transfer in articular cartilage. Magn Reson Med 1993; 29:211-215.
122. Lattanzio PJ, Marshall KW, Damyanovich AZ, Peemoeller H. Macromolecule and water magnetization exchange modeling in articular cartilage. Magn Reson Med 2000; 44:840-851.
123. Seo GS, Aoki J, Moriya H, et al. Hyaline cartilage: in vivo and in vitro assessment with magnetization transfer imaging. Radiology 1996; 201:525-530.
124. Toffanin R, Mlynarik V, Russo S, et al. Proteoglycan depletion and magnetic resonance parameters of articular cartilage. Arch Biochem Biophys 2001; 390:235-242.
125. Potter K, Butler JJ, Horton WE, Spencer RG. Response of engineered cartilage tissue to biochemical agents as studied by proton magnetic resonance microscopy. Arthritis Rheum 2000; 43:1580-1590.
126. Laurent D, O'Byrne E, Wasvary J, Pellas TC. In vivo MRI of cartilage pathogenesis in surgical models of osteoarthritis. Skeletal Radiol 2006; 35:555-564.
127. Laurent D, Wasvary J, O'Byrne E, Rudin M. In vivo qualitative assessments of articular cartilage in the rabbit knee with high-resolution MRI at 3 T. Magn Reson Med 2003; 50:541-549.
128. Laurent D, Wasvary J, Yin J, et al. Quantitative and qualitative assessment of articular cartilage in the goat knee with magnetization transfer imaging. Magn Reson Imaging 2001; 19:1279-1286.
129. Wachsmuth L, Juretschke HP, Raiss RX. Can magnetization transfer magnetic resonance imaging follow proteoglycan depletion in articular cartilage? Magma 1997; 5:71-78.
130. Lehner KB, Rechl HP, Gmeinwieser JK, et al. Structure, function, and degeneration of bovine hyaline cartilage: assessment with MR imaging in vitro. Radiology 1989; 170:495-499.
131. Liess C, Lusse S, Karger N, et al. Detection of changes in cartilage water content using MRI T2-mapping in vivo. Osteoarthritis Cartilage 2002; 10:907-913.
132. Lusse S, Claassen H, Gehrke T, et al. Evaluation of water content by spatially resolved transverse relaxation times of human articular cartilage. Magn Reson Imaging 2000; 18:423-430.
133. Lusse S, Knauss R, Werner A, et al. Action of compression and cations on the proton and deuterium relaxation in cartilage. Magn Reson Med 1995; 33:483-489.
134. Shapiro EM, Borthakur A, Kaufman JH, et al. Water distribution patterns inside bovine articular cartilage as visualized by 1H magnetic resonance imaging. Osteoarthritis Cartilage 2001; 9:533-538.
135. Fragonas E, Mlynarik V, Jellus V, et al. Correlation between biochemical composition and magnetic resonance appearance of articular cartilage. Osteoarthritis Cartilage 1998; 6:24-32.
136. Nieminen MT, Toyras J, Rieppo J, et al. Quantitative MR microscopy of enzymatically degraded articular cartilage. Magn Reson Med 2000; 43:676-681.
137. Watrin A, Ruaud JP, Olivier PT, et al. T2 mapping of rat patellar cartilage. Radiology 2001; 219:395-402.

138. Watrin-Pinzano A, Ruaud JP, Cheli Y, et al. T2 mapping: an efficient MR quantitative technique to evaluate spontaneous cartilage repair in rat patella. Osteoarthritis Cartilage 2004; 12:191-200.
139. Grunder W, Wagner M, Werner A. MR-microscopic visualization of anisotropic internal cartilage structures using the magic angle technique. Magn Reson Med 1998; 39:376-382.
140. Xia Y, Farquhar T, Burton-Wurster N, et al. Diffusion and relaxation mapping of cartilage-bone plugs and excised disks using microscopic magnetic resonance imaging. Magn Reson Med 1994; 31:273-282.
141. Xia Y. Relaxation anisotropy in cartilage by NMR microscopy (muMRI) at 14-microm resolution. Magn Reson Med 1998; 39:941-949.
142. Xia Y, Farquhar T, Burton-Wurster N, Lust G. Origin of cartilage laminae in MRI. J Magn Reson Imaging 1997; 7:887-894.
143. Goodwin DW, Dunn JF. High-resolution magnetic resonance imaging of articular cartilage: correlation with histology and pathology. Top Magn Reson Imaging 1998; 9:337-347.
144. Mlynarik V, Degrassi A, Toffanin R, et al. A method for generating magnetic resonance microimaging T2 maps with low sensitivity to diffusion. Magn Reson Med 1996; 35:423-425.
145. Kim DJ, Suh JS, Jeong EK, et al. Correlation of laminated MR appearance of articular cartilage with histology, ascertained by artificial landmarks on the cartilage. J Magn Reson Imaging 1999; 10:57-64.
146. Xia Y. Heterogeneity of cartilage laminae in MR imaging. J Magn Reson Imaging 2000; 11:686-693.
147. Nieminen MT, Rieppo J, Toyras J, et al. T2 relaxation reveals spatial collagen architecture in articular cartilage: a comparative quantitative MRI and polarized light microscopic study. Magn Reson Med 2001; 46:487-493.
148. Xia Y, Moody JB, Alhadlaq H. Orientational dependence of T2 relaxation in articular cartilage: a microscopic MRI (microMRI) study. Magn Reson Med 2002; 48:460-469.
149. Goodwin DW, Wadghiri YZ, Zhu H, et al. Macroscopic structure of articular cartilage of the tibial plateau: influence of a characteristic matrix architecture on MRI appearance. AJR Am J Roentgenol 2004; 182:311-318.
150. Shinar H, Seo Y, Ikoma K, et al. Mapping the fiber orientation in articular cartilage at rest and under pressure studied by 2H double quantum filtered MRI. Magn Reson Med 2002; 48:322-330.
151. Keinan-Adamsky K, Shinar H, Navon G. The effect of detachment of the articular cartilage from its calcified zone on the cartilage microstructure, assessed by 2H-spectroscopic double quantum filtered MRI. J Orthop Res 2005; 23:109-117.
152. Xia Y. Magic-angle effect in magnetic resonance imaging of articular cartilage: a review. Invest Radiol 2000; 35:602-621.
153. Krasnosselskaia LV, Fullerton GD, Dodd SJ, Cameron IL. Water in tendon: orientational analysis of the free induction decay. Magn Reson Med 2005; 54:280-288.
154. Bydder M, Rahal A, Fullerton GD, Bydder GM. The magic angle effect: a source of artifact, determinant of image contrast, and technique for imaging. J Magn Reson Imaging 2007; 25:290-300.
155. Cameron IL, Hunter KE, Ord VA, Fullerton GD. Relationships between ice crystal size, water content and proton NMR relaxation times in cells. Physiol Chem Phys Med NMR 1985; 17:371-386.
156. Xia Y. Averaged and depth-dependent anisotropy of articular cartilage by microscopic imaging. Semin Arthritis Rheum 2008; 37:317-327.
157. Moger CJ, Barrett R, Bleuet P, et al. Regional variations of collagen orientation in normal and diseased articular cartilage and subchondral bone determined using small angle X-ray scattering (SAXS). Osteoarthritis Cartilage 2007; 15:682-687.
158. Driessen NJ, Wilson W, Bouten CV, Baaijens FP. A computational model for collagen fibre remodelling in the arterial wall. J Theor Biol 2004; 226:53-64.
159. Wilson W, Driessen NJ, van Donkelaar CC, Ito K. Prediction of collagen orientation in articular cartilage by a collagen remodeling algorithm. Osteoarthritis Cartilage 2006; 14:1196-1202.
160. Shirazi R, Shirazi-Adl A. Deep vertical collagen fibrils play a significant role in mechanics of articular cartilage. J Orthop Res 2008; 26:608-615.
161. Korhonen RK, Julkunen P, Wilson W, Herzog W. Importance of collagen orientation and depth-dependent fixed charge densities of cartilage on mechanical behavior of chondrocytes. J Biomech Eng 2008; 130:021003.
162. Julkunen P, Korhonen RK, Nissi MJ, Jurvelin JS. Mechanical characterization of articular cartilage by combining magnetic resonance imaging and finite-element analysis—a potential functional imaging technique. Phys Med Biol 2008; 53:2425-2438.
163. Bae WC, Wong VW, Hwang J, et al. Wear-lines and split-lines of human patellar cartilage: relation to tensile biomechanical properties. Osteoarthritis Cartilage 2008; 16:841-845.
164. Federico S, Herzog W. On the anisotropy and inhomogeneity of permeability in articular cartilage. Biomech Model Mechanobiol 2007; 7:367-378.
165. Xia Y, Moody JB, Burton-Wurster N, Lust G. Quantitative in situ correlation between microscopic MRI and polarized light microscopy studies of articular cartilage. Osteoarthritis Cartilage 2001; 9:393-406.
166. Alhadlaq HA, Xia Y. The structural adaptations in compressed articular cartilage by microscopic MRI (microMRI) T(2) anisotropy. Osteoarthritis Cartilage 2004; 12:887-894.

167. Xia Y. Averaged properties of articular cartilage from multidisciplinary microscopic imaging study. Conf Proc IEEE Eng Med Biol Soc 2005; 3:3161-3164.
168. Regatte RR, Kaufman JH, Noyszewski EA, Reddy R. Sodium and proton MR properties of cartilage during compression. J Magn Reson Imaging 1999; 10:961-967.
169. Wayne JS, Kraft KA, Shields KJ, et al. MR imaging of normal and matrix-depleted cartilage: correlation with biomechanical function and biochemical composition. Radiology 2003; 228:493-499.
170. Watrin-Pinzano A, Ruaud JP, Olivier P, et al. Effect of proteoglycan depletion on T2 mapping in rat patellar cartilage. Radiology 2005; 234:162-170.
171. Mosher TJ, Chen Q, Smith MB. ^{1}H magnetic resonance spectroscopy of nanomelic chicken cartilage: effect of aggrecan depletion on cartilage T2. Osteoarthritis Cartilage 2003; 11:709-715.
172. Mosher TJ, Dardzinski BJ. Cartilage MRI T2 relaxation time mapping: overview and applications. Semin Musculoskelet Radiol 2004; 8:355-368.
173. Babyn PS, Kim HK, Lemaire C, et al. High-resolution magnetic resonance imaging of normal porcine cartilaginous epiphyseal maturation. J Magn Reson Imaging 1996; 6:172-179.
174. Olivier P, Loeuille D, Watrin A, et al. Structural evaluation of articular cartilage: potential contribution of magnetic resonance techniques used in clinical practice. Arthritis Rheum 2001; 44:2285-2295.
175. Vogel HG. Influence of maturation and aging on mechanical and biochemical properties of connective tissue in rats. Mech Ageing Dev 1980; 14:283-292.
176. Aszodi A, Hunziker EB, Olsen BR, Fassler R. The role of collagen II and cartilage fibril-associated molecules in skeletal development. Osteoarthritis Cartilage 2001; 9(Suppl A):S150-S159.
177. Bank RA, Bayliss MT, Lafeber FP, et al. Ageing and zonal variation in post-translational modification of collagen in normal human articular cartilage: the age-related increase in non-enzymatic glycation affects biomechanical properties of cartilage. Biochem J 1998; 330:345-351.
178. Verzijl N, DeGroot J, Bank RA, et al. Age-related accumulation of the advanced glycation endproduct pentosidine in human articular cartilage aggrecan: the use of pentosidine levels as a quantitative measure of protein turnover. Matrix Biol 2001; 20:409-417.
179. Brama PA, van den Boom R, DeGroott J, et al. Collagenase-1 (MMP-1) activity in equine synovial fluid: influence of age, joint pathology, exercise and repeated arthrocentesis. Equine Vet J 2004; 36:34-40.
180. Woodfield TB, Van Blitterswijk CA, De Wijn J, et al. Polymer scaffolds fabricated with pore-size gradients as a model for studying the zonal organization within tissue-engineered cartilage constructs. Tissue Eng 2005; 11:1297-1311.
181. Foster JE, Maciewicz RA, Taberner J, et al. Structural periodicity in human articular cartilage: comparison between magnetic resonance imaging and histological findings. Osteoarthritis Cartilage 1999; 7:480-485.
182. Lanzer WL, Komenda G. Changes in articular cartilage after meniscectomy. Clin Orthop Relat Res 1990; (252):41-48.
183. Pfander D, Rahmanzadeh R, Scheller EE. Presence and distribution of collagen II, collagen I, fibronectin, and tenascin in rabbit normal and osteoarthritic cartilage. J Rheumatol 1999; 26:386-394.
184. Rogart JN, Barrach HJ, Chichester CO. Articular collagen degradation in the Hulth-Telhag model of osteoarthritis. Osteoarthritis Cartilage 1999; 7:539-547.
185. Bi X, Yang X, Bostrom MP, et al. Fourier transform infrared imaging and MR microscopy studies detect compositional and structural changes in cartilage in a rabbit model of osteoarthritis. Anal Bioanal Chem 2007; 387:1601-1612.
186. Maroudas A, Venn M. Chemical composition and swelling of normal and osteoarthrotic femoral head cartilage: II. Swelling. Ann Rheum Dis 1977; 36:399-406.
187. Mow VC, Holmes MH, Lai WM. Fluid transport and mechanical properties of articular cartilage: a review. J Biomech 1984; 17:377-394.
188. David-Vaudey E, Ghosh S, Ries M, Majumdar S. T2 relaxation time measurements in osteoarthritis. Magn Reson Imaging 2004; 22:673-682.
189. Gahunia HK, Lemaire C, Cross AR, et al. Osteoarthritis in rhesus macaques: assessment of cartilage matrix quality by quantitative magnetic resonance imaging. Agents Actions Suppl 1993; 39:255-259.
190. Gahunia HK, Babyn P, Lemaire C, et al. Osteoarthritis staging: comparison between magnetic resonance imaging, gross pathology and histopathology in the rhesus macaque. Osteoarthritis Cartilage 1995; 3:169-180.
191. Spandonis Y, Heese FP, Hall LD. High resolution MRI relaxation measurements of water in the articular cartilage of the meniscectomized rat knee at 4.7 T. Magn Reson Imaging 2004; 22:943-951.
192. Watrin-Pinzano A, Ruaud JP, Cheli Y, et al. Evaluation of cartilage repair tissue after biomaterial implantation in rat patella by using T2 mapping. Magma 2004; 17:219-228.
193. Gahunia HK, Lemaire C, Babyn PS, et al. Osteoarthritis in rhesus macaque knee joint: quantitative magnetic resonance imaging tissue characterization of articular cartilage. J Rheumatol 1995; 22:1747-1756.
194. Beltran J, Marty-Delfaut E, Bencardino J, et al. Chondrocalcinosis of the hyaline cartilage of the knee: MRI manifestations. Skeletal Radiol 1998; 27:369-374.

195. Mosher TJ, Smith H, Dardzinski BJ, et al. MR imaging and T2 mapping of femoral cartilage: in vivo determination of the magic angle effect. AJR Am J Roentgenol 2001; 177:665-669.
196. Smith HE, Mosher TJ, Dardzinski BJ, et al. Spatial variation in cartilage T2 of the knee. J Magn Reson Imaging 2001; 14:50-55.
197. Van Breuseghem I, Bosmans HT, Elst LV, et al. T2 mapping of human femorotibial cartilage with turbo mixed MR imaging at 1.5 T: feasibility. Radiology 2004; 233:609-614.
198. Dardzinski BJ, Laor T, Schmithorst VJ, et al. Mapping T2 relaxation time in the pediatric knee: feasibility with a clinical 1.5-T MR imaging system. Radiology 2002; 225:233-239.
199. Dardzinski BJ, Mosher TJ, Li S, et al. Spatial variation of T2 in human articular cartilage. Radiology 1997; 205:546-550.
200. Welsch GH, Mamisch TC, Weber M, et al. High-resolution morphological and biochemical imaging of articular cartilage of the ankle joint at 3.0 T using a new dedicated phased array coil: in vivo reproducibility study. Skeletal Radiol 2008; 37:519-526.
201. Watanabe A, Boesch C, Siebenrock K, et al. T2 mapping of hip articular cartilage in healthy volunteers at 3T: a study of topographic variation. J Magn Reson Imaging 2007; 26:165-171.
202. Nishii T, Tanaka H, Sugano N, et al. Evaluation of cartilage matrix disorders by T2 relaxation time in patients with hip dysplasia. Osteoarthritis Cartilage 2008; 16:227-233.
203. Lazovic-Stojkovic J, Mosher TJ, Smith HE, et al. Interphalangeal joint cartilage: high-spatial-resolution in vivo MR T2 mapping—a feasibility study. Radiology 2004; 233:292-296.
204. Mosher TJ, Liu Y, Yang QX, et al. Age dependency of cartilage magnetic resonance imaging T2 relaxation times in asymptomatic women. Arthritis Rheum 2004; 50:2820-2828.
205. Eckstein F, Burstein D, Link TM. Quantitative MRI of cartilage and bone: degenerative changes in osteoarthritis. NMR Biomed 2006; 19:822-854.
206. Mendlik T, Faber SC, Weber J, et al. T2 quantitation of human articular cartilage in a clinical setting at 1.5 T: implementation and testing of four multiecho pulse sequence designs for validity. Invest Radiol 2004; 39:288-299.
207. Moody JB, Xia Y. Analysis of multi-exponential relaxation data with very short components using linear regularization. J Magn Reson 2004; 167:36-41.
208. Xia Y. Resolution “scaling law” in MRI of articular cartilage. Osteoarthritis Cartilage 2007; 15:363-365.
209. Quaia E, Toffanin R, Guglielmi G, et al. Fast T2 mapping of the patellar articular cartilage with gradient and spin-echo magnetic resonance imaging at 1.5 T: validation and initial clinical experience in patients with osteoarthritis. Skeletal Radiol 2008; 37:511-517.
210. Goebel JC, Watrin-Pinzano A, Bettembourg-Brault I, et al. Age-related quantitative MRI changes in healthy cartilage: preliminary results. Biorheology 2006; 43:547-551.
211. Mosher TJ, Dardzinski BJ, Smith MB. Human articular cartilage: influence of aging and early symptomatic degeneration on the spatial variation of T2—preliminary findings at 3 T. Radiology 2000; 214:259-266.
212. Mosher TJ, Collins CM, Smith HE, et al. Effect of gender on in vivo cartilage magnetic resonance imaging T2 mapping. J Magn Reson Imaging 2004; 19:323-328.
213. Kight AC, Dardzinski BJ, Laor T, Graham TB. Magnetic resonance imaging evaluation of the effects of juvenile rheumatoid arthritis on distal femoral weight-bearing cartilage. Arthritis Rheum 2004; 50:901-905.
214. Stahl R, Blumenkrantz G, Carballido-Gamio J, et al. MRI-derived T2 relaxation times and cartilage morphometry of the tibio-femoral joint in subjects with and without osteoarthritis during a 1-year follow-up. Osteoarthritis Cartilage 2007; 15:1225-1234.
215. Dunn TC, Lu Y, Jin H, et al. T2 relaxation time of cartilage at MR imaging: comparison with severity of knee osteoarthritis. Radiology 2004; 232:592-598.
216. King KB, Lindsey CT, Dunn TC, et al. A study of the relationship between molecular biomarkers of joint degeneration and the magnetic resonance-measured characteristics of cartilage in 16 symptomatic knees. Magn Reson Imaging 2004; 22:1117-1123.
217. Welsch GH, Mamisch TC, Domayer SE, et al. Cartilage T2 assessment at 3-T MR imaging: in vivo differentiation of normal hyaline cartilage from reparative tissue after two cartilage repair procedures—initial experience. Radiology 2008; 247:154-161.
218. Domayer SE, Kutscha-Lissberg F, Welsch G, et al. T2 mapping in the knee after microfracture at 3.0T: correlation of global T2 values and clinical outcome—preliminary results. Osteoarthritis Cartilage 2008; 16:903-908.
219. Trattnig S, Mamisch TC, Welsch GH, et al. Quantitative T2 mapping of matrix-associated autologous chondrocyte transplantation at 3 Tesla: an in vivo cross-sectional study. Invest Radiol 2007; 42:442-448.
220. Trattnig S, Millington SA, Szomolanyi P, Marlovits S. MR imaging of osteochondral grafts and autologous chondrocyte implantation. Eur Radiol 2007; 17:103-118.
221. White LM, Sussman MS, Hurtig M, et al. Cartilage T2 assessment: differentiation of normal hyaline cartilage and reparative tissue after arthroscopic cartilage repair in equine subjects. Radiology 2006; 241:407-414.
222. Kangarlu A, Gahunia HK. Magnetic resonance imaging characterization of osteochondral defect repair in a goat model at 8 T. Osteoarthritis Cartilage 2006; 14:52-62.
223. Kaufman JH, Regatte RR, Bolinger L, et al. A novel approach to observing articular cartilage deformation in vitro via magnetic resonance imaging. J Magn Reson Imaging 1999; 9:653-662.

224. Neu CP, Hull ML. Toward an MRI-based method to measure non-uniform cartilage deformation: an MRI-cyclic loading apparatus system and steady-state cyclic displacement of articular cartilage under compressive loading. J Biomech Eng 2003; 125:180-188.
225. Eckstein F, Adam C, Sittek H, et al. Non-invasive determination of cartilage thickness throughout joint surfaces using magnetic resonance imaging. J Biomech 1997; 30:285-289.
226. Li G, Wan L, Kozanek M. Determination of real-time in-vivo cartilage contact deformation in the ankle joint. J Biomech 2008; 41:128-136.
227. Wan L, de Asla RJ, Rubash HE, Li G. In vivo cartilage contact deformation of human ankle joints under full body weight. J Orthop Res 2008; 26:1081-1089.
228. Eckstein F, Tieschky M, Faber SC, et al. Effect of physical exercise on cartilage volume and thickness in vivo: MR imaging study. Radiology 1998; 207:243-248.
229. Eckstein F, Reiser M, Englmeier KH, Putz R. In vivo morphometry and functional analysis of human articular cartilage with quantitative magnetic resonance imaging—from image to data, from data to theory. Anat Embryol (Berl) 2001; 203:147-173.
230. Eckstein F, Lemberger B, Stammberger T, et al. Patellar cartilage deformation in vivo after static versus dynamic loading. J Biomech 2000; 33:819-825.
231. Eckstein F, Lemberger B, Gratzke C, et al. In vivo cartilage deformation after different types of activity and its dependence on physical training status. Ann Rheum Dis 2005; 64:291-295.
232. Kessler MA, Glaser C, Tittel S, et al. Recovery of the menisci and articular cartilage of runners after cessation of exercise: additional aspects of in vivo investigation based on 3-dimensional magnetic resonance imaging. Am J Sports Med 2008; 36:966-970.
233. Kersting UG, Stubendorff JJ, Schmidt MC, Bruggemann GP. Changes in knee cartilage volume and serum COMP concentration after running exercise. Osteoarthritis Cartilage 2005; 13:925-934.
234. Eckstein F, Hudelmaier M, Putz R. The effects of exercise on human articular cartilage. J Anat 2006; 208:491-512.
235. Gratzke C, Hudelmaier M, Hitzl W, et al. Knee cartilage morphologic characteristics and muscle status of professional weight lifters and sprinters: a magnetic resonance imaging study. Am J Sports Med 2007; 35:1346-1353.
236. Hudelmaier M, Glaser C, Hausschild A, et al. Effects of joint unloading and reloading on human cartilage morphology and function, muscle cross-sectional areas, and bone density: a quantitative case report. J Musculoskelet Neuronal Interact 2006; 6:284-290.
237. Ruckstuhl H, Krzycki J, Petrou N, et al. A quantitative study of humeral cartilage in individuals with spinal cord injury. Spinal Cord 2008; 46:129-134.
238. Song Y, Greve JM, Carter DR, et al. Articular cartilage MR imaging and thickness mapping of a loaded knee joint before and after meniscectomy. Osteoarthritis Cartilage 2006; 14:728-737.
239. Guilak F, Ratcliffe A, Mow VC. Chondrocyte deformation and local tissue strain in articular cartilage: a confocal microscopy study. J Orthop Res 1995; 13:410-421.
240. Kim KW, Wong ME, Helfrick JF, et al. Biomechanical tissue characterization of the superior joint space of the porcine temporomandibular joint. Ann Biomed Eng 2003; 31:924-930.
241. Herberhold C, Faber S, Stammberger T, et al. In situ measurement of articular cartilage deformation in intact femoropatellar joints under static loading. J Biomech 1999; 32:1287-1295.
242. Grunder W, Kanowski M, Wagner M, Werner A. Visualization of pressure distribution within loaded joint cartilage by application of angle-sensitive NMR microscopy. Magn Reson Med 2000; 43:884-891.
243. Neu CP, Hull ML, Walton JH, Buonocore MH. MRI-based technique for determining nonuniform deformations throughout the volume of articular cartilage explants. Magn Reson Med 2005; 53:321-328.
244. Neu CP, Hull ML, Walton JH. Error optimization of a three-dimensional magnetic resonance imaging tagging-based cartilage deformation technique. Magn Reson Med 2005; 54:1290-1294.
245. Neu CP, Walton JH. Displacement encoding for the measurement of cartilage deformation. Magn Reson Med 2008; 59:149-155.
246. Hardy PA, Ridler AC, Chiarot CB, et al. Imaging articular cartilage under compression—cartilage elastography. Magn Reson Med 2005; 53:1065-1073.
247. Lopez O, Amrami KK, Manduca A, Ehman RL. Characterization of the dynamic shear properties of hyaline cartilage using high-frequency dynamic MR elastography. Magn Reson Med 2008; 59:356-364.
248. Lopez O, Amrami KK, Manduca A, et al. Developments in dynamic MR elastography for in vitro biomechanical assessment of hyaline cartilage under high-frequency cyclical shear. J Magn Reson Imaging 2007; 25:310-320.
249. Othman SF, Xu H, Royston TJ, Magin RL. Microscopic magnetic resonance elastography (microMRE). Magn Reson Med 2005; 54:605-615.
250. Filidoro L, Dietrich O, Weber J, et al. High-resolution diffusion tensor imaging of human patellar cartilage: feasibility and preliminary findings. Magn Reson Med 2005; 53:993-998.
251. Deng X, Farley M, Nieminen MT, et al. Diffusion tensor imaging of native and degenerated human articular cartilage. Magn Reson Imaging 2007; 25:168-171.
252. Meder R, de Visser SK, Bowden JC, et al. Diffusion tensor imaging of articular cartilage as a measure of tissue microstructure. Osteoarthritis Cartilage 2006; 14:875-881.
253. de Visser SK, Crawford RW, Pope JM. Structural adaptations in compressed articular cartilage measured by diffusion tensor imaging. Osteoarthritis Cartilage 2008; 16:83-89.

254. Stammberger T, Herberhold C, Faber S, et al. A method for quantifying time dependent changes in MR signal intensity of articular cartilage as a function of tissue deformation in intact joints. Med Eng Phys 1998; 20:741-749.
255. Alhadlaq HA, Xia Y. Modifications of orientational dependence of microscopic magnetic resonance imaging T(2) anisotropy in compressed articular cartilage. J Magn Reson Imaging 2005; 22:665-673.
256. Kaab MJ, Ito K, Clark JM, Notzli HP. Deformation of articular cartilage collagen structure under static and cyclic loading. J Orthop Res 1998; 16:743-751.
257. Nag D, Liney GP, Gillespie P, Sherman KP. Quantification of T(2) relaxation changes in articular cartilage with in situ mechanical loading of the knee. J Magn Reson Imaging 2004; 19:317-322.
258. Mosher TJ, Smith HE, Collins C, et al. Change in knee cartilage T2 at MR imaging after running: a feasibility study. Radiology 2005; 234:245-249.

Chapter 9

MOLECULAR IMAGING OF RHEUMATOID ARTHRITIS AND OSTEOARTHRITIS

Sandip Biswal

What is *molecular imaging?* The term certainly has been used to describe a wide variety of imaging approaches. For our purpose, we limit it to a definition so elegantly put forth by Massoud and Gambhir as "the visual representation, characterization, and quantification of biological processes at the cellular and subcellular levels within intact living organisms. It is a novel multidisciplinary field, in which the images produced reflect cellular and molecular pathways and in vivo mechanisms of disease present within the context of physiologically authentic environments."[1] With molecular imaging techniques we can study the spatiotemporal distribution of specific molecular entities, such as antibodies and cytokines, or we can track specific cell populations. We can study the expression of specific genes or the augmentation of certain gene products, such as proteases.

So, why do we need molecular imaging? Using tried-and-true methods of radiography, MRI, computed tomography, or a combination of these, we can usually establish the diagnosis, or so it seems. The current methods, however, have weaknesses with regard to the assessment of chronic diseases, detection of acute-on-chronic changes (whether related to disease recurrence or post-therapeutic effects), and identification of hyperacute phases of disease. It is in this arena of uncertainty that molecular imaging may prove very useful, providing information not discernible by current clinical imaging techniques.

Furthermore, the fusion of functional and molecular imaging procedures with conventional, anatomic imaging methods will no doubt add to the specificity and sensitivity of imaging diagnosis, just as 2-deoxy-2-(^{18}F)fluoro-D-deoxyglucose (FDG)-positron emission tomography (PET)/CT has done for general tumor screening and staging. Molecular imaging procedures should be viewed as important complementary tools to an already powerful armamentarium of clinical imaging devices. For the near future, hybrid imaging technologies such as PET/CT, single photon emissions computed tomography/CT (SPECT/CT), and, eventually, PET/MRI will be the workhorses for the molecular imager. New molecular "contrast agents" for MRI and ultrasonography will further enhance their potential. Additionally, commonly used optical imaging methods used in preclinical animal models of disease, namely, fluorescence and bioluminescence molecular imaging, will also make strides into the clinical realm.

Perhaps another important reason to increase one's understanding of this evolving discipline of molecular imaging is that in this era of molecular medicine, therapies, including gene therapy and cell-based therapies, can be directly and indirectly studied using molecular imaging procedures and techniques. Basic scientists and molecular imagers are combining forces to find better ways to design and monitor such therapy in living subjects. Ultimately, clinical imagers will be asked to determine whether a certain gene or cell therapy is working in the targeted location in the manner in which it was designed.

Although the application of molecular imaging procedures runs the gamut of musculoskeletal diseases, our discussion of molecular imaging procedures and techniques in this chapter relates its application to two important chronic musculoskeletal disease entities: rheumatoid arthritis (RA) and osteoarthritis (OA).

RHEUMATOID ARTHRITIS

Current Imaging Challenges

Despite the improved sensitivity of newer methods, conventional radiography remains the dominant imaging method for RA evaluation. Radiography can provide excellent detail of osseous erosions, joint space narrowing, and periarticular osteopenia, but only after the clinical symptoms have been present for several months or even years. Furthermore, radiography is considered a relatively insensitive means to measure changes of RA.[2,3] Conventional radiography may appear negative for a period of 6 to 12 months after the onset of disease, and in as many as 25% of RA patients no radiographic erosions are seen for as long as 5 years.[3] The lack of radiologic erosions has unfortunately been used to exclude patients from clinical trials or the initiation of antirheumatic drugs.

Patients suffering from RA would greatly benefit from early detection and treatment of disease. MRI and ultrasonography are being used successfully to detect early RA-related changes in patients and preclinical animal models. MRI allows early detection of osseous and soft tissue changes in RA, including joint effusions, synovitis, tenosynovitis, tendon/ligament damage, bone marrow signal changes, and cartilage destruction; and it is currently considered the superior method in the evaluation of this disease.[4-7] MRI can be applied to the analysis of relatively early changes and chronic periods of the disease. Gadolinium-enhanced MRI allows detection of synovitis with great sensitivity and aids in the differentiation of soft tissue inflammation and a joint effusion.

High-frequency ultrasonography (7.5-10 MHz for conventional studies and 20 MHz for fine detail musculoskeletal work), which can detect synovial thickening, and power Doppler ultrasonography, which indirectly measures hyperemia related to capillary flow, have been used to assess the thickened, hypervascularized synovium of the inflamed small joints of the hands and feet in RA. Ultrasound evaluation is believed to have superior sensitivity to MRI with regard to the detection of effusions and tenosynovial fluid but is inferior to MRI in the assessment of synovitis, tendon/ligament damage, and bone erosions.[8] Ultrasonography is particularly useful during earlier stages of disease and serves as a relatively accessible and inexpensive procedure using nonionizing radiation to assess small joints.

Radionuclide techniques can also be used to detect early changes of RA. By specifically "tagging" or labeling important cellular and protein mediators, RA can be "visualized" from a cellular or molecular context (see later). The white blood cell (WBC) or leukocyte scan, for example, is a classic assay for studying the migration and trafficking of these specialized cells to sites of inflammation. Studies of rheumatoid arthritic wrists have shown that MR measurements of synovial volume correlated with the metabolic rate of the inflamed tissue as measured by FDG-PET ($r > .86$; $P < .0001$).[9] Further details on the utility of FDG-PET have been provided in Chapter 7.

Ultimately, the conventional imaging methods just described can only demonstrate abnormalities that are relatively downstream to the inciting event, that is, activation of the T cell. Effusions, hypervascularity, erosions, and synovial proliferation are changes seen only after the activation of T cells and macrophages. Molecular imaging protocols, as discussed later in this chapter, attempt to image these cells and related acute mediators of disease (Fig. 9-1A).

Pathogenesis

Despite extensive reviews on the subject, the cause of RA remains a mystery.[10,11] Presumably, an unidentified arthritogenic antigen stimulates or activates $CD4^+$ T cells that normally reside in synovium. Neighboring cells, such as dendritic cells, monocytes, synovial fibroblasts, and macrophages, are induced to produce the proinflammatory cytokines, interleukin (IL)-1 (IL-1), tumor necrosis factor-α (TNF-α) and IL-6. These same cells are also stimulated to secrete the matrix metalloproteinases, which cause degradation of the synovium and cartilaginous and osseous extracellular matrix tissue. Activated T cells also stimulate B cells to produce immunoglobulins, the most notorious of which is rheumatoid factor (RF). RF may play a role in the pathogenesis of RA by binding and activating complement, which further contributes to the inflammatory process. Furthermore, activated T cells also possess the ability to directly activate osteoclasts, which are cells that are responsible for the bone erosions typical of the disease. Angiogenesis, an eventual prominent feature in the synovial tissues, can be attributed to activated macrophages, lymphocytes, and fibroblasts. It is this proliferation of vascular elements that gives rise to the synovial enhancement seen with gadolinium-enhanced MRI and power Doppler ultrasonography. Endothelial cells that populate both the newly created and preexisting vessels produce proinflammatory proteins (e.g., certain receptors) and adhesion molecules under inflammatory conditions. It is these increased cytokines, proteinases, immunoglobulins, inflammatory mediators, adhesion molecules, and other molecules that molecular imaging protocols exploit for generating image contrast.

Molecular Imaging

A fundamental explanation for the frustration of clinicians in defining appropriate therapeutic options in patients with RA is the variable clinical manifestations and responses to treatment. Adding to the complexity of this disease are the seemingly uncoupled events of synovitis and bone destruction.[12] For these reasons, clinicians and molecular imagers alike are interested in finding consistent, reliable biomarkers of RA. Identifying common cellular and molecular denominators of disease that can be applied broadly during the course of disease is of great importance. Rather than focusing on anatomic changes of the disease, molecular imaging attempts to detect cellular and molecular perturbations by exploiting the stereotypic changes seen in this disease. Inflammatory cells, for example, are recruited to an affected joint, an event that, in turn, is followed by a cascade of inflammation-related biochemical processes such as the upregulation of certain cell surface receptors. By specifically "tagging" inflammatory cells or carefully selected ligands, one may be able to define specific and discrete aspects of the inflammatory process. Furthermore, by tailoring molecular imaging protocols in light of current molecular therapies, we may be able to better assist our colleagues who are designing therapies specifically to deal with the action of T cells, autoantibodies, cytokines, or other effector cells. A summary of both conventional and molecular methods to image RA is provided in Table 9-1.

TRACKING INFLAMMATORY CELLS AND SPECIFIC SUBPOPULATIONS

Cell trafficking of specific cell populations to inflamed joints is a common strategy to image RA and related autoimmune diseases. This concept is the underlying premise for many long-established radionuclide-based techniques such as the

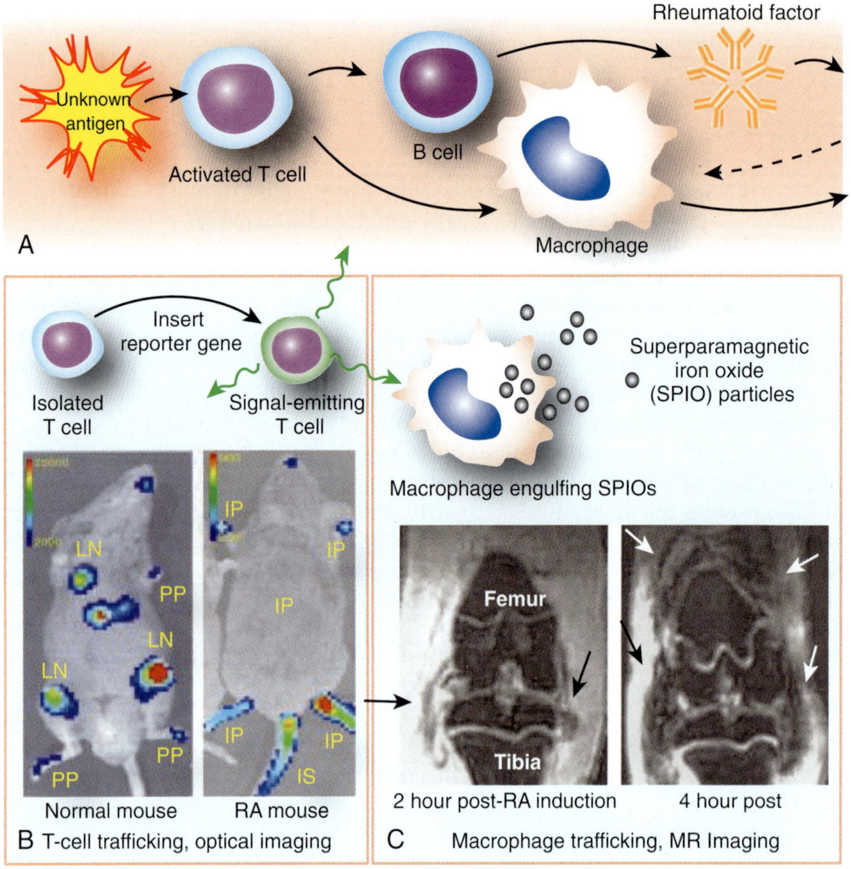

FIGURE 9-1. Molecular imaging of rheumatoid arthritis. **A,** Schematic of RA pathogenesis. T-cell activation by an undetermined antigen causes the subsequent activation of B cells and macrophages, resulting in the elaboration of antibodies and inflammatory cytokines, respectively. Leukocytes, including polymorphonuclear cells, are subsequently recruited and activated in the affected joint as well, producing a number of proteases, such as metalloproteinases and collagenases. These enzymes are responsible for much of the destruction and lytic changes seen in RA. **B,** T cells play a major role in the initiation and progression of RA. They are found in the affected joints and have been labeled by a variety of radionuclide, optical, and MRI-based techniques. In this example, they have been isolated from the peripheral blood and labeled with a light-emitting gene, firefly luciferase, and then systemically reintroduced into experimental animals.[18] Using a cooled, optical, charged couple device (CCD) camera designed for optical imaging, images obtained from nonarthritic, control animals showed that optically labeled T cells resided in axillary and inguinal lymph nodes. By comparison, animals with polyarticular inflammation showed that the specially marked cells migrated out of the lymph nodes and into the inflamed joints. **C,** Macrophages isolated from a subject can be loaded with dextran-coated superparamagnetic iron oxide particles (SPIO) and reintroduced into the subject, which is then scanned. On gradient-echo sequences, cells carrying this contrast agent appear low in signal intensity owing to the large susceptibility effect generated by the sequestered SPIO particles. Investigators have successfully shown the temporal-dependent migration of SPIO-labeled macrophages to the synovium of a rat knee model of RA.[31] Note the characteristic increase in thickening and signal dropout in the synovium when SPIO-labeled cells infiltrate the inflamed joint.

gallium-67 (^{67}Ga) scan and the WBC scan. How PET-, optical-, and MRI-based methods compare with standard methods (e.g., the WBC scan) remains to be seen because head-to-head comparisons have not been performed. Generalized methods for improving radiolabeling of T lymphocytes and monocytes for PET imaging have been described.[13,14]

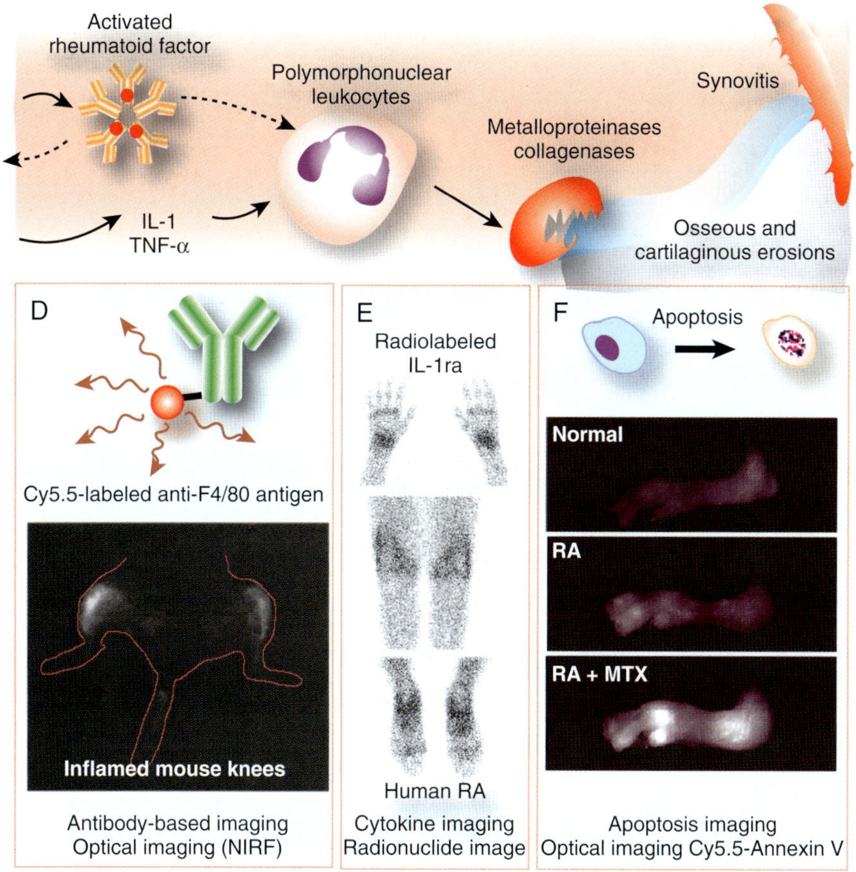

FIGURE 9-1. cont'd **D,** Using a fluorescently labeled (Cy5.5) monoclonal antibody to F4/80 antigen, investigators have demonstrated localization of this antibody in inflamed mouse joints using optical imaging strategies.[41] The antigen F4/80 is present on the surface of macrophages infiltrating an inflamed joint, and thus targeted imaging of these macrophages via antibodies presents yet another approach to RA imaging. **E,** Just as antibodies can be labeled, so can cytokines and other inflammation-related proteins. In this example, a receptor antagonist to the interleukin-1 receptor has been labeled with ^{123}I and the tracer has been tested in humans. Gamma camera images show localization of the tracer to affected joints of the hand, knee, and feet in patients with RA.[44] **F,** The near-infrared fluorochromes have been covalently attached to annexin V and have been successfully utilized to image apoptosis in an animal model of RA.[56] Images of the hind paw show slightly increased fluorescence in joints of RA animals, indicating that some apoptosis was occurring in the joints of the experimental model. RA animals treated with methotrexate (MTX), a standard disease-modifying antirheumatic drug (DMARD), show increased Cy5.5/annexin V fluorescence in the joints and correspondingly increased apoptosis in the joints as determined by terminal deoxynucleotidyl transferase–mediated UTP nick-end labeling (TUNEL). The increased apoptosis seen in MTX-treated RA animals is most likely due to the cytotoxic effects of MTX on the hyperplastic synovium. Normal subjects, in contrast, did not show this accumulation of tracer material.

T-Cell Trafficking

One particularly exciting method to monitor the pathogenesis of RA will be to track one of the main cellular culprits associated with this autoimmune disease, namely, the reactive $CD4^+$ T-cell lymphocytes.[15] There are means of isolating and purifying such cells from a subject using sophisticated cell-sorting techniques. Once isolated from peripheral blood, these cells can be "marked" with a contrast agent and then reintroduced into the same subject. After a period of incubation, the subject can undergo serial imaging to determine the distribution of the cells. Traditional cell-labeling techniques are based on radionuclide methods (e.g., ^{111}In-oxime,

TABLE 9-1. Imaging of Rheumatoid Arthritis

Targeted Pathology	Temporal Pattern	Modality and Specific Methods	Clinical vs. Preclinical	References
T-cell infiltration	Hyperacute to acute	NM: ^{99m}Tc-HMPAO-labeled T cells	Clinical	16
		PET reporter genes	Preclinical	16
		Optical: luciferase reporter genes	Preclinical	18
		MRI: CLIO-Tat	Preclinical	26
Antibody-based Imaging	Hyperacute to chronic	NM: ^{64}Cu-labeled anti-GPI	Preclinical	37
		^{111}In- or ^{99m}Tc-labeled nonspecific IgG	Clinical	109
		^{99m}Tc-labeled anti-CD3	Clinical	110
		^{99m}Tc-labeled anti-CD4	Clinical	111
		^{111}In- or 99mTc-labeled anti-E-selectin Fab	Clinical	112
		Radiolabeled anti-TNF-α, anti-IL-1, anti-IL-2, and anti-IL-6	Preclinical	35
		^{123}I-antileukoproteinase	Preclinical	113
		^{99m}Tc-labeled anti-CD15 immunoglobulin M (IgM)	Clinical	114
		Optical: NIRF-labeled anti-F4/80 macrophage surface antigen	Preclinical	41
Macrophage recruitment	Hyperacute to chronic	MRI: Superparamagnetic iron oxide particles (SPIO)	Clinical	31
		Ultrasmall SPIO (USPIO)	Preclinical	115
		NM: ^{99m}Tc-folic acid (EC20; folate receptor imaging agent)	Preclinical	32
		Optical: NIRF-labeled folate (NIR2-folate)	Preclinical	34
Leukocyte recruitment	Hyperacute to chronic	NM: ^{99m}Tc-HMPAO-labeled WBCs	Clinical	36
		^{111}In-labeled WBC	Clinical	36
		^{67}Ga-citrate	Clinical	36
Cytokine production	Hyperacute to chronic	NM: ^{123}I-labeled interleukin-1 receptor antagonist (IL-1ra)	Clinical	44
Activated nuclear factor-κB (NF-κB)	Hyperacute to CHRONIC	Optical: NF-κB reporter mouse	Preclinical	47, 48
Matrix-degrading enzymes	Hyperacute to chronic	Optical: cathepsin and matrix metalloproteinase-sensitive NIRFs	Preclinical	49, 50
Synovitis/ tenosynovitis	Acute to chronic	US: Gray-scale sonography Power Doppler	Clinical	116
		MRI: Nonenhanced and gadolinium-enhanced MRI	Clinical	116
Joint effusion	Acute to chronic	Ultrasonography	Clinical	117
		MRI	Clinical	117
		Radiography	Clinical	117
Soft tissue swelling	Acute to chronic	Ultrasonography	Clinical	117
		MRI	Clinical	117
		Radiography	Clinical	117
Bone marrow changes	Acute to chronic	MRI	Clinical	117
		NM: ^{99m}Tc-methylene diphosphonate (MDP)	Clinical	118
Increased metabolism	Acute to chronic	NM: ^{18}F-FDG-PET	Clinical	119

TABLE 9-1. Imaging of Rheumatoid Arthritis—cont'd

Targeted Pathology	Temporal Pattern	Modality and Specific Methods	Clinical vs. Preclinical	References
Cell stress/ apoptosis	Acute to chronic	NM: ^{99m}Tc-, ^{123}I-, ^{124}I, ^{125}I-, ^{18}F-, ^{11}C-, ^{64}Cu-, ^{67}Ga-, and ^{68}Ga-labeled annexin V	Clinical	84
		MRI: CLIO-labeled annexin V	Clinical	89
		Optical: Cy5.5-labeled annexin V	Clinical	56
Vascular inflammation angiogenesis	Acute to chronic	NM: ^{99m}Tc-anti-E-selectin-Fab	Preclinical	65
		Power Doppler ultrasonography	Clinical	116
		MRI: gadolinium-enhanced	Clinical	116
Osseous or cartilaginous erosions	Intermediate to chronic	Radiography	Clinical	117
		CT	Clinical	117
		MRI	Clinical	117
Tendon damage	Intermediate to chronic	Ultrasonography	Clinical	117
		MRI	Clinical	117
Subluxations and dislocations	Chronic	Radiography	Clinical	117
		CT	Clinical	117
		MRI	Clinical	117
Secondary OA	Chronic	Radiography	Clinical	117
		CT	Clinical	117
		MRI	Clinical	117

NM, nuclear medicine; HMPAO, hexamethylpropyleneamine oxime; WBCs, white blood cells; GPI, glucose-6-phosphate isomerase; NIRF, near infrared fluorochromes; CLIO, crosslinked iron oxide particles.

^{111}In-tropolonate, and ^{99m}Tc-HMPAO)[16,17]; however, a number of PET, optical, and MR-compatible methods are currently available.

In animal models of collagen-induced RA, the localization of collagen-reactive CD4$^+$ cells has been shown through imaging assays in living mice. To track the cells, the investigators transfected reactive CD4$^+$ T-cell hybridomas with a recombinant retroviral vector encoding green fluorescent protein (GFP) and firefly luciferase optical-based reporter genes.[18] A detailed review of in-vivo reporter genes is beyond the scope of this chapter but can be found elsewhere.[1,19] Briefly, cells such as the T cells have been genetically re-engineered to express fluorescent or bioluminescence proteins, which give these "labeled" cells the ability to emit light under the appropriate conditions. Light emission from the T cells can be detected with a highly sensitive cooled, optical, charged couple device (CCD) camera, resulting in images that give the general spatial location of these optically labeled T cells. Images obtained from nonarthritic, control animals showed that optically labeled T cells resided in axillary and inguinal lymph nodes (see Fig. 9-1B). By comparison, animals with polyarticular inflammation showed that the specially marked cells migrated from the lymph nodes to the inflamed joints. Investigators also used these cells to specifically deliver anti-inflammatory gene therapy to the joints in the form of cytokine antagonist IL-12 p40. Injection of collagen-specific IL-12 p40–producing T cells retarded the development of collagen-induced arthritis.[18]

Another method to monitor T-cell traffic has been developed for MRI. T cells isolated from a subject can be loaded with dextran-coated superparamagnetic iron oxide particles (SPIO) or similar dextran-coated crosslinked iron oxide particles (CLIO).[20,21] When exposed to SPIO, T-cells will engulf the 30-nm particles by endocytosis. The T cells are eventually reintroduced into the subject, and the subject is scanned. On gradient-echo sequences, cells carrying this contrast agent appear low in signal intensity owing to the large susceptibility effect generated by the sequestered SPIO particles. In rat models of cardiac, renal, and lung allograft rejection, migration of SPIO-labeled T cells to the allograft has been found during rejection.[22-24]

Recently, this cell-labeling contrast agent has undergone a modification that facilitates its entry into target cells. The superparamagnetic core of the iron oxide particle has been linked with peptide sequences of the transactivator protein (Tat) of human immunodeficiency virus-1 (HIV-1), resulting in CLIO-Tat particles.[25,26] The HIV-1 Tat protein is an 86-amino acid protein required for replication of the virus. It appears to be involved in translocating the viral particle freely across cellular and nuclear membranes. A short segment of the peptide, amino acid residues 48-57, is largely responsible for this transport phenomenon, and when this short peptide segment is attached to a CLIO particle it increases the cell labeling efficiency 100-fold. This agent has been tested in animals, in which the expected migration of CLIO-Tat–labeled T cells to the reticuloendothelial system is seen, and in an animal model of autoimmune diabetes, in which labeled T cells traffic to the pancreas.[27] Other recent cell-labeling techniques involve directly labeling cells with technetium-99m (^{99m}Tc) or with MRI-detectable DNA-binding chelates.[28-31] Many of these methods have not yet been applied to arthritic models but have great potential.

Macrophage Trafficking

SPIO can also be used to monitor monocytic/macrophage migration patterns in the setting of RA. After intravenous injection of SPIO particles, cells that reside in the reticuloendothelial syndrome, including macrophages, engulf the agent. Because macrophages are recruited to inflamed joints, monitoring their distribution by SPIO-based techniques can be helpful, especially during early phases of the disease. MRI can be used to study the migration of these cells from the reticuloendothelial syndrome to inflamed joints. Investigators have successfully documented the migration of SPIO-labeled macrophages to the synovium of a rat model of RA (see Fig. 9-1C).[32]

Activated macrophages are also known to express a large number of folic acid receptors, and this characteristic has been exploited by several investigators as a means to study the distribution of macrophages in the inflamed joints of animals. The ligand for the receptor, folic acid, has been coupled to a variety of optical and radionuclide labels, and early studies with the intravenously administered, labeled folate in animal models have shown localization of the tracer in inflamed joints.[33-35]

Leukocyte Trafficking

Leukocytes include neutrophils, basophils, eosinophils, monocytes, macrophages, and lymphocytes. They participate in a host of inflammatory reactions in disease such as RA, infection, and trauma. Imaging leukocyte trafficking has been a staple procedure among the radionuclide-based imaging examinations for the past few decades. Better known as a WBC scan, a variety of methods have been developed that can successfully label leukocytes with ^{99m}Tc, ^{67}Ga, and indium-111 (^{111}In), and these methods have been specifically applied to the study of RA.[36] Because of its relatively low cost, ease of use, low radiation burden, general accessibility, and high sensitivity and the significant correlation of accumulated activity at sites of active disease (as measured by the swollen joint count), ^{99m}Tc-hexamethylpropyleneamine oxime (HMPAO)–labeled leukocyte scintigraphy is one of the methods of choice to study migration of these cells into inflamed joints.[37]

ANTIBODY-BASED AND CYTOKINE-BASED IMAGING

Autoantibodies that develop during the course of RA have been labeled and injected, and their distribution has been studied. Additionally, specific antibodies to T cells, general leukocytes, cytokines, and receptors have also been utilized in this manner. A variety of specific and nonspecific antibodies of interest have been radiolabeled or fluorescently labeled and imaged in animal models of RA (see Table 9-1). One example is an antibody to the glycolysis enzyme glucose-6-phosphate isomerase (GPI), which has been the subject of intense interest, because 50% of RA patients have serum antibodies to GPI. By labeling anti-GPI immunoglobulin G (IgG) with the positron emitter copper-64 (^{64}Cu), investigators have studied the biodistribution of this antibody in animal models of RA. PET imaging reveals accumulation of the labeled antibody in the front paws, hind ankles, and rear feet of animals with RA, while control animals showed negligible articular uptake.[38] Other antibodies, including polyclonal, nonspecific IgG, have been similarly interrogated using scintigraphic methods.[39-41] Whereas the exact mechanism remains poorly understood, the use of nonspecific antibodies is encouraged by its high sensitivity. However, the lack of specificity (<50%) and the relative high cost compared with more conventional scintigraphic techniques (e.g., leukocyte scintigraphy) probably prevent the routine utilization of radiolabeled antibody–based techniques at the current time.

Another way to track antibodies is through fluorescence labeling. Using a fluorescently labeled (Cy5.5) monoclonal antibody to F4/80 antigen, investigators have demonstrated the localization of this antibody in the inflamed joints of mice using optical imaging strategies (see Fig. 9-1D).[42] The antigen F4/80 is present on the surface of macrophages that infiltrate an inflamed joint, and targeted imaging of these macrophages via antibodies represents yet another approach to RA imaging. Numerous other antibodies (see Table 9-1) have been developed to bind to the various mediators of disease, including T cells, cytokines, and receptors. Recent evidence, however, suggests that the use of antibody-based imaging techniques may be problematic, because only a fraction of the radiolabeled monoclonal antibodies (directed CD4$^+$ T lymphocytes) actually bind to target cells while a majority of the dose gets trapped in the reticuloendothelial system such as the liver.[43] Modifications to antibodies (i.e., diabodies, tetrabodies, and minibodies) are currently being studied to avoid such problems in the future.[44]

Just as antibodies can be labeled, so can inflammatory cytokines or receptor antagonists. Investigators have labeled a receptor antagonist to the interleukin-1 receptor (IL-1ra) with iodine-123, and the tracer has been tested in humans. Gamma camera images show localization of the tracer to affected joints in patients with RA (see Fig. 9-1E).[45]

ACTIVATED NUCLEAR FACTOR-κ B (NF-κB) IMAGING

NF-κB is a rapid-acting transcription factor found in nearly all cell types and is a major proinflammatory mediator. Activation of NF-κB stimulates or regulates transcription of over 150 genes, including monocyte chemotactic protein 1, intracellular adhesion molecule (ICAM-1), TNF-α, IL-1β, IL-6, inducible nitric oxide synthase (iNOS), IL-8, matrix metalloproteinases, and cyclooxygenase 2 (COX-2), which are necessary for the initialization and persistence of chronic inflammation, including that seen in RA.[46,47] Prior to modulating the expression of these genes, activation of NF-κB requires enzymatic action with the IkB kinase (IKK) complex. After activation, NF-κB translocates into the nucleus and binds to a 10-base-pair DNA sequence. Under the control of the NF-κB–inducible promoter, transgenic mice have been developed that express luciferase under the control of an activated NF-κB, permitting real-time, in-vivo longitudinal, optical imaging of NF-κB activity in living animals.[48] This "NF-κB reporter mouse" has already demonstrated its prowess as an important tool in monitoring multicellular inflammatory responses in models of arthritis and studies of drug action. Through its selective inhibitory effect on the IKK complex, ML120B, a potent, small molecule, for example, has been shown to reduce

NF-κB activity and concomitantly reduce the expression of multiple inflammation genes in the NF-κB pathway in an antibody-induced arthritis model.[49]

Protease-Specific Activated Near-Infrared Probes

The production of matrix metalloproteinases (MMP) and cathepsins is also enhanced in active stages of joint inflammation. In the optical imaging world, a recently developed "smart" fluorescent probe has been developed to detect elevated levels of MMP and cathepsins.[50] This probe, or contrast agent, will emit light only when cleaved by its specific target enzyme; otherwise, the probe is optically invisible. This breed of fluorescent probe is dependent on the close proximity of multiple Cy5.5 near-infrared fluorochromes (NIRF), which are bound to a synthetic graft copolymer backbone (partially methoxypoly[ethylene glycol] modified poly-L-lysine).[51]

When placed in close proximity, a pair of these fluorochromes will "quench" each other and, therefore, be "invisible." Once the fluorochromes achieve a minimal physical separation, they will begin to fluoresce. The basis of this physical phenomenon is called mutual fluorescence energy transfer (FRET). When cathepsin B, which has lysine-lysine substrate specificity, interacts with the Cy5.5-loaded NIRF "contrast agent," the lysine backbone is cleaved and the Cy5.5 fluorochromes spatially dissociate to fluoresce. These contrast agents are "red shifted," and, thus, fluoresce in the near-infrared portion of the electromagnetic spectrum (excitation wavelength of 673 nm; emissions wavelength of 689 nm). Red-shifted fluorochromes are ideal fluorescent agents for use in intact organisms, because longer wavelengths penetrate tissues such as bone better than green-fluorescing agents.

Because many of the arthritides (as well as tumors) during stages of progression and angiogenesis necessarily elaborate certain matrix-digesting proteases, these clever, or "smart," biocompatible autoquenched near-infrared fluorescent probes can potentially be used to detect a variety of arthritic processes (including OA), as well as cancers. The successful application of a cathepsin B–sensitive probe has been demonstrated in an animal model of RA.[52,53] After intravenous administration of the NIRF probe, light was seen to arise from the inflamed knees and ankles of animals with RA but not from the joints of normal animals.

Cell Stress/Apoptosis Imaging

The inflammation of RA is an event that is stressful to cells involved in the process. Furthermore, there appears to be an abnormal rate of apoptosis occurring in synovial tissue in RA. Whether the level of apoptosis is excessive or reduced remains a matter of debate.[54] Imaging of cell stress and apoptosis is now possible in living subjects using an endogenous molecule called annexin V. Annexin V recognizes a cell membrane component that presents itself during times of increased metabolic stress, apoptosis, and necrosis (see later).

In the collagen-induced arthritis model, increased uptake of radiolabeled ^{99m}Tc-HYNIC-annexin V is seen in the paws of arthritic animals when compared with controls.[55] Steroid treatment of the arthritic model not only alleviates clinical manifestations of collagen-induced arthritis but also results in diminished uptake of annexin V, suggesting that the steroids provided some type of cytoprotective effect. In another example, near-infrared fluorescence (NIRF) imaging with Cy5.5-annexin V showed no significant imaging differences between collagen-induced arthritis models and controls (see Fig. 9-1F).[56] When methotrexate was administered to both groups, an increased accumulation of Cy5.5-annexin V was observed in the joints of both models, with substantially more seen in the collagen-induced arthritis model.

Vascular Markers

Vascular endothelial cells associated with the area of inflammation, whether related to trauma, infection, arthritis, or other causes, become "activated," and their activation is integral to the process of leukocytic recruitment and ensuing synovitis. These stimulated endothelial cells necessarily amplify a number of cellular adhesion molecules, including selectins (e.g., P-selectin, E-selectin), integrins (e.g., β_4, β_1), immunoglobulins (e.g., ICAM-1), vascular cellular adhesion molecule-1 (VCAM-1), and cadherins (e.g., E-cadherin, cadherin-11), to attract and bind inflammatory cells.[57-59] Additionally, the endothelial cell–specific vascular endothelial growth factor (VEGF), which has been well characterized in hypoxic stress models and tumor angiogenesis, has also been found to be augmented in aggressive synovitis and strongly correlates with RA activity.[60]

In efforts to improve detection of vasculitic processes, a number of contrast agents that target endothelial epitopes have been developed for ultrasonography, MRI, and radionuclide-based imaging. For example, echogenic microbubbles have been conjugated to antibodies for ICAM-1, fibrinogen, or P-selectin.[61,62] These agents will localize to the endothelium of an organ that has sustained an ischemia-reperfusion injury. Alternatively, these agents will diffusely localize to the endothelium when systemic tumor TNF-α is administered. Echogenic liposomal agents have also been coated with anti–ICAM-1, resulting in their localization to atheromatous plaques during ultrasound imaging.[63,64] Radionuclide approaches that employ a ^{99m}Tc-radiolabeled E-selectin–binding peptide have also been attempted with some success.[65] Optical approaches have employed highly fluorescent quantum dots that have antibodies directed against adhesion molecules conjugated to its surface. This contrast agent has successfully highlighted retinal vascular inflammation seen in a rat model of diabetes.[66]

MR researchers have also created agents for cellular adhesion molecules. One group of investigators has produced liposomes containing a gadolinium lipid chelator that becomes paramagnetic in the presence of gadolinium.[67] By biotinylating these paramagnetic liposomes, biotinylated antibodies can be conjugated to the liposomes via an avidin linker, creating an antibody-conjugated paramagnetic liposome (ACPL). In an animal model of experimental autoimmune encephalitis (EAE), localization of ICAM-1 ACPL in the brain leads to increased signal intensity. Another MR-based imaging agent involves the conjugation of monocrystalline iron oxide nanoparticles to anti–human E-selectin.[68] In cell culture, umbilical vein endothelial cells avidly bind this MR contrast agent compared with controls when exposed to the inflammatory mediator IL-1β.

Imaging of VEGF receptors (VEGFRs) has been successfully performed in living murine hindlimb ischemia models using radiolabeled vascular endothelial growth factor-121 (VEGF121) and ^{64}Cu-VEGF121 PET.[69] Microvessel density as measured with laser Doppler imaging correlated strongly with uptake of VEGF121 radiotracer. Imaging of integrin $\alpha_V\beta_3$ has been successfully performed using ^{18}F-labeled PEGylated tetrameric RGD peptide in tumor angiogenesis models.[70] The application of such tracers to arthritis models may prove to be an important biomarker of aggressive forms of synovitis.

OSTEOARTHRITIS

Current Challenges

Articular cartilage, menisci, bones, synovium, and ligaments are among the tissues affected during the progression of OA. Of these, derangement of hyaline articular cartilage appears fundamental to the initiation and progression of disease. Although articular cartilage is generally believed to be unsalvageable after substantial deterioration, there is increasing evidence that early localized changes may be rescued through well-timed medical or gene/cell therapeutic interventions. As a result, the cartilage damage in OA is being recharacterized by an earlier dynamic phase, which is potentially reversible, followed by an irreversible pathologic phase that ultimately leads to joint pain and immobility. The point at which cartilage damage is deemed irreversible has not been defined but probably depends on the size of lesion, age of the patient, underlying cause, comorbid factors, activity level, joint stabilizers, genetic predisposition, health of the subchondral bone and synovium, and other factors.

A majority of those persons with early disease are asymptomatic or have only minor clinical problems. Thus, only a small proportion of those persons seek medical attention, whereas most will seek medical assistance only after they have entered the irreparable phase of disease. The impetus to detect early lesions is to allow timely intervention so as to prevent the eventual evolution of radiographically evident joint space narrowing, osteophytosis, subchondral sclerosis, and cyst formation. Various MRI methods have evolved to better characterize early articular cartilage lesions, a number of which have been discussed in detail in preceding chapters of this book. Other attempts to better characterize these small and early cartilage lesions from a molecular and cellular imaging approach are discussed in the remainder of this chapter. Imaging assays that monitor the contribution from other joint-related tissues toward the progression of OA, such as synovium and subchondral bone, are also discussed.

Pathogenesis

To detect early cartilage damage, molecular imaging research has focused on either the identification of finding better ways to visualize extracellular matrix depletion or measurements of events that are associated with cartilage damage, such as chondrocyte death and the elaboration of matrix-degrading enzymes. In OA, there is a general acceptance that abnormal chondrocyte apoptosis is a pivotal event in the eventual destruction of articular cartilage.[71,72]

The major constituents of articular cartilage are water (75% by weight), collagen (predominantly type II; 20% by weight), aggrecan (5% by weight), and a variety of other extracellular matrix molecules, all of which are maintained by resident chondrocytes. From a mechanical standpoint, collagen acts as rebar contributing to the tensile strength of cartilage whereas aggrecan, a macromolecule consisting of negatively charged glycosaminoglycans, acts as electrostatic springs, providing the compressive strength of cartilage. Chondrocytes maintain a very intimate relationship with the extracellular matrix through a variety of adhesion molecules and proteins; they are integral to homeostasis of the extracellular matrix, and their survival dictates the health of the tissue.

In fact, a focal cartilage injury, complete with matrix derangement, matrix depletion, and chondrocyte apoptosis, can be viewed as the beginning of a vicious cycle. The natural history of OA-related cartilage loss seen in serial joints studies is a reflection of this downward course. Trauma results in matrix disruption or chondrocyte apoptosis or a combination of both. Chondrocytic apoptosis is thought to arise from abnormal acute or chronic mechanical loads.[73] In the setting of trauma or microtrauma, there are two fundamental means of chondrocytic apoptosis: (1) traumatic events that directly result in a significant mechanical load on the chondrocyte itself can cause apoptosis; and (2) traumatic loads disrupt the extracellular matrix, causing the chondrocyte to be physically isolated from its immediate surroundings. For reasons not entirely clear, chondrocyte detachment causes the cell to undergo programmed cell death. With regard to the latter phenomenon, investigators have proposed that the denuded, exposed chondrocyte is vulnerable to Fas-mediated killing or nitric oxide toxicity once it has been released from its protective surroundings.[74,75]

Chondrocyte apoptosis leads to matrix dysregulation and an inability to sufficiently regenerate the matrix, causing local mechanical deficiencies. Chondrocytes that have survived the local insult attempt to proliferate and synthesize new matrix elements; but if the injury is too great, cartilage repair will be outpaced by chondral loss. Injured areas also produce active degradative enzymes, matrix metalloproteinases (MMPs), aggrecanase, and cathepsins; interestingly, these enzymes may reside in an inert state in the extracellular matrix and become activated once cartilage injury ensues.[76] Increased level of production of the proteinases, including the metalloproteinases (MMP-1, MMP-3, MMP-8 and MMP-13) and the aggrecanases (a disintegrin and metalloproteinase with thrombospondin [ADAMTS]-4 and -5; also known as aggrecanase-1 and aggrecanase-2), have been identified in OA cartilage.[77] Additionally, both injured chondrocytes as well as other joint tissues, such as synovium, have been found to elaborate proinflammatory cytokines IL-1 and TNF-α in early and late OA. Because chondrocytes also express IL-1 receptors and other proteins responsive to IL-1–mediated inflammatory cascade, injured chondrocytes have the ability to autostimulate the production of catabolic proteinases described earlier as well as other proinflammatory mediators, including cyclooxygenase-2 and nitrous oxide synthase.

Once the injured area of cartilage becomes mechanically insufficient, loads are transferred to the more normal peripheral regions of the injured area. Subsequently, viable chondrocytes at the border of an injured area are subject to abnormal forces and undergo apoptosis. These "border" chondrocytes eventually undergo apoptosis themselves once abnormal forces become excessive, perpetuating the paradigm between matrix loss and chondrocyte apoptosis and resulting in an expanded area of matrix decomposition. The cycle of apoptosis and matrix loss is perpetuated over time, resulting in the progressive changes seen either as joint space loss with serial radiographs as joint space narrowing or as actual cartilage loss seen with MRI. Imaging research and development are focused on the detection of very early cartilage derangement, protease elaboration, and chondrocyte apoptosis.

Molecular and Functional Techniques for Early OA

Charge-Based Methods

Hyaline cartilage, with its intricate network of negatively charged, hydrophilic glycosaminoglycan (GAG) molecules, possesses a fixed charge density. Diseased, GAG-depleted areas of osteoarthritic cartilage correlate with areas of diminished fixed charge density. Methods to measure changes in charge density distribution are possible through the use of charged contrast agents.

As one example, delayed gadolinium-enhanced MRI of cartilage (dGEMRIC) utilizes the negatively charged T1-shortening agent gadopentetate dimeglumine (Gd-DTPA).[78] Because it is similar in charge to the fixed charge density, Gd-DTPA is repulsed by normal, intact cartilage and found in extracartilaginous tissue such as the synovial fluid or subchondral bone after its intravenous administration. Injured cartilage, which contains GAG-deficient areas, permit penetration of Gd-DTPA within the cartilage proper, and, thus, the local concentration of Gd-DTPA is *inversely* related to the fixed charge density. T1 relaxation measurements of damaged cartilage show redistribution of the contrast agent in specific GAG-depleted areas. Thus, with dGEMRIC imaging, T1 relaxation times are lower in areas of cartilage damage than in normal, intact cartilage. The clinical application of this method is not without challenge, namely, a requirement for intra-articular injection of Gd-DTPA, a 30-minute to 3-hour time delay after injection before imaging can be performed, and a requirement for exercise of the joint, but this technique has already proved useful in the evaluation of early OA in dysplastic hips (Fig. 9-2).[79,80]

Another method that takes advantage of the fixed charge density of cartilage is MR sodium-23 (^{23}Na) spectroscopy. The local concentration of positively charged ^{23}Na atoms *directly* correlates with fixed charge density; thus, local concentrations of ^{23}Na are decreased in GAG-depleted cartilage specimens. Although proving to be a sensitive measure of GAG content, the clinical application of this method is limited by specialized hardware requirements that are not widely available.

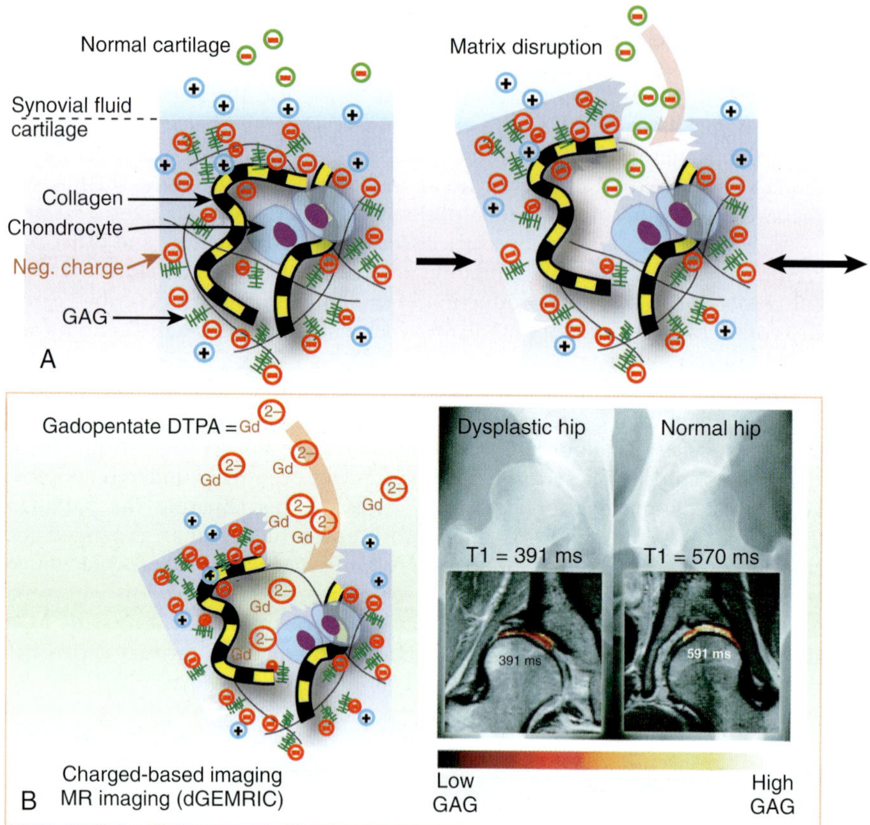

FIGURE 9-2. Molecular imaging of osteoarthritis. **A,** Simplistic schematic of OA pathogenesis. Matrix derangement and chondrocyte apoptosis as the results of trauma or excessive mechanical loads are believed central to the cause of early cartilage degeneration and subsequent OA. Cartilage damage begets more cartilage damage, because viable chondrocytes surrounding a focal cartilage injury are now subject to abnormal loads, resulting in further apoptosis and matrix loss/dysregulation. **B,** Charge-based methods. Hyaline cartilage, with its intricate network of negatively charged, hydrophilic GAG molecules, possesses a fixed charge density. Diseased, GAG-depleted areas of osteoarthritic cartilage correlate to areas of diminished fixed charge density. "Fissures" or openings in the cartilage matrix allow for other negatively charged ions to enter the cartilage, when it would otherwise be repelled from like charges. This is the basis of MRI-based dGEMRIC, and matrix-depleted areas (specifically, GAG-deficient areas) permit penetration of Gd-DTPA within cartilage; thus, the local concentration of Gd-DTPA is *inversely* related to the fixed charge density. After intra-articular administration, MR images show increased T1 signal in the articular cartilage of dysplastic hip.[80]

Imaging Apoptosis

Apoptotic chondrocytes have been found in the mechanically injured cartilage.[71,72] Programmed cell death (PCD), also known as apoptosis, is a normal, physiologic phenomenon required for biologic growth and development, homeostasis, and immune surveillance. Many disease processes, however, can be characterized as having too much or too little apoptosis. Diseases with excessive cell death include neurodegenerative disorders, myelodysplastic syndromes, ischemia/reperfusion injury, viral infections, transplant rejection, and OA. Diseases exemplified by a paucity of apoptosis include cancer (uncontrolled cell growth and proliferation) and autoimmune diseases such as RA, although the latter association is controversial.

Most procedures and techniques that directly assay cell death require tissue sampling and employ histologic and other in-vitro techniques. Recently, a method has

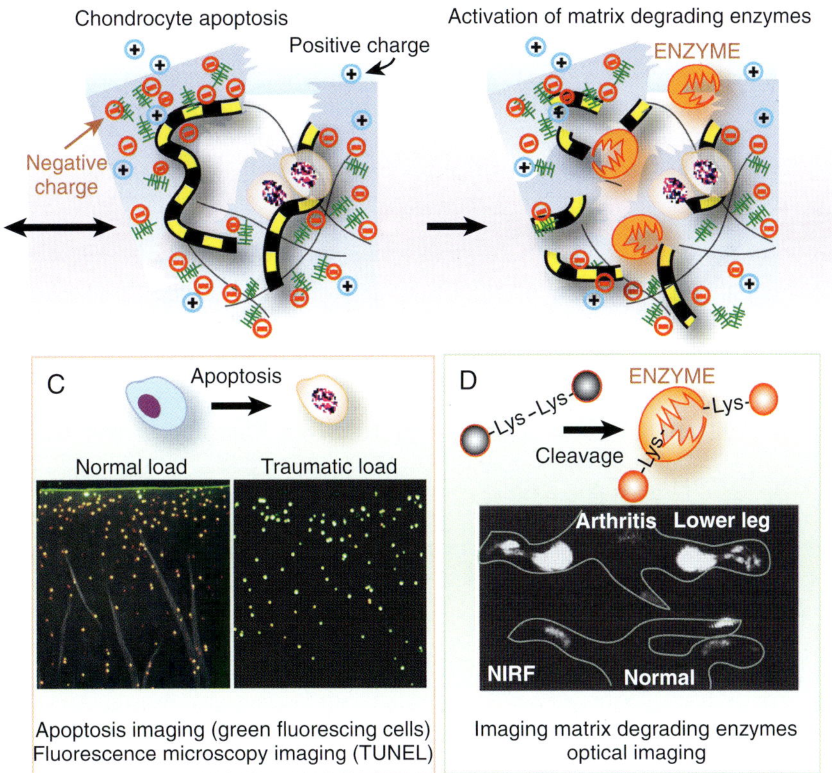

FIGURE 9-2. cont'd **C,** Imaging apoptosis. A histologic section through normal and mechanically traumatized cartilage that has been processed with an in-vitro method for apoptosis called terminal deoxynucleotidyl transferase–mediated UTP nick-end labeling (TUNEL). Apoptotic chondrocytes (shown as green fluorescing cells) can be found in the mechanically injured cartilage. Normal cartilage, on the other hand, had significantly fewer apoptotic cells.[71,72] Such preclinical results are driving the need for the development of tracers, such as annexin V, which have the potential to detect such events in living subjects. **D,** Imaging matrix-degrading enzymes. Damaged cartilage appears to activate hibernating proteases such as matrix metalloproteinases and cathepsins. Using a cathepsin B–sensitive near-infrared fluorescent probe, researchers have found a significant amount of signal arising from an arthritic knee when compared with normal knees in an animal model of OA.[96]

become available for the study in living subjects. This method takes advantage of an endogenous protein, annexin V, whose function is not clearly understood but is thought to have a role in coagulation.[81] Annexin V has an extremely strong affinity for the cell membrane phospholipid phosphatidylserine (PS), which is "externalized" or "expressed" to the outer surface of the cell membrane during the apoptotic cascade. Annexin V, a 35-kD *extracellular* protein, binds the negatively charged, externalized PS with an extremely high affinity (10^{-9} M). It is this interaction that is the basis for PCD imaging.[82-84] Under normal conditions, healthy cells have relatively little annexin V bound to the cell membrane, because most PS molecules are located in the inner leaflet. In contrast, a cell undergoing apoptosis externalizes its PS, thereby increasing annexin V binding approximately 100- to 1000-fold. The use of annexin V, labeled with either a radioisotope or a fluorescent marker, provides an excellent opportunity to image PCD. To date, annexin V has been labeled with ^{99m}Tc, iodine (^{125}I, ^{124}I, ^{123}I), ^{111}In, ^{11}C, ^{67}Ga, ^{68}Ga, and ^{18}F, making it appropriate for either SPECT or PET imaging.[84-88] Annexin V has also been conjugated with CLIO particles for use with MRI and with Cy5.5 fluorescent dye for use with optical techniques.[84,89] Any organ or structure demonstrating increased annexin V uptake is thought to be experiencing substantial apoptosis or tremendous metabolic stress.

Annexin V imaging has yet to be applied to the assessment of human OA. In part, the clinical use of this tracer faces challenges with regard to crossing the blood/synovium barrier. Perhaps direct intra-articular injection of the agent with arthroscopic evaluation will be needed. Alternatively, mutants or modifications of annexin V may be designed to cross such barriers. Radiolabeled annexin V has been studied in animal models of collagen-induced RA.[55] The use of radiolabeled annexin V as an imaging agent has been applied in human clinical trials dealing with myocardial ischemia, cardiac transplant rejection, and cancer chemotherapy.[90-93]

Annexin V imaging will face other challenges as well. The externalization of PS to the outer leaflet is not limited to apoptotic cells. Viable cells under severe stress or those undergoing necrosis will also present PS molecules to the outer membrane for annexin V binding. Because of this, annexin V imaging loses specificity. Also, there appears to be a biphasic, temporally dependent pattern of PS externalization following an apoptotic signal, which restricts the timing of optimal imaging periods.[94] A better understanding of annexin V biology will help determine specific imaging requirements in the future. Additionally, other techniques to image apoptosis, including lipid ^{1}H magnetic resonance spectroscopy (MRS), anti-annexin V monoclonal antibodies, anti-PS monoclonal antibodies, and radiolabeled caspase inhibitors/substrates, are being explored as imaging agents (see Fig. 9-2).[84,95]

Imaging Proteases

Details of this method are provided in the earlier section dealing with RA. Just as occurs in RA, certain proteases are elaborated during the course of OA. As mentioned earlier, damaged cartilage appears to activate hibernating proteases such as matrix metalloproteinases and cathepsins. Using a cathepsin B–sensitive near-infrared fluorescent probe, researchers have found significant amounts of signal arising from an arthritic knee when compared with normal knees in an animal model of OA (see Fig. 9-2).[96]

Cyclooxygenase-2

Cyclooxygenase-2 (COX-2) is considered a major facilitator of tissue inflammation because of its role in prostanoid production from the metabolism of arachidonic acid into prostaglandin H (PGH); PGH is eventually converted into prostaglandin E_2 (PGE_2) by catalytic enzymes. The success of COX-2 inhibitors among patients with chronic osteoarthritic pain is evidence of its importance in the inflammatory cascade. A few, selective COX-2 inhibitors have been radiolabeled and may potentially be useful in imaging that type of inflammation that is characterized by increased COX-2 enzyme expression. To date, such tracers as ^{99m}Tc-Celebrex, ^{18}F-SC51825, and ^{18}F-desbromo-DuP-697 have been developed and studied in a preliminary fashion.[97-99] Planar images with ^{99m}Tc-Celebrex showed the localization of this tracer to xenografts in tumor-bearing animals. Imaging with ^{18}F-desbromo-DuP-697 and ^{11}C-rofecoxib has been attempted in an animal models of inflammation with little success, in part owing to the relatively low level of COX-2 enzyme generated in this model.[100] Additional studies will be needed to verify whether COX-2 can serve a marker for arthritis.

Subchondral Bone Metabolism

The role of subchondral bone in the progression of cartilage damage has been gaining more attention. In OA, repetitive mechanical loads or repetitive traumatic injury results in increases in trabecular volume, mineral deposition, and osteophytosis in the subchondral bone. This architectural alteration results in a more rigid subchondral bone, leading to an elevated stiffness gradient across the articular cartilage.[101]

Transmitted loads across the articular subsequently become harsher, resulting in fibrillation of articular cartilage. The ability to detect increasing mineralization of the subchondral bone may have important therapeutic implications, because a number of therapies have been designed to target the pathologic bony changes associated OA.

In routine clinical practice, the "bone scan" (i.e., ^{99m}Tc-labeled methylene diphosphonate [MDP]) has long been used to examine bone metabolism. Advantages of this study include its relative availability and affordability, but disadvantages stem from the low resolution and lack of specificity of the radionuclide technique (i.e., ^{99m}Tc may dissociate from the MDP tracer in bone tissues).[102] An alternative method utilizes a positron-emitting isotope, fluoride-18 (^{18}F), which has a high affinity for bone.[103] After capillary diffusion into the bone, ^{18}F exchanges with hydroxyl groups in bone crystal to form fluoroapatite; it becomes naturally incorporated into cortical bone.[104] Turnover of ^{18}F in bone is thought to be related to the physiologic responsibility of osteoblasts and osteoclasts to maintain bone matrix. Thus, the ^{18}F can be used as a tracer (FDG) for the evaluation of bone metabolism using PET. Advantages of this method are that it offers a means to scan living subjects in a fully quantitative, noninvasive, and repetitive manner. FDG-PET also allows for higher sensitivity and possible higher resolution when compared with ^{99m}Tc-labeled MDP bone scintigraphy; it is potentially a "super bone scan," if you will. Still, bone scanning with either gamma camera/SPECT or PET usually results in imaging characteristics that are relatively nonspecific, and thus there is the philosophy that bone scans should usually accompany radiography, CT, or MRI. FDG-PET to date has not been applied to the evaluation of early osteoarthritic changes but has been shown to be more accurate in detection of early aseptic loosening of total knee arthroplasty when compared with standard clinical techniques, as well as to aid in the identification of causes of back pain in adolescents.[105-107]

An alternative to radionuclide-based bone scanning employs the optical imaging agent Pam78, which is a near-infrared fluorescent biphosphonate derivative.[108] Pam78 possesses excitation and emission maxima at 771 nm and 796 nm, respectfully. Early studies have been performed in mice utilizing imaging with a CCD camera.

SUMMARY

A wide array of molecular imaging tools for the evaluation of musculoskeletal diseases is now available. There is hope that these particular tools will advance the understanding and management of a variety of chronic musculoskeletal diseases, including not only OA and RA but also cancer, musculoskeletal pain, fracture healing, bone metabolism, chronic osteomyelitis, and, possibly, osteoporosis.

It is likely, in the next decade, that PET/CT, SPECT/CT, PET/MRI and advanced molecular MR techniques, such as hyperpolarized MRI, will be the major workhorses for molecular imaging. PET-based technologies have an advantage, given their greater sensitivity as well as the ability to use biologic molecules that nearly simulate the structure and interactions of the native molecule and can be radiolabeled. Future technical improvements are certain to aid optical and MR-based protocols for human application. Increasing alliance between molecular biologists, rheumatologists, orthopedic surgeons, engineers, chemists, physicists, and pharmacologists will develop during the next generation of molecular imaging technologies and expand their capabilities in the diagnosis and treatment of arthritis. The current research and clinical environment provides a great opportunity for the continued study of molecular imaging protocols and the application of these protocols to the analysis of a large variety of musculoskeletal disorders.

References

1. Massoud TF, Gambhir SS. Molecular imaging in living subjects: seeing fundamental biological processes in a new light. Genes Dev 2003; 17:545-580.
2. Foley-Nolan D, Stack JP, et al. Magnetic resonance imaging in the assessment of rheumatoid arthritis—a comparison with plain film radiographs. Br J Rheumatol 1991; 30:101-106.
3. Taylor PC. The value of sensitive imaging modalities in rheumatoid arthritis. Arthritis Res Ther 2003; 5:210-213.
4. Kirwan JR. The effect of glucocorticoids on joint destruction in rheumatoid arthritis. The Arthritis and Rheumatism Council Low-Dose Glucocorticoid Study Group. N Engl J Med 1995; 333:142-146.
5. Stenger AA, Van Leeuwen MA, et al. Early effective suppression of inflammation in rheumatoid arthritis reduces radiographic progression. Br J Rheumatol 1998; 37:1157-1163.
6. Lipsky PE, van der Heijde DM, et al. Infliximab and methotrexate in the treatment of rheumatoid arthritis. Anti-Tumor Necrosis Factor Trial in Rheumatoid Arthritis with Concomitant Therapy Study Group. N Engl J Med 2000; 343:1594-1602.
7. Goldbach-Mansky R, Woodburn J, et al. Magnetic resonance imaging in the evaluation of bone damage in rheumatoid arthritis: a more precise image or just a more expensive one? Arthritis Rheum 2003; 48:585-589.
8. Hoving JL, Buchbinder R, et al. A comparison of magnetic resonance imaging, sonography, and radiography of the hand in patients with early rheumatoid arthritis. J Rheumatol 2004; 31:663-675.
9. Palmer WE, Rosenthal DI, et al. Quantification of inflammation in the wrist with gadolinium-enhanced MR imaging and PET with 2-[F-18]-fluoro-2-deoxy-D-glucose. Radiology 1995; 196:647-655.
10. Choy EH, Panayi GS. Cytokine pathways and joint inflammation in rheumatoid arthritis. N Engl J Med 2001; 344:907-916.
11. Arend WP, Gabay C. Cytokines in the rheumatic diseases. Rheum Dis Clin North Am 2004; 30:41-67, v-vi.
12. Conaghan PG, O'Connor P, et al. Elucidation of the relationship between synovitis and bone damage: a randomized magnetic resonance imaging study of individual joints in patients with early rheumatoid arthritis. Arthritis Rheum 2003; 48:64-71.
13. Adonai N, Nguyen KN, et al. Ex vivo cell labeling with 64Cu-pyruvaldehyde-bis(N4-methylthiosemicarbazone) for imaging cell trafficking in mice with positron-emission tomography. Proc Natl Acad Sci U S A 2002; 99:3030-3035.
14. Paik JY, Lee KH, et al. Use of insulin to improve [18 F]fluorodeoxyglucose labelling and retention for in vivo positron emission tomography imaging of monocyte trafficking. Nucl Med Commun 2002; 23:551-557.
15. Panayi GS, Corrigall VM, et al. Pathogenesis of rheumatoid arthritis: the role of T cells and other beasts. Rheum Dis Clin North Am 2001; 27:317-334.
16. Jorgensen C, Couret I, et al. Radiolabelled lymphocyte migration in rheumatoid synovitis. Ann Rheum Dis 1995; 54:39-44.
17. Peters AM. The use of nuclear medicine in infections. Br J Radiol 1998; 71:252-261.
18. Nakajima A, Seroogy CM, et al. Antigen-specific T cell-mediated gene therapy in collagen-induced arthritis. J Clin Invest 2001; 107:1293-1301.
19. Biswal S. Molecular imaging of musculoskeletal diseases. Semin Musculoskelet Radiol 2003; 7:317-350.
20. Dodd SJ, Williams M, et al. Detection of single mammalian cells by high-resolution magnetic resonance imaging. Biophys J 1999; 76:103-109.
21. Josephson L, Kircher MR, et al. Near-infrared fluorescent nanoparticles as combined MR/optical imaging probes. Bioconjug Chem 2002; 13:554-560.
22. Kanno S, Lee PC, et al. A novel approach with magnetic resonance imaging used for the detection of lung allograft rejection. J Thorac Cardiovasc Surg 2000; 120:923-934.
23. Zhang Y, Dodd SJ, et al. Magnetic resonance imaging detection of rat renal transplant rejection by monitoring macrophage infiltration. Kidney Int 2000; 58:1300-1310.
24. Kanno S, Wu YJ, et al. Macrophage accumulation associated with rat cardiac allograft rejection detected by magnetic resonance imaging with ultrasmall superparamagnetic iron oxide particles. Circulation 2001; 104:934-938.
25. Josephson L, Tung CH, et al. High-efficiency intracellular magnetic labeling with novel superparamagnetic-Tat peptide conjugates. Bioconjug Chem 1999; 10:186-191.
26. Dodd CH, Hsu HC, et al. Normal T-cell response and in vivo magnetic resonance imaging of T cells loaded with HIV transactivator-peptide-derived superparamagnetic nanoparticles. J Immunol Methods 2001; 256:89-105.
27. Moore A, Sun PA, et al. MRI of insulitis in autoimmune diabetes. Magn Reson Med 2002; 47:751-758.
28. Harrison LH Jr, Schwarzenberger PO, et al. Gene-modified PA1-STK cells home to tumor sites in patients with malignant pleural mesothelioma. Ann Thorac Surg 2001; 70:407-411.
29. Bogdanov A Jr, Tung CH, et al. DNA binding chelates for nonviral gene delivery imaging. Gene Ther 2001; 8:515-522.

30. Colombo FR, Torrente Y, et al. Biodistribution studies of 99mTc-labeled myoblasts in a murine model of muscular dystrophy. Nucl Med Biol 2001; 28:935-940.
31. Min JJ, Gambhir SS. Gene therapy progress and prospects: noninvasive imaging of gene therapy in living subjects. Gene Ther 2004; 11:115-125.
32. Beckmann N, Falk R, et al. Macrophage infiltration into the rat knee detected by MRI in a model of antigen-induced arthritis. Magn Reson Med 2003; 49:1047-1055.
33. Turk MJ, Breur GJ, et al. Folate-targeted imaging of activated macrophages in rats with adjuvant-induced arthritis. Arthritis Rheum 2002; 46:1947-1955.
34. Paulos CM, Turk MJ, et al. Folate receptor-mediated targeting of therapeutic and imaging agents to activated macrophages in rheumatoid arthritis. Adv Drug Deliv Rev 2004; 56:1205-1217.
35. Chen WT, Mahmood U, et al. Arthritis imaging using a near-infrared fluorescence folate-targeted probe. Arthritis Res Ther 2005; 7:R310-R317.
36. de Bois MH, Pauwels EK, et al. New agents for scintigraphy in rheumatoid arthritis. Eur J Nucl Med 1995; 22:1339-1346.
37. Gaal J, Mezes A, et al. 99mTc-HMPAO labelled leukocyte scintigraphy in patients with rheumatoid arthritis: a comparison with disease activity. Nucl Med Commun 2002; 23:39-46.
38. Wipke BT, Wang Z, et al. Dynamic visualization of a joint-specific autoimmune response through positron emission tomography. Nat Immunol 2002; 3:366-372.
39. Breedveld FC, van Kroonenburgh MJ, et al. Imaging of inflammatory arthritis with technetium-99m-labeled IgG. J Nucl Med 1989; 30:2017-2021.
40. Pons F, Moya F, et al. Detection and quantitative analysis of joint activity inflammation with 99Tcm-polyclonal human immunoglobulin G. Nucl Med Commun 1993; 14:225-231.
41. Pons F, Sanmarti R, et al. Scintigraphic evaluation of the severity of inflammation of the joints with 99TCm-HIG in rheumatoid arthritis. Nucl Med Commun 1996; 17:523-528.
42. Hansch A, Frey O, et al. In vivo imaging of experimental arthritis with near-infrared fluorescence. Arthritis Rheum 2004; 50:961-967.
43. Kinne RW, Wolski A, et al. Minimal contribution of cell-bound antibodies to the immunoscintigraphy of inflamed joints with 99mTc-anti-CD4 monoclonal antibodies. Nuklearmedizin 2002; 41:129-134.
44. Wu AM, Yazaki PJ. Designer genes: recombinant antibody fragments for biological imaging. Q J Nucl Med 2002; 44:268-283.
45. Barrera P, van der Laken CJ, et al. Radiolabelled interleukin-1 receptor antagonist for detection of synovitis in patients with rheumatoid arthritis. Rheumatology (Oxford) 2000; 39:870-874.
46. Pahl HL. Activators and target genes of Rel/NF-kappaB transcription factors. Oncogene 1999; 18:6853-6866.
47. Murphy G, Knauper V, et al. Matrix metalloproteinases in arthritic disease. Arthritis Res 2002; 4(Suppl 3):S39-S49.
48. Carlsen H, Moskaug JO, et al. In vivo imaging of NF-kappa B activity. J Immunol 2002; 168:1441-1446.
49. Izmailova ES, Paz N, et al. Use of molecular imaging to quantify response to IKK-2 inhibitor treatment in murine arthritis. Arthritis Rheum 2007; 56:117-128.
50. Ntziachristos V, Bremer C, et al. Fluorescence imaging with near-infrared light: new technological advances that enable in vivo molecular imaging. Eur Radiol 2003; 13:195-208.
51. Weissleder R, Tung CH, et al. In vivo imaging of tumors with protease-activated near-infrared fluorescent probes. Nat Biotechnol 1999; 17:375-378.
52. Ji H, Ohmura K, et al. Arthritis critically dependent on innate immune system players. Immunity 2002; 16:157-168.
53. Wunder A, Tung CH, et al. In vivo imaging of protease activity in arthritis: a novel approach for monitoring treatment response. Arthritis Rheum 2004; 50:2459-2465.
54. Mountz JD, Zhang HG. Regulation of apoptosis of synovial fibroblasts. Curr Dir Autoimmun 2001; 3:216-239.
55. Post AM, Katsikis PD, et al. Imaging cell death with radiolabeled annexin V in an experimental model of rheumatoid arthritis. J Nucl Med 2002; 43:1359-1365.
56. Wunder A, Schellenberger E, et al. Methotrexate-induced accumulation of fluorescent annexin V in collagen-induced arthritis. Mol Imaging 2005; 4:1-6.
57. Dayton PA, Ferrara KW. Targeted imaging using ultrasound. J Magn Reson Imaging 2002; 16:362-377.
58. Lindner JR. Detection of inflamed plaques with contrast ultrasound. Am J Cardiol 2002; 90:32L-35L.
59. Agarwal SK, Brenner MB. Role of adhesion molecules in synovial inflammation. Curr Opin Rheumatol 2006; 18:268-276.
60. Taylor PC. VEGF and imaging of vessels in rheumatoid arthritis. Arthritis Res 2002; 4(Suppl 3):S99-S107.
61. Lindner JR, Song J, et al. Ultrasound assessment of inflammation and renal tissue injury with microbubbles targeted to P-selectin. Circulation 2001; 104:2107-2112.
62. Lindner JR. Evolving applications for contrast ultrasound. Am J Cardiol 2002; 90(Suppl 10A):72J-80J.
63. Demos SM, Alkan-Onyuksel H, et al. In vivo targeting of acoustically reflective liposomes for intravascular and transvascular ultrasonic enhancement. J Am Coll Cardiol 1999; 33:867-875.

64. Demos SM, Onyuksel H, et al. In vitro targeting of antibody-conjugated echogenic liposomes for site-specific ultrasonic image enhancement. J Pharm Sci 1997; 86:167-171.
65. Zinn KR, Chaudhuri TR, et al. Specific targeting of activated endothelium in rat adjuvant arthritis with a 99mTc-radiolabeled E-selectin-binding peptide. Arthritis Rheum 1999; 42:641-649.
66. Jayagopal A, Russ PK, et al. Surface engineering of quantum dots for in vivo vascular imaging. Bioconjug Chem 2007; 18:1424-1433.
67. Sipkins DA, Gijbels K, et al. ICAM-1 expression in autoimmune encephalitis visualized using magnetic resonance imaging. J Neuroimmunol 2000; 104:1-9.
68. Kang HW, Josephson L, et al. Magnetic resonance imaging of inducible E-selectin expression in human endothelial cell culture. Bioconjug Chem 2002; 13:122-127.
69. Willmann JK, Chen K, et al. Monitoring of the biological response to murine hindlimb ischemia with 64Cu-labeled vascular endothelial growth factor-121 positron emission tomography. Circulation 2008; 117:915-922.
70. Wu Z, Li ZB, et al. microPET of tumor integrin alphavbeta3 expression using 18F-labeled PEGylated tetrameric RGD peptide (18F-FPRGD4). J Nucl Med 2007; 48:1536-1544.
71. D'Lima DD, Hashimoto S, et al. Human chondrocyte apoptosis in response to mechanical injury. Osteoarthritis Cartilage 2001; 9:712-719.
72. D'Lima DD, Hashimoto S, et al. Cartilage injury induces chondrocyte apoptosis. J Bone Joint Surg Am 2001; 83(Suppl 2):19-21.
73. Loening AM, James Ie, et al. Injurious mechanical compression of bovine articular cartilage induces chondrocyte apoptosis. Arch Biochem Biophys 2000; 381:205-212.
74. Hashimoto S, Setareh M, et al. Fas/Fas ligand expression and induction of apoptosis in chondrocytes. Arthritis Rheum 1997; 40:1749-1755.
75. Grodzicky T, Elkon KB. Apoptosis in rheumatic diseases. Am J Med 2000; 108:73-82.
76. DiMicco MA, Patwari P, et al. Mechanisms and kinetics of glycosaminoglycan release following in vitro cartilage injury. Arthritis Rheum 2004; 50:840-848.
77. Goldring MB. Update on the biology of the chondrocyte and new approaches to treating cartilage diseases. Best Pract Res Clin Rheumatol 2006; 20:1003-1025.
78. Bashir A, Gray ML, et al. Gd-DTPA2- as a measure of cartilage degradation. Magn Reson Med 1996; 36:665-673.
79. Burstein D, Velyvis J, et al. Protocol issues for delayed Gd(DTPA)(2-)-enhanced MRI (dGEMRIC) for clinical evaluation of articular cartilage. Magn Reson Med 2001; 45:36-41.
80. Kim YJ, Jaramillo D, et al. Assessment of early osteoarthritis in hip dysplasia with delayed gadolinium-enhanced magnetic resonance imaging of cartilage. J Bone Joint Surg Am 2003; 85:1987-1992.
81. Reutelingsperger CP, van Heerde WL. Annexin V, the regulator of phosphatidylserine-catalyzed inflammation and coagulation during apoptosis. Cell Mol Life Sci 1997; 53:527-532.
82. Blankenberg FG, Strauss HW. Will imaging of apoptosis play a role in clinical care? A tale of mice and men. Apoptosis 2001; 6:117-123.
83. Reutelingsperger CP. Annexins: key regulators of haemostasis, thrombosis, and apoptosis. Thromb Haemost 2001; 86:413-419.
84. Lahorte CM, Vanderheyden JL, et al. Apoptosis-detecting radioligands: current state of the art and future perspectives. Eur J Nucl Med Mol Imaging 2004; 31:887-919.
85. Blankenberg FG, Katsikis PD, et al. In vivo detection and imaging of phosphatidylserine expression during programmed cell death. Proc Natl Acad Sci U S A 1998; 95:6349-6354.
86. Russell J, O'Donoghue JA, et al. Iodination of annexin V for imaging apoptosis. J Nucl Med 2002; 43:671-677.
87. Glaser M, Collingridge DR, et al. Iodine-124 labelled annexin-V as a potential radiotracer to study apoptosis using positron emission tomography. Appl Radiat Isot 2003; 58:55-62.
88. Zijlstra S, Gunawan J, et al. Synthesis and evaluation of a 18F-labelled recombinant annexin-V derivative, for identification and quantification of apoptotic cells with PET. Appl Radiat Isot 2003; 58:201-207.
89. Schellenberger EA, Bogdanov A Jr, et al. Annexin V-CLIO: a nanoparticle for detecting apoptosis by MRI. Mol Imaging 2002; 1:102-107.
90. Hofstra L, Liem IH, et al. Visualisation of cell death in vivo in patients with acute myocardial infarction. Lancet 2002; 356:209-212.
91. Belhocine T, Steinmetz N, et al. Increased uptake of the apoptosis-imaging agent (99m)Tc recombinant human Annexin V in human tumors after one course of chemotherapy as a predictor of tumor response and patient prognosis. Clin Cancer Res 2002; 8:2766-2774.
92. Reutelingsperger CP, Dumont E, et al. Visualization of cell death in vivo with the annexin A5 imaging protocol. J Immunol Methods 2002; 265:123-132.
93. Thimister PW, Hofstra L, et al. In vivo detection of cell death in the area at risk in acute myocardial infarction. J Nucl Med 2003; 44:391-396.
94. Blankenberg F. To scan or not to scan, it is a question of timing: technetium-99m-annexin V radionuclide imaging assessment of treatment efficacy after one course of chemotherapy. Clin Cancer Res 2002; 8:2757-2758.
95. Bauer C, Bauder-Wuest U, et al. ^{131}I-labeled peptides as caspase substrates for apoptosis imaging. J Nucl Med 2005; 46:1066-1074.

96. Lai WF, Chang CH, et al. Early diagnosis of osteoarthritis using cathepsin B sensitive near-infrared fluorescent probes. Osteoarthritis Cartilage 2004; 12:239-244.
97. McCarthy TJ, Sheriff AU, et al. Radiosynthesis, in vitro validation, and in vivo evaluation of 18F-labeled COX-1 and COX-2 inhibitors. J Nucl Med 2002; 43:117-124.
98. de Vries EF, van Waarde A, et al. Synthesis and in vivo evaluation of 18F-desbromo-DuP-697 as a PET tracer for cyclooxygenase-2 expression. J Nucl Med 2003; 44:1700-1706.
99. Yang DJ, Bryant J, et al. Assessment of cyclooxygense-2 expression with 99mTc-labeled Celebrex. Anticancer Drugs 2004; 15:255-263.
100. de Vries EF, Doorduin J, et al. Evaluation of [(11)C]rofecoxib as PET tracer for cyclooxygenase 2 overexpression in rat models of inflammation. Nucl Med Biol 2008; 35:35-42.
101. Radin EL, Rose RM. Role of subchondral bone in the initiation and progression of cartilage damage. Clin Orthop Relat Res 1986; 213:34-40.
102. Schwartz Z, Shani J, et al. Uptake and biodistribution of technetium-99m-MD32P during rat tibial bone repair. J Nucl Med 1993; 34:104-108.
103. Berger F, Lee YP, et al. Whole-body skeletal imaging in mice utilizing microPET: optimization of reproducibility and applications in animal models of bone disease. Eur J Nucl Med Mol Imaging 2002; 29:1225-1236.
104. Ishiguro K, Nakagaki H, et al. Distribution of fluoride in cortical bone of human rib. Calcif Tissue Int 1993; 52:278-282.
105. Lim R, Fahey FH, et al. Early experience with fluorine-18 sodium fluoride bone PET in young patients with back pain. J Pediatr Orthop 2007; 27:277-282.
106. Ovadia D, Metser U, et al. Back pain in adolescents: assessment with integrated 18F-fluoride positron-emission tomography-computed tomography. J Pediatr Orthop 2007; 27:90-93.
107. Sterner T, Pink R, et al. The role of [18F]fluoride positron emission tomography in the early detection of aseptic loosening of total knee arthroplasty. Int J Surg 2007; 5:99-104.
108. Zaheer A, Lenkinski RE, et al. In vivo near-infrared fluorescence imaging of osteoblastic activity. Nat Biotechnol 2001; 19:1148-1154.
109. Cindas A, Gokce-Kustal Y, et al. Scintigraphic evaluation of synovial inflammation in rheumatoid arthritis with (99m)technetium-labelled human polyclonal immunoglobulin G. Rheumatol Int 2001; 20:71-77.
110. Marcus C, Thakur ML, et al. Imaging rheumatic joint diseases with anti-T lymphocyte antibody OKT-3. Nucl Med Commun 1994; 15:824-830.
111. Becker W, Emmrich F, et al. Imaging rheumatoid arthritis specifically with technetium 99m CD4-specific (T-helper lymphocytes) antibodies. Eur J Nucl Med 1990; 17:156-159.
112. Jamar F, Houssiau FA, et al. Scintigraphy using a technetium 99m-labelled anti-E-selectin Fab fragment in rheumatoid arthritis. Rheumatology (Oxford) 2002; 41:53-61.
113. Meyer P, Burkhardt H, et al. ^{123}I-antileukoproteinase scintigraphy reveals microscopic cartilage alterations in the contralateral knee joint of rats with "monarticular" antigen-induced arthritis. Arthritis Rheum 2000; 43:298-310.
114. Boerman OC, Dams ET, et al. Radiopharmaceuticals for scintigraphic imaging of infection and inflammation. Inflamm Res 2001; 50:55-64.
115. Dardzinski BJ, Schmithorst VJ, et al. MR imaging of murine arthritis using ultrasmall superparamagnetic iron oxide particles. Magn Reson Imaging 2001; 19:1209-1216.
116. Taylor PC, Steuer A, et al. Comparison of ultrasonographic assessment of synovitis and joint vascularity with radiographic evaluation in a randomized, placebo-controlled study of infliximab therapy in early rheumatoid arthritis. Arthritis Rheum 2004; 50:1107-1116.
117. Resnick D. Rheumatoid arthritis and the seronegative spondylarthropathies: radiographic and pathologic concepts. In Resnick D (ed) Diagnosis of Bone and Joint Disorders. Philadelphia, WB Saunders, 2002, vol 2, pp 837-890.
118. McQueen FM. A vital clue to deciphering bone pathology: MRI bone oedema in rheumatoid arthritis and osteoarthritis. Ann Rheum Dis 2007; 66:1549-1552.
119. Beckers C, Ribbens C, et al. Assessment of disease activity in rheumatoid arthritis with (18)F-FDG PET. J Nucl Med 2004; 45:956-964.

INDEX

Note: Page numbers followed by b, f, and t indicate boxes, figures and tables, respectively.